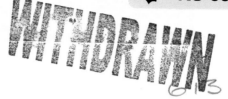
Nursing concepts
for health promotion

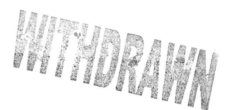
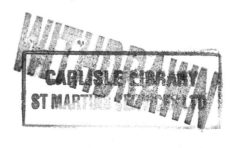

# Nursing concepts for health promotion

RUTH BECKMANN MURRAY R.N., M.S.N., Ed.D.
*St Louis University School of Nursing*

JUDITH PROCTOR ZENTNER R.N., M.A., C.S.N.P.
*Carson Furniture Industries, Valdese, North Carolina*

Adapted for the United Kingdom by
CINDY HOWELLS R.G.N., N.D.N., R.N.T., Cert. Ed. (F.E.)
*Warwickshire School of Nursing*

Prentice Hall
New York    London    Toronto    Sydney    Tokyo    Singapore

First published 1989 by
Prentice Hall International (UK) Ltd,
66 Wood Lane End, Hemel Hempstead,
Hertfordshire, HP2 4RG
A division of
Simon & Schuster International Group

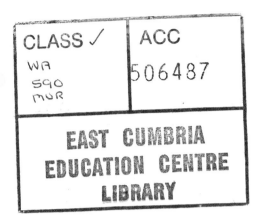

Original edition published by Appleton & Lange

Printed and bound in Great Britain by
BPCC Wheatons Ltd, Exeter

British Library Cataloguing-in-Publication Data

Murray, Ruth Beckmann
    Nursing concepts for health promotion,
    1. Health education
    I. Title   II. Zentner, Judith Proctor
    613'.07

    ISBN 0-13-627662-8

3 4 5   93 92

# Contents

# Unit II   Factors influencing health in a pluralistic society

# To the reader

We believe the nurse must consider the total health of the person and family. The physical, mental, emotional, sociocultural and spiritual-moral needs are interrelated. Increasingly your emphasis must be on comprehensive health promotion rather than on patchwork remedies.

Often nurses study some of the topics presented in isolated courses with little or no application to the care of the client, the family and the community. Therefore, an integral part of this book is the nursing application of such material, interwoven when appropriate, and emphasized in special sections at other times.

Your role in nursing is changing from that of working primarily for the physician or agency to that of being an advocate for the patient, client or family. Today's physicians are often so specialized that the client feels fragmented and unable to understand how a specific disease process – the avoidance, modification, or elimination of it – will affect life and wellbeing. The person is afraid to ask, thinking that the physician is too busy and too engrossed in medical terminology. Most of us have been taught to seek the physician's help for illness and treatment rather than to maintain good health. Thus *your* response to the client and to a family is crucial, whether they are well or ill. You are the one caring person who can interpret health-care services, serve as a liaison between the physician, other health-team members, and the client, and prevent fragmentation of health services.

Comprehensive health promotion is no longer a dream of only a few people. The good-health movement and self-care concepts are now woven into the nursing curriculum. Also we have seen the emergence of nursing as a profession that can stand on its own with its own body of knowledge and practice capabilities. Finally, the patient/consumer/client is no longer always afraid to ask questions of the medical profession.

Before reading any chapter, you should orient yourself by studying the organization chart shown here, which illustrates the many facets that must be considered in nursing for health promotion. Next, read the Introduction. You can gain further orientation by looking at the objectives listed at the beginning of each chapter.

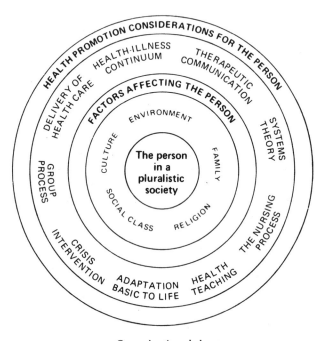

Organizational chart

We invite you to be an active participant as you read. The ideas are presented with conviction and directness, but we want you to integrate and modify these ideas to your specific circumstances. Each of you will have to adapt this information to your setting – be it independent practice, health maintenance, hospital, clinic or home.

# General introduction

This text on nursing in a pluralistic society is divided into two units. Unit I (Chapters 1–6) establishes a framework for health promotion in a complex society. As society becomes more complicated, nursing increasingly requires a framework – a set of concepts and tools – that can be used in any setting with a variety of people. Chapters 1–6 present topics whose sequential arrangement does not necessarily indicate that one subject must follow another. Rather, these topics are just important components of nursing knowledge, gathered from various sources and placed together into one unit for convenient reference.

Chapter 1 introduces the reader to the concept of health and its many meanings. Basic definitions of and variables influencing health and illness are examined. *Systems theory* is introduced as a framework relating all of the concepts presented in this book.

Chapter 2 explores the meaning of therapeutic communication. Since you will observe and talk with persons and their families before, during and after giving care, how you affect these people through your communication pattern will establish a basis for the nursing process, the topic of Chapter 3. Here the five steps of the nursing process, assessment, nursing diagnosis, planning, intervention and evaluation, are described as a systematic method of providing health service to a person or group of persons, and the nurse-client relationship is explored as the basic unit of interaction in this process. The changing role of the nurse is also examined.

To help you learn and teach more effectively as a nurse, health teaching principles are discussed in Chapter 4. Attention is given to the creative process, the difference between child and adult learning and methods that you may employ in teaching others to maintain or regain health.

Chapters 5 and 6 provide two theories, along with suggestions for their practical application. The first, *Adaptation theory*, considers how each aspect of the person or group must continually be adjusted to maintain wellbeing. The second, *Crisis theory*, gives direction for helping the person, family, group or community during crises, since many of the people you work with will be in some phase of crisis.

Unit II (Chapters 7–10) discusses factors influencing health development and use of the nursing process. In the past, the person's health status has usually been considered apart from the many factors that help define him/her-factors, moreover, that are an integral part of health (or lack of it). Health-care systems rip the person out of his/her environment, often disregarding sociocultural, religious or spiritual background and practices and family life. Then we wonder why the client seems overwhelmed or disorientated in the health-care setting.

Unit II takes a cosmopolitan view. Environmental pollution is considered as a world problem. Types of cultures and religions are examined. The individual's family life is discussed. You need to understand the physical climate from which he/she comes and the working and living conditions. Knowledge of the person's background will help you better plan the environment in which to work with him/her and the family. You need to know whether the culture emphasizes trust or mistrust in the medical profession. You need to understand the basis for and importance of religious rituals. You can better plan for care if you know the sociocultural values. You can also work more effectively with the whole family if you know whether it is an extended or a nuclear family. A knowledge of all these various background factors will enable you to treat each individual and his/her significant others or family with the special understanding that they deserve.

# UNIT I

A framework for health
promotion in a pluralistic society

# 1

# Basic considerations in health and illness

**Study of this chapter will enable you to:**

1. Define *health* and *illness* and explain the meaning of the health-illness continuum.

2. Define *system* and identify characteristics of a system.

3. Describe the person and health-care business as systems and the implications for nursing.

4. Identify needs that influence behaviour and that must be met to maintain health.

5. Describe the external environmental and internal variables that affect behaviour and health.

6. Examine measures that promote health of the individual and family unit.

7. Discuss nursing measures that are conducive to health promotion – well being, considering factors that influence preventive health behaviour.

'Bob, are you ill?'
'No, why?'
'Your face looks a little puffy.'

Bob, who thought he was well, suddenly decides he hasn't had his usual energy for several weeks. He thinks he'll make an appointment to see the doctor.

'I wish I knew what you mean by being ill. Sometimes I feel so bad I could curl up and die, but I have to go on because the kids have to be taken care of. Some people can go to bed any time with anything, but most of us can't take the time to be ill – even when we need to be.'

These expressions immediately portray the difficulty in defining health and illness. Each person's definition is affected by cultural concepts, economic level, the value system of self and others, ethnic background, customs, and past experiences.

Subjectivity may be intensified by identifying three ways in which a person defines himself as ill: (a) feeling 'bad', (b) having distressing symptoms, such as pain, and (c) being unable to carry on daily activities. Thus both illness and health are what the person says they are. Person A may have the same symptoms as person B; but while A says 'I'm well,' B says 'I'm ill'.

The well person usually has some small degree of illness – physical or mental. And the person who is physically very ill, even near death, may still have some health potential. Similarly, the emotionally ill person will manifest some health or appropriate behaviour.

Although *health* and *illness* are subjective and relative terms, such qualities as hope, purpose and direction in life can produce and maintain wellbeing, even in the face of stress. Similarly, demoralization through daily struggle for existence can help produce illness.

As a nurse, your concern, knowledge and skill are directed to the health needs of persons from many different kinds of backgrounds and in various settings. It is essential, therefore, to understand the physical, mental, emotional, spiritual and social aspects of wellbeing and illness; the factors influencing health and illness; and the basic regulatory mechanisms in the human body that normally maintain a state of health. The use of this information will assist you in helping others to maintain as well as regain health.

## DEFINITIONS OF HEALTH AND ILLNESS

Working definitions of *health* and *illness*, although generalized, can give perspective. Traditionally they have been defined as opposites. An example is the definition given by the United Nations World Health Organization: *Health* is a 'state of complete physical, mental and social wellbeing and not merely the absence of disease'. The only option in the absence of complete physical, mental and social wellbeing, according to such a definition, is illness. No allowance is made for degrees of illness and health.

R. Dubois views *health* as adaptation, a function of adjustment. He believes a utopian state of health can never be reached because a person is never so perfectly adapted to the environment that life does not involve struggle, failure, and suffering.[1]

H. S. Hayman defines *health* as a state of feeling sound in body, mind and spirit, with a sense of reserve power. This perception of health is based on normal functioning of the body's physiological processes, understanding the principles of healthful living, and an attitude that regards health not as an end of survival and self-fulfilment in itself but as a means to a creative social adjustment and a richer, fuller life as measured in constructive service to humans.[2]

H. Blum defines *health* as the person's capacity to function to the greatest capacity; to maintain a balance appropriate to age and social needs; to be reasonably free of gross dissatisfaction, discomfort, disease, or disability; and to behave in ways that promote survival as well as self-fulfilment or enjoyment.[3]

Dunn defines *health* and *illness* on a graduated scale or continuum. Each person has neither absolute health nor illness but is in a relative and ever changing state of being, ranging from peak to 'high-level' health to extreme poor health with death imminent.[4]

**High-level health** refers *to the person's ability to (a) function in one or more domains at or above the expected norm, and (b) use inner potential continually in order to meet the demands of everyday life.* This definition involves a holistic approach that considers developmental levels, past experience, present situation, disabilities, and environment.

*Health-wellbeing* and *disease-illness* are now thought of as complex, dynamic processes on a continuum that includes physical, psychological (emotional, cognitive, and developmental), spiritual and social components and adaptive behavioural responses to internal and external stimuli. Health depends on genetic, environmental, sociocultural and spiritual influences that either help or hinder an individual in actively fulfilling the basic needs and reaching the highest health potential.

The emotionally healthy person generally shows behaviour congruent with events within or around him/her. Key concepts in health-wellbeing include homeostasis, adaptation, dynamic nature of health-illness continuum, influence of internal and external environment, state of harmony with nature and people, comfort, safety, social relationships and prevention of disease, disability, and social decay.

Men and women are socialized to define health and illness differently. Statistics show that women report more illnesses and disabilities, visit the physician more, and are hospitalized more often, including for emotional illnesses. Physicians are also more likely to prescribe drugs for women than for men, especially the mood-changing drugs. Often the physician does not take a complete history or learn of underlying problems that can be corrected other than through use of medication. Yet women have longer life expectancies than men and there is no difference between men and women in the incidence of psychosis. Perhaps the seeking of more health care by women reflects: (a) a different perception of illness or disability; (b) different cultural norms about health-care behaviour for men and women; (c) sex-role conflicts for women, which result in more illness, and (d) differences in diagnostic and treatment services for men and women. All these factors may be operating. The longer life expectancy of women may be the result of early diagnosis and treatment of disease, of inherent sex-linked resistance to disease, or of different exposure or response to noxious physical and social stressors.[5]

A person's age influences the definition of health. Children define health as feeling good and being able to participate in desired activities. Children's ideas about health progress from a specific, concrete concern for health practices to future-oriented interests in optimal development and societal problems. Six-year-olds view health as completely different from illness and as a series of specific health practices, such as eating nutritional foods, getting exercise and keeping clean. Nine-year-olds are less concerned with specific health practices and more concerned with total body states, such as feeling good or being 'in shape'. To them, health means being physically fit to do the activities of daily living; it is impossible to be partly healthy and partly unhealthy. Twelve-year-olds view health as long-term feeling good, not being sick, participating in desired activities, and as including mental as well as physical components. Some children include a fit environment as part of health. In contrast, adults typically define health as a state enabling them to perform at least minimal daily activities and including physical, mental, spiritual, and social components. The adult's perception, as well as life situation, influences the definition of health.

As used in this book, **health** *is a state of wellbeing in which the person is able to use purposeful, adaptive responses and processes, physically, mentally, emotionally, spiritually and socially, in response to internal and external stimuli (stressors) in order to maintain relative stability and comfort and to strive for personal objectives and cultural goals.*

**Emotional and social health** *means that the feelings, emotions, interests, motivations, attitudes and values of the person continue to mature and change over a lifetime, as the person engages in transactions with other people and the broader environment, manifests both flexibility and stability in adaptive abilities, accomplishes the developmental tasks appropriate to the life era and age, and fulfils social roles with a maximum of effectiveness and happiness.*

The definition of 'disease' has progressed through several stages. Primitive people saw disease as an independent force that dominated and eventually overtook the victim. Next, the medical-physiological view interpreted the human being as an active being with the ability to resist disease attack. The ecological definition looks at the environmental influence on health, whereas the equilibrium view emphasizes ineffective attempts to maintain homeostasis or adaptation. Finally, the social approach defines illness in terms of whether the person is performing expected cultural norms and social functions.

Illness is more than signs and symptoms. It is a process and an experience. **Illness** *is the failure of the person's adaptive powers to maintain physical and emotional balance and to use the usual health-promoting resources in the face of internal or external stressors. It is an experience that exists when there is disturb-*

*ance or failure in the bio-psychosocial development or adaptation of the person, with observable or felt changes, discomforts, or impaired ability to carry out minimal physical, psychological, or social behavioural expectations appropriate to customary roles and status.* The person who has a disease may not consider the self ill; the person who considers the self ill may not have a disease or pathological state. The person does not consider the self ill or is not cognizant of disease unless the condition is considered significantly deviant from family, community or ethic standards, regional customs, class values, or occupational attitudes.

Mental or emotional illness may be defined as inappropriate interpersonal behaviour or behaviour that is inadequate for the social context. Each person may have some small degree of illness – physical or emotional – even when feeling good and looking well. The illness may be minor aches, temper flares, inappropriate forgetfulness or overuse of certain defence mechanisms such as rationalization or forgetfulness. Similarly the emotionally ill person, including the psychotic patient, manifests some degree of health – some appropriate thinking and behaviour – some of the time.

## GENERAL SYSTEMS THEORY: UNDERSTANDING HUMANS, HEALTH AND THE HEALTH-CARE SYSTEM

Nothing can be studied as a lone entity: the macroenvironment, sociocultural components; politico-legal, religious, educational and other social institutions; the person, family, groups or community; or the health-care delivery organization. All are interrelated. A theory to help you gain a comprehensive point of view and a holistic or interdisciplinary view of the person is *General systems theory.* According to this theory, there is probably nothing that is determined by a single cause or explained by a single factor.

*A* **system** *is an assemblage of interdependent parts, persons, or objects that are united by some form or order into a recognizable unit and that are in equilibrium.*

People satisfy their needs within social systems. The **social system** *consists of groups of people joined cooperatively to achieve certain common goals of the individual or group, using an organized set of practices to regulate behaviour.* The person occupies various positions and has defined roles in the social system. The person and his/her health are shaped by the system; in turn, people create and change social systems.

### Characteristics of a system

The following elements or components are common to all systems; a given entity is not a system unless these characteristics are present:

1. **Parts** *are the system's components and they are interdependent units.* None can operate without the other. Change in one part affects the entire unit. The person as a whole system, for example, is made up of physical, emotional, mental, spiritual and social aspects. Physically, he/she is made up of the body systems – neurological, cardiovascular, and so on. The health agency is one part of the health-care system and it, in turn, is made up of parts: the physical plant, employees, clients, departments that give services.

2. **Attributes** *are characteristics of the parts,* such as temperament or health of the person or the roles, education, or age of hospital emloyees.

3. **Information** *or* **communication,** *the sending of messages and getting feedback or the exchange of energy,* varies with the system but is essential to achieve goals.

4. **Boundary** *is a barrier or area of demarcation that limits or keeps a system distinct from its environment* and within which information is exchanged. The skin of the person, home of the family, or walls of the health agency are boundaries. Yet the boundary is not always rigid. Relatives outside the home are part of the family. The boundary may be an imaginary line, such as the feeling that comes from belonging to a certain racial or ethnic group.

5. **Organization** *is the formal or informal arrangement of parts to form a whole entity so that the organism or institution has a working order that results in established hierarchy, rules or customs.* The person is organized into a physical structure, basic needs, cognitive stages and achievement of developmental tasks. Hierarchy in the family or health agency provides organization that is based on power (ability to control others) and responsibility. Nursing care may be organized into primary or team nursing, which is a way of differentiating services. The specialization of medical practice is also a way of organizing care. Organization in an institution is also maintained by norms, roles, and customs that each member must learn.

6. **Goals** *are the purposes of or reasons for the system to exist.*

7. **Environment** *refers to the social and physical world outside the system, boundaries or the community in which the system exists.* A constant exchange of energy and information must exist with the surrounding specified environment if the system is to be open, useful and creative. If this information or energy exchange does not occur, the system becomes closed and ineffective.

*A person as a social system*

Every person is an open social system consisting physically of a hierarchy of such components as cells, organs and organ systems; emotionally of levels of needs and feelings; and socially of a relative rank in a hierarchy of prestige, such as boss, worker, adult or child. While internal stimuli are at work, such as those governed by the nervous and endocrine systems, outer stimuli also affect the person – for example, the feelings of others or the external environment. The boundaries or environment – such as one's skin, the limits set by others, one's status, home and community – influence the person's needs and goal achievement. To remain healthy, the person must have feedback: the condition of the skin tells about temperature; an emotional reaction signifies a job well done or a failure; a pain signifies malfunction or injury.

A person is an open system, receiving stimuli from the outer world and, in turn, influencing that world through personal behaviour.

Other social systems are the family; church; economic; politico-legal, and educational institutions; and health-care agencies.

**Linkage** *occurs when two systems exchange energy across their boundaries.* Industry, the church, or the health agency, for example, draws energy from its linkage to the family. In return, industry is willing to contribute to family welfare funds, mental-health campaigns or ecological improvements. The church maintains its role as prime defender of family stability. The health agencies set the standards for health care.

*Health care as a system*

Although much care to maintain health and overcome illness is given by a nurturing person in the home, formal health care can be thought of as a system having various subsystems – for instance, hospitals in the private and public sector, clinics, GP's surgeries and group practices.

The goal of any health-care agency is to provide health, medical and nursing care by providing a variety of services related to health for a specifically defined population. How this goal is achieved depends on how the agency is organized.

In a highly organized system, such as a hospital, what one department does is crucial to another department. Action in one health centre may have little effect on any other health agency. Hierarchy is obvious and rigid in some agencies. For example, in some hospitals a staff nurse cannot take certain actions without obtaining permission from the sister. In other agencies the nurses are peers.

Social controls exist in each health agency and these controls create either coercion or cooperation. A nurse, for instance, may enlist the cooperation of a patient in establishing an oral drug routine or may quickly inject a medication when the patient refuses the oral medicine – a form of coercion.

Because each agency serves a specifically defined population, the subject of boundary becomes significant. Sometimes the environment is distinct. Or the environment may be diffuse: patients may come for hundreds of miles to a hospital for open-heart surgery. The hospital or home-health agency may also relate with other health-care subsystems in the environment, such as a nursing home, mental-health association, Alcoholics Anonymous, or the Red Cross. Maintaining communication with and obtaining feedback from the community served are essential in serving the people's needs – the goal of the system.

Health-care agencies can be categorized as being either authoritarian or democratic. In the authoritarian system one person is in charge; other people follow. Ideas originate with the person at the top, flow down and go unquestioned. People who are lower in rank have no power and little room for creativity. In the democratic system members are peers and all members are involved in decision making. Members arrive at a solution by discussion and consensus. Anyone may originate an idea and that person receives either negative or positive feedback about his ideas and behaviour. All relationships in an agency are affected by the dominant pattern.

A health-care agency may be one or the other, but typically it combines characteristics of these two ends of the continuum. Some nurses like to work in an informal but non-changing atmosphere, they like to feel part of a big happy family. Other nurses are frustrated by this system, they enjoy a formal efficient atmosphere. They feel they should concentrate on nursing as a job, they are not especially interested in the personal problems or joys of other workers.

An understanding of your own basic preference and a careful study of the philosophy and characteristics of the agency you plan to work for are useful in selecting a satisfying work position. Much of the mobility in nursing may be the result of one personality type being employed by another agency type, so that the person's emotional and social needs cannot be met. Economic rewards are always important, but some people have strong needs for peer approval, individual recognition for a job well done or an affectionate relationship with the person in charge.

*Application of systems theory for nursing*

Appreciating the complexity and interrelationships of the people, social institutions and organizations giving health care will enable you to understand your role in giving health care. As a nurse, you will have a twofold purpose: to adjust at times to the system as it exists and at other times to work with people to produce necessary changes. The public increasingly expects you to do the latter to meet their needs.

*Systems theory* takes the major responsibility for change from you as an individual person and recognizes the importance of the total situation in creating and maintaining problems that hinder change and are beyond the power of the individual to correct. Each aspect of life is so interrelated and people are so interdependent that you are unlikely to make much change in a situation unless you work with others and consider many factors.

Fundamental changes come from within the individual or system. They cannot be imposed from without, although an outsider can be an influence. The push for maintaining the status quo and the push for change exist simultaneously. If you strive for better conditions in a health agency, you may find that they can only be achieved by pressures for policy and administrative change on a high level. Through your educational preparation, understanding of communication patterns, and experiences as a nurse, you will be in a position to promote changes in the health-care system.

As a member of various health, education, welfare and regulatory agencies in the community, you may function in the health-care system in the following ways:

1. As an advocate for the person or family needing health services.
2. As a concerned, active community member.
3. As an expert in health affairs.
4. As a consumer of health services.

If you understand and are comfortable with Systems theory, you can work more effectively for furtherance of health. You can also better understand the relationships that exist within the person you care for, in the agency where you work, and in the total health-care field. The hospitalized patient may appear as a complex of unrelated parts while various specialists are examining the patient's/client's lungs, heart, head or kidneys. You can help other health professionals perceive the patient as a whole. Disease affects the whole person, not just a single part. Community surveys, assessments, and demographic studies are tools that will help you use the nursing process in the social system of the community and specific health agency.

Intervention on the systems level includes talking with the nursing supervisor, clinical specialists, or dietitian about cold food at mealtimes or getting a wheelchair so that a patient can get out of the confining four walls of the room. You may be instrumental in creating a patient action group that has at least some effect on improving the environment of a unit.

Outside the institution you can participate in starting organizations for older or disabled persons that help to meet their individual needs and have an impact on the political life of their community or you may be instrumental in establishing a holistic health programme for employees in the workplace or for athletes on a sports team as illustrated in fig 1.1.

Although you will not always strive for big institutional upheavals, avoid accepting the present situation as an unalterable fact. Frequently when working at the same place for some time, you adapt to distressing situations so that you do not even notice them, even though they cause considerable discomfort or suffering for the patient. Periodically survey your work environment as if you were a stranger to it. You might keep a diary of your reactions to the work setting when you are first employed and then refer to it periodically to determine changes you wish to initiate. In this way, you can better work as your patient's/client's advocate and as an advocate for nursing.

You may not always be able to make constructive changes in the system. Some changes take longer than others, but you should keep trying. Often an idea must be proposed several times before it gains acceptance by others.

*Systems framework* helps you to remember that each patient/client is a system, interrelates with other systems, and is a part of a family, various groups and organizations, a job, and a community. In turn, the patient/client is affected by the various systems in which he/she participates. Therefore while you directly care for one system, you are indirectly caring for other systems as well.

Keep Systems theory in mind as you read the rest of this book. The systems surrounding the person affect behaviour and ultimately health. Nursing is a system because it consists of elements in interaction – the patient/client, family, nurse – communicating or exchanging information, engaging in the teaching-learning process or group work. A system must be adaptive to survive. Chapters 5 and 6 describe adaptation as a concept and crisis intervention as one way to help a troubled person or family system. Unit II looks at a variety of systems: the macroenvironment, the cultural, social and religious groups, the family, and the relationship of these entities to health, illness, and the nursing process.

## VARIABLES THAT AFFECT BEHAVIOUR AND HEALTH

### Basic needs

**Behaviour** *is the observable response to environmental stimuli, including verbal reports about emotional state, perceptions and thoughts.* The primary purpose of behaviour is to meet the needs of the person or the group.[6]

*Human needs* are those aspects of the individual that must be satisfied for life to continue and that can be divided into three broad categories: physiological, libidinal (sensual and affectional) and ego developmental. *Physiological needs* are cyclic, perpetual and imperative for survival. They include the need for oxygen, water, food, elimination, sleep, temperature control or shelter, safety or movement.

*Libidinal needs* refer to sensual-sexual and affectional-emotional needs. *Sensual-sexual* needs are not uniformly rhythmic in humans, although hormonal rhythms of the menstrual cycle are correlated with affective and behavioural changes in some women. The basis of sensual-sexual needs is organic, but these needs take on psychologic meanings.

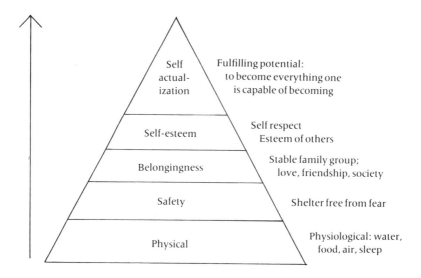

*Fig. 1.1    Maslow's hierarchy of human needs*

*Affectional-emotional* needs are constant and are at the core of normal psychic dependence. The person must be given love, security, approval, respect, support, care and protection for emotional and physical development.

*Ego-developmental* needs refer to the need for cognitive, perceptual and memory development (training and education). The person must have opportunity for and help with mastery of age-adequate behaviours, including motor coordination; emotional autonomy, independence and self-identity; social skills; communication skills (speech, reading, writing, nonverbal); adaptive mechanisms; moral development; control of drives; problem solving; work skills; and the opportunity for development of creative and self-actualization behaviour.

Libidinal- and ego-developmental needs emerge together; they influence each other and are equally significant for psychic and physical well-being. Ego development proceeds from mastery of simple to complex tasks.

Humans are very adaptable in meeting their needs, but adaptive potentials are not unlimited. In prehistoric evolution humans met many stresses, but their genetic constitutions were able to adapt over time. Now humans face threats created by modern technology that have no precedent in their evolutionary past. The rate of biological evolution is too slow to keep up with the effects of technological and social changes. Thus certain needs may not be met as well; other needs may be created. Unmet needs affect health status.

In countries where the population continues to increase rapidly, there is a strain on all social and human resources, including economic and educational development, and many people will have unmet needs. In such countries, health promotion is an ideal; preventing starvation and providing shelter are already consuming the resources of many nations. When physiological needs are not met, the other needs described previously cannot be met. It is a challenge to international nursing to foster the meeting of basic needs, disease prevention and health in the people of all nations.

### External environmental variables

The external environment includes all stimuli, objects, and people impinging on the person.

The *physical environment* contains a wide variety of potential stimuli: gravity, light and sound waves, and meteorological stimuli, such as temperature variation, wind velocity, atmospheric pressure, humidity, solar radiation, air pollutants, ozone, oxygen, carbon-dioxide and carbon-monoxide levels, electromagnetic fields, day-night and seasonal periodicity, and infectious microorganisms.[7] The physical environment, such as housing and sanitation facilities, affects health. Air, food, water and other pollutants are directly or indirectly the cause of one-half of all cancers. Cigarette smoke is a form of indoor pollution for nonsmokers. Maternal smoking increases the risk of respiratory infection and asthma in the child. Nonsmokers who are chronically exposed to cigarette smoke in the workplace have pulmonary function similar to that of light smokers and poorer than nonsmokers in a smoke-free environment. Lung cancer is increased in nonsmoking wives of heavy smokers.

Migrants moving from one environment to another develop the cancer pattern of the new geographic area. Mortality rates from cancer, as well as other diseases differ according to geographic region.

*Meteorological stimuli* are mediated primarily by the thermo-regulatory centres of the hypothalamus and the autonomic nervous system. Seasonal variations affect every physiological system. In winter, calcium, magnesium and phosphate blood levels are lowered; thyroid and adrenocorticord activities are elevated; hemoglobin levels are increased; and gastric acid secretion is high. These changes are gradual and reflect the thermostatic properties of the hypothalamus in conserving heat and energy during cold winter months.

Daily variations in *thermal stimuli* simultaneously affect the person. Responses to an approaching cold front include diuresis without increased fluid intake, increased thyrotropin production, elevated leucocyte and thrombocyte levels, elevated hemoglobin, lowered erythrocyte sedimentation rate and increased fibrinolysis. The opposite changes occur during a heat wave.[8] Any extreme fluctuation in environmental conditions results in a temporary disruption of internal environment and requires more energy to restore physiological adaptation.

*Sociocultural attributes of climate and weather* are reflected in the person's lifestyle, the kind of clothing worn, the food eaten, or the activities engaged in.

*Psychological attributes of climate and weather* relate to personal preference and symbolic interpretation. Some people have optimal performance in cold weather; others in warm weather. Some people associate fog and rain with depression; to others such weather symbolizes security.[9]

Although weather and climatic conditions affect the person in a given geographical setting, the *immediate physical environment* also provides multiple sensory stimuli. Room design and colour, combinations of light and sound, and the arrangement of objects and persons in the room all form a *gestalt*, a whole pattern that may be perceived as either pleasant or unpleasant. One is sensitive to the physical and chemical stimuli in the environment that are of sufficient intensity and interest; some stimuli will not be perceived.

The *psychological environment* surrounding someone is difficult to ascertain because it has a specific meaning to that person; the person's perception of the environment is a major determinant of behaviour. The reactions of others contribute to the development of self-concept and self-esteem, foster support to and involvement with the person, stimulate maturity, and convey limits on behaviour.[10]

To remain emotionally healthy, it is necessary to be with people who are healthy and in a group climate that contributes to developing one's optimal potential. Emotional health implies the capacity to love, learn, live fully and share with others in the adventure of life. The emotionally ill person comes from an environment in which there is excessive tension, a barrier to emotional communication, an isolation between people, and in which emotional and social needs are not met. The emotional illness of one person in the family or group spills over so that all members are unhealthy to some degree.

Married and unmarried persons differ in their health status. Married men and women have lower morbidity rates for physical illness, use health services less frequently, and live longer than unmarried people. Although married women have a higher incidence of emotional illness than married men, single women have less incidence of emotional illness than single men. Married, employed women exhibit fewer physical and psychiatric symptoms than married, nonemployed women. Single men are at a greater risk for both physical and emotional illness. Sex-role expectations and lifestyle, as well as resultant emotional states, may be factors behind these statistics.

Today, more women, married and unmarried, are employed than ever before. Many working women also bear the major responsibility of child care. Women are exposed to the same physical and emotional hazards of the work environment as men, plus the pressures created by multiple roles and conflicting expectations.[11]

The *sociocultural environment* includes the historical era, family, and other people and groups; social institutions, such as government, schools and church; all sorts of social events; and shared values and moral, ethical and religious beliefs. All groups have developed rules and regulations that assist an individual in the specific historical time in the process of becoming a useful and valued member of the group and that serve to constrain certain behaviours. Society helps an individual decide on the rules applicable in a particular situation, but it also grants the privilege of ignoring the rule if he/she so chooses. Punishment will be established for deviancy by the group if the rule is essential for the group's survival. Change occurs so rapidly in our society that old values and relationships no longer have the same importance or meaning. Social instability produces conflict and alienation between groups, creates lack of direction for members and contributes to illness.[12]

The family contributes not only to genetic predisposition but also to the actual etiology of specific diseases through lack of hygiene measures, nutritional imbalance, transmission of social values, the socialization process of the child and the family pattern of daily living and behaviour. The family may also contribute to long-term health problems in its members through physical or emotional abuse or through sexual assault or incest.

*Population density* affects social behaviour in animal studies and parallels human behaviour in crowded conditions. Studies on small mammals show that uncontrolled population growth causes specific behaviours as population density increases: aggression, confusion as the number of social roles in the animal colony decreases, social withdrawal and avoidance of other animals, and loss of interest in tending young.

Socioeconomic class, occupation and social roles influence behaviour at various times of the day, preventive health measures practised, and susceptibility to disease. Socioeconomic level influences health-care accessibility. More affluent urban people can afford housing, food and regular medical examinations that can promote health. Yet more affluent people may also be in executive positions or occupations or social roles that are highly stressful or that encourage overeating or social use of drugs or alcohol, thus predisposing the person to chemical dependency. The poorer rural person may not have an annual physical examination but may eat a diet composed primarily of simple carbohydrates, fish and homegrown fruits and vegetables, which will contribute to health. Social roles are significant to health because they place various demands on the person and call for shifts and flexibility in attitude and behaviour, which may be demanding to the point of illness. The occupational role is important. Whether the person is a farmer, nurse, coal miner, physician, executive or clerk predisposes to different stressors and illnesses. The worker in an industrial plant may be exposed to carcinogenic materials. The miner living in poverty develops respiratory disease; he may realize his work is making him ill, but he is financially unable to change jobs or geographic locations. The middle-class person may work in a clean office, have conveniences to assist with housework, and see the dentist twice yearly for a checkup. The higher the socioeconomic class and occupational position, the greater is the variety of behavioural choices available to specific goals. When availability of resources becomes restricted because of economic or geographical reasons, lifestyle and behaviour are restricted.[13]

*Internal variables*

*Genetic inheritance* influences the physical characteristics, innate temperament, the activity level and intellectual potential of the person. Physical characteristics include sex and such features as skin and eye colour, hair colour and degree of curl, facial structure and height. The physical characteristics influence the response of others as well as the person's response to the environment. The positive reinforcement and the interaction from the environment that a child or adult with desirable physical characteristics receives affect that person's self-concept development and relationship to others.[14]

**Intelligence,** *the ability to deal with complex, abstract material*, is influenced by inheritance, environment and sociocultural influences. The test score reflecting intelligence is influenced by many factors: motivation at the time of testing, what the test means to the person, level of anxiety, cultural and social-class background of the person, physical environment of the testing situation, and the race and other characteristics of the tester.[15]

*Circadian and psychobiological rhythms* are part of the internal processes of the person, are interdependent with the time-space aspects of the environment and help to organize behaviour.[16] **Biological rhythms** *are self-sustaining repeating patterns* or inner clocks. They help explain why some people are mentally sharp at 6.00 a.m. while others work to full capacity at 10.00 p.m. Biological rhythms may be **exogenous,** *dependent on the rhythm of external environmental events, such as sunlight, or* **endogenous,** *arising within the organism and uninfluenced by the environment.*[17] Biological rhythms are classified according to the length or occurrence of the rhythmic pattern (oscillation) as diurnal, circadian, ultradian and infradian.[18] The terms *diurnal* and *circadian* were used in the past to mean a rhythm occurring once a day. The term *diurnal rhythm*, however, is ambiguous when applied to diurnal animals; so **diurnal** *rhythm is used to describe fluctuations in body processes confined to the working day, whereas* **circadian** *rhythm describes fluctuations occurring every 20 to 28 hours. The terms* **ultradian** and

**infradian**, coined by Franz Halberg, *refer to rhythmic processes occurring less frequently than every 24 hours* and *on a weekly or monthly basis, respectively.*[19]

*Gender* of the person affects disease susceptibility: certain genetic and acquired diseases are more common in one sex than in the other. *Sexual identity*, determined embryologically and moulded through the influences of sociocultural environment, affects patterns of behavioural responses developed by that person. Cross-cultural studies show that division of labour is made on the basis of sex, although not all cultures designate home and child care as female functions. The environment makes distinctions in the expected and valued behaviours for each sex as well as to indicate which sex is more valuable.

*Age and developmental level* influence illness susceptibility as well as behaviour. Response patterns and capabilities are minimal for the first few years of life and near the end of life. The infant has few response patterns available because of two factors: lack of experience and a state of physiological and psychological immaturity. The aged person has limited responses because of declining sensory-perceptual monitoring of the environment and declining physical abilities. The periods of greatest availability of responses to environmental and social demands are in young and middle adulthood; the peak years vary with each person and with occupational groups. Athletes peak earlier than physicians, for example.[20]

*Race* of the person is related to cultural and ethnic experiences, values and attitudes, as well as responses of others to the person. Behavioural patterns may vary with the race, as does susceptibility to illness. Descendants of African and Mediterranean people, for instance, are more prone to sickle cell trait and sickle cell anaemia.[21]

**Self-concept** *is the person's perception of self physically, emotionally, and socially, based on the internalized reactions of others to self.* The self-concept, self-expectations, perceived abilities, values, attitudes, habits and beliefs affect how that person will handle situations and relate to others. How the person behaves depends on whether he/she feels positively or negatively and on how the person feels others expect him/her to behave in a specific situation. Additionally, the person discloses different aspects of self in various situations, depending on personal needs, what is considered socially acceptable, how others react, and past experience with self-disclosure. Thus the hospitalized patient's behaviour may be different from the usual pattern; the person may behave according to others' expectations instead of how he/she desires. These variables also affect health practices and treatment sought. The incidence of cancer has been linked to geographical or environmental factors. For example, in the United Staes, Seventh Day Adventists have half as much cancer as the national average and rural Mormons in Utah have 60 to 75 per cent less, apparently because of their lifestyle, which is related to their religion.

The feelings of the person may be related to internal neuroendocrine processes, but they are also related to events in the external environment, including stressful events. A sense of hopelessness, despair or extreme fear may cause death as well as disease. Many human and animal studies confirm this fact and the death that results from a hex being placed on a member is documented in various societies. When the person becomes an outcast and has nothing to live for, physiological processes stop and death occurs.[22]

Although responses to stressful situations vary, anxiety is a common one. **Anxiety**, *a state of mental discomfort or uneasiness related to a feeling of helplessness or threat to self-image*, occurs in everyone, well or ill. Often there is no objective cause. The ill or hospitalized person may experience anxiety because of environmental changes. The individual exhibits signs of anxiety about the unknown: the outcome of surgery, the stability of job and family income, and possible death. The anxious person may experience the physical and behavioural effects that are described in Chapter 5 and Table 5.1. Other responses to stress include grief, mourning and denial. These concepts will be covered in later chapters. Should the felt mental, emotional, or even physical disequilibrium become severe, mental or physical illness may result. Therefore the health of persons is directly related to and affected by their reactions to both the internal and external environment.

The **mind–body relationship,** *the effect of emotional responses to stress on body function, and the emotional reactions to body conditions*, has been established through research and experience. Emotional factors are important in the precipitation or exacerbation of nearly every organic disease and may increase susceptibility to infections. Stress and emotional distress, including depression, may influence function of the immunologic system via the central nervous system and endocrine mediation, which is related to incidence of cancer, infections and autoimmune diseases. Apparently adrenal cortical steroid hormones may be immunosuppressive. Recurring or chronic emotional stress has a cumulative physiologic effect and eventually may produce chronic dysfunction, such as hypertension or gastric ulcers. The dynamics involve repression of certain feelings, such as rage or guilt, fooling the mind into thinking the feelings have disappeared. But the body's physiological functions respond to the feelings or perception of the effect (stressor). *When physical or organic symptoms or disease result from feeling states, the process is called* **psychosomatic**. The opposite process, *feeling states of depression or worry in response to physical disease states, is called* **somato-psychic**.

Feelings are often related to the person's perception of the event. Certain life events, especially undesirable ones, are perceived by most people as stressful or as crises because of the amount of change or extent of readjustment required. Because change is stressful, and stress is a causative factor in illness, a relationship exists between the amount of recent change, number of crises encountered, and onset of illness. Stressful events may even speed up death.

The determinants of behaviour, health and illness are multiple. Using knowledge from a variety of disciplines is useful in gaining a comprehensive view of the person under your care.

## ROLE OF THE NURSE: PROMOTION AND MAINTENANCE OF HEALTH

*Personal health promotion*

Until recently most of the focus in health care was on disease and death. Now more emphasis is being placed on how to achieve, measure or maintain health. The goal of health promotion is to raise the levels of health in individuals, families and communities. Health and illness may exist simultaneously with each of us; you must relate to both aspects of the person. If each person is to reach the goal of optimum health, you must place more emphasis on the fulfilment of health for you and your client through health education, preventive measures and continuity of care. Since health is a purposeful, adaptive, total body response to internal and external stimuli to maintain stability and comfort, **health promotion** *includes those factors that help the person to maintain this necessary stability, to foster ongoing development,* and has been defined by Pender as *developing the resources that maintain or enhance wellbeing.* [23]

The following are considered factors that promote health for you and others:

1. Assessing present health status regularly through periodic health examinations, including dental checkups, and participating in mass screening programmes in the community.
2. Learning preventive measures and warning signals of disease, such as those published by the Health Education Authority and The British Heart Foundation.
3. Learning safety measures to prevent injury and emergency treatment to avoid excessive or unnecessary tissue damage if an accident or illness occurs.
4. Securing anticipatory guidance for potential crises and for stresses related to developmental stage or lifestyle. See Chapters 2 and 6 for communication measures that promote anticipatory guidance.
5. Caring for the body functions, including those factors affecting the skin, mucous membranes, teeth, elimination, and sensory organs.
6. Avoiding products harmful to health – for instance, excess in caffeine, tobacco, any kind of drugs, alcohol or food. Caffeine consumption has been linked to breast cancer and other diseases. Nicotine, excessive intake of most drugs, alcohol, and obesity are each linked to various diseases. Excessive or inappropriate use of prescribed or over-the-

counter drugs frequently has serious consequences. A majo
involves overuse and inappropriate prescription of antibiotic
ing in resistant strains of microorganisms and inadequate trea
infections. The excessive and careless prescribing of mood-c
drugs may result in loss of behavioural control and even in p ,sical
and psychological addiction.

Taking a combination of many prescribed or unprescribed drugs
may result in interactive effects that are toxic to the body. Alcohol is a
major cause of many accidental injuries and deaths as well as of other
diseases. Refer to Chapter 7 for discussion of other agents that are
harmful to health.

7. Avoiding extreme stress, fatigue or exhaustion, providing for adequate relaxation, rest and sleep, and using relaxation techniques if necessary.

8. Maintaining essential nutrition and staying within 10 pounds of normal body weight. Nutritionists, in general, agree that the best diet is high in fibre, moderate in protein and fat and low in sugar and salt. High-fibre foods include bran and other whole grains, raw fruits and vegetables. These foods prevent constipation and apparently other gastrointestinal diseases, including cancer. Red meat should not be the main source of protein. Sources of saturated fats, such as red meat, butter or whole milk, should be limited because they impair the body's ability to reverse cholesterol build-up. Processed foods should not be the mainstay of a diet. Coffee, tea and cola intake should be limited, for excessive caffeine intake has been linked to feelings of increased stress. Cooking with herbs or using lemon juice, vinegar, or other condiments can decrease the need to use salt as a flavouring.

9. Using safety measures or devices, such as seat belts in cars, safety equipment in power machines, and sturdy ladders, to prevent injury.

10. Using principles of body mechanics can prevent injury. When you are moving or lifting objects, do the following to prevent muscle strain or musculoskeletal injury: (a) roll or slide the object rather than lift; (b) move objects on a flat or level surface if possible; (c) keep objects close to the centre of gravity in the body; (d) use the largest and strongest muscles to apply forces – for instance, thighs, legs, arms, and shoulders; (e) use leverage to apply force or move an object when possible rather than relying on body weight; and (f) reduce friction if possible when moving an object. Injury is also prevented by using the proper chair in the workplace. The back of the chair should be high enough to come about 2 inches above the lower tip of the shoulder blades and should tilt backward about 10 degrees. The back of the seat should be 3 degrees higher than the front edge. This will place you forward a bit so that you can lean back to maintain balance, thus putting your body in a good natural position. The depth of the seat should be such that the front edge comes to within 1 inch of the back of your knee, allowing

your thighs to rest on it without putting pressure on your knees or calves. Feet should rest on the floor. The person should also be advised not to cross knees which interferes with circulation. The aches and strains that develop in workers who sit or stand in poor posture daily can finally result in feeling ill and even in injury.

11. Preventing, when possible, and attending to any infection or injury that occurs. First-aid measures can be obtained from the Red Cross, St John Ambulance or a nursing text.

12. Securing necessary immunization for the children and adults in the family, especially with outdoor exercise and athletic programmes, wide travel and resurgence of communicable diseases.

13. Maintaining a regular, moderate exercise programme to enhance physical and emotional health. The exercise should involve large muscle groups in dynamic movement for about 20 minutes three or more days a week and should require 60 per cent or more of a person's cardiorespiratory capacity. The exertion should be within limits appropriate to the physical status and needs of the person and should also be accompanied by a sense of excitement, flexibility, strength, and energy. At the end of exercise the person should feel replenished rather than bored, burned out, or excessively fatigued. Furthermore, the personal need to increase exercise to the point of competitive winning or achievement of maximal physical performance may contribute to eventual anatomical, physiological and psychological breakdown.

There is no evidence that running is better than other aerobic physical exercise, such as fast walking, swimming, bicycling or dancing. The benefits of running are that it allows for psycho-motor expression without the hazards of contact sports and is adaptable to a wide range of weather or geographical conditions, time schedules, personalities and body types. Running can be social or asocial or organized or unorganized as an activity.

Running, or any strenuous physical exercise, also has some hazards. It can become addictive because release of endorphins in the body causes the person to feel euphoric and oblivious to pain or injury while running and very anxious when the exercise is omitted or delayed. The person who engages in intense exercise may either engage in other health-promotion measures, or may feel invulnerable to disease and death. That myth may prevent engaging in other health-promotion measures. The long-term effects on joints and organs or regular, long-distance running is currently unknown; some orthopaedic physicians report musculoskeletal damage resulting from the 'pounding' effects. Some physicians also report that breast tissue is damaged if inadequately supported by a brassiere, and pelvic organs in women may suffer prolapse from excessive long-distance running. Other physicians disagree.

14. Taking time for play, leisure or diversional activities and spiritual pursuits that are (a) rewarding emotionally; (b) done voluntarily rather than out of obligation; (c) outside of ordinary life routines; (d) absorbing in attention; (e) are not necessarily productive in earnings, and (f) have definite time and space boundaries.

Many forces are in play as a person decides for or against what has been defined as health-promotion or illness-prevention behaviour. Internal (personality), external (environmental), and various knowledge and emotional forces, some unknown to the person, all contribute.

Sometimes health-promotion behaviour is motivated by other than health factors. White teeth and a slim body are regarded as sexually attractive, for example. A person may brush teeth and lose weight for this reason rather than to delay tooth decay and cardiovascular failure. On the other hand, a person may know that losing 100 pounds will increase the life span by 6 years and allow a better functioning cardiovascular system and yet be unable to forego the immediate reward system of high-calorie, low carbohydrate desserts.

*Preventive health behaviour* is related to subjective ideas about vulnerability and present health state, the value placed on health and early detection of illness, and the sense of internal versus external control.

Pender defines **prevention** as *activities that protect from potential or actual health threats and their harmful consequences.*[24]

Family history is important; the greater the incidence of specific illness within the family and the closer the blood relationship of the affected persons to an individual, the more likely the person will feel vulnerable. Feeling weak or fatigued, having been ill within the year, or identifying self as part of a high-risk group also increases the sense of personal vulnerability. Anticipating a health problem can motivate the person to do something to prevent it.

Four factors contribute to the perceived seriousness of any given health problem: (1) degree of threat; (2) overt visibility of illness or disability; (3) degree of interference with a person's lifestyle, family or occupational roles, and (4) communicability of disease to others. The person's concern for the welfare of others may be greater than for personal health. Thus preventive measures are more likely to be followed for communicable disease than for those that affect only the individual.[25]

The person chooses the preventive services that are perceived as being most effective in lowering the threat of illness. The higher the educational or socioeconomic levels, the more will people be aware of the entire range of preventive health alternatives available.

The person who feels powerless or unable to control the environment is not likely to try preventive health behaviour. The person who feels able to control the self internally perceives self as less vulnerable to ill health and usually takes preventive health actions.

Four key factors influence the decision to seek preventive health services. First, the person may seek health care because of family encouragement. Second, patterns of using preventive services are learned in the family. The level of the mother's education correlates highly with preventive practices because the mother is often the decision maker in this area. Third, expectations of friends are powerful motivators to seek preventive health care, for parents especially want to fulfil the expectation of peers, neighbours or friends about what 'good parents should do'. Fourth, information and respectful care from health professionals also increase the readiness to engage in preventive health behaviour especially if the health professional is seen as knowledgeable and caring. The small-group approach to giving information is more effective than teaching only one person. However, knowing what is healthy is no guarantee that the person will follow healthy patterns of living.

Situational determinants that influence the decision to practise preventive measures include cultural values on health and prevention, group norms and pressures, and information from mass media.

Yet various barriers impede a person's action even after the decision to take action: high costs, inconvenience, unpleasantness of treatment measures or facilities, pain, fear of findings from early detection measures, inability to decide which course of action would be best, psychological needs that are fulfilled by the illness or prescribed changes in lifestyle that are perceived as undesirable.[26]

You should do everything possible within the agency to structure policies and the environment to meet the needs of those who present themselves for preventive health care. Unnecessary waiting; cold, harsh manner; excessive noise, heat, or cold in the waiting area; architectural barriers that impede movement by persons with wheelchairs, walkers or canes can be eliminated or minimized in order to avoid discouraging those who come or who might return for care. Some services could be taken to the clients' homes, places of employment, and schools. Additionally, churches, playgrounds and shopping centres could be viewed as centres to provide certain teaching or screening services periodically.

The nurse-client relationship must be viewed differently than previously. The client becomes pivotal in all interactions whereas the nurse functions as an encourager, facilitator, teacher, counsellor or assistant who promotes adaptation and self-care by the client. Both parties must agree to the plan of care and responsibilities in the relationship.[27]

*Good-health programmes*

Traditionally the main health concern for employees in the workplace was that of safety and accident prevention. A yearly physical examination was also included in many industries.

Today industries and some hospitals and other work settings are a programmes for their employees that generally include emphasis in areas: stress reduction, exercise, smoking cessation, and nutritional weight guidance, particularly for obesity and sodium and cholesterol reduction. Some employers also run schemes to prepare for retirement.

*Health education*

**Health education** *is the learning process by which persons and groups learn to promote, maintain, or restore health.* Health education should be a constant part of people's lives. It is important for them to understand the impact that such factors as stress, smoking, exercise, excess weight, chronic disease, air pollution, recreation and occupation have on health. Once a person has been exposed to a health-education programme, the desired outcome is a change in health behaviour or attitude.[28]

Health education must be adjusted to learning levels and directed to situations of immediate interest for the particular age group. For example, a 10-year-old boy is concerned with increasing muscular prowess via proper food and exercise whereas the 16-year-old is concerned with the effects of smoking, drugs and alcohol consumption. Adults are increasingly concerned about the effects of stress, pollutants, smoking and drugs on long-term health.

As a health educator, you must learn about the health and health needs of each person by determining knowledge, values, attitudes, and practices related to personal health promotion, plans for health protection, and present mental and emotional health status. The individual who has a positive self-concept and who feels a sense of control over health and personal life is more likely to practise health-education beliefs and preventive measures. All these points must be considered before the actual planning and during implementation of any health-education programme.

You also play an important part in health education by promoting control of infection and disease through mass screening or immunization and by supporting and promoting community projects for improved housing, adequate sanitation facilities, vermin control, slum clearance, and control of leaded paint and petrol. You may also be involved in the use of mass media for health education. Turnbull found that television publicity about disease and disease prevention can increase use of health-promotion measures, such as breast self-examination.[29] Or you may help people explore less traditional forms of health promotion or healing, such as concepts used in Oriental or other folk medicine.

Teaching parents about child care, nutrition, normal patterns of development, how to manage given budgetary and other limitations, and realistic expectations for themselves and their children can promote adaptation to the ordinary stresses of family living and childrearing.

Helping parents to feel 'good' or positive about themselves and their children is basic to any teaching. By promoting the adaptive capacities of parents, you can help prevent child abuse. All these items are interrelated to enhance the health – physically, mentally, emotionally and socially – of the person, family and community.

In the past, health education was handled mainly by nurses. Today health educators, social workers, dietitians and others are contributing to this process. Teaching about healthy lifestyles is one of our most effective techniques of fostering health promotion. More and more the consumer from all backgrounds expects a holistic or total approach to health care and prevention. The client increasingly expects a good-health orientation that includes body, mind, spirit and cultural background considerations. The balance of lifestyle, environment and relationships must be considered. Traditional and nontraditional methods of health care must be used. A holistic approach respects the right of the person to make choices about health care and to assume responsibility for those choices. Positive attitudes are promoted in a holistic health practice. The result of holistic health is an ever higher expression of potential and fulfilment.

The remainder of this book explores in greater depth the information that you can use to promote the wellbeing of yourself and others in a **pluralistic society** – *a society containing diverse groups of people distinctive in environmental setting, racial or ethnic origins, sociocultural patterns, and religion, who maintain independent lifestyles within the confines of a common civilization.* Information about developmental norms that will assist you in understanding people in a pluralistic society is also available.[30]

REFERENCES

1. Dubois, Rene, 'Man Overadapting', *Psychology Today*, vol. 4 no. 9.
2. Hayman, H.S., 'An Ecological View of Health and Health Education', *Journal of School Health*, vol. 35 (1965) no. 3.
3. Blum, Henrik L., *Planning for Health: Genetics for the Eighties* (Human Sciences Press, 2nd edition, New York, 1981).
4. Dunn, Halbert J., *High Level Wellness* (Mount Vernon Publishing Co. Inc., Washington DC, 1961).
5. Briscoe, M., 'Sex Differences in Perception of Illness and Expressed Life Satisfaction', *Psychological Medicine*, vol. 8 no. 2 (1978), pp. 339–45.
6. See note 2, above.
7. See note 1, above.
8. Porter, Dawn and Judith Shamien 'Self-care in Theory and Practice', *The Canadian Nurse*, vol. 79 no. 8 (1983), pp. 21–3.
9. Ibid.; see also, Griffith, W., 'Environmental Effects on Interpersonal Affective Behaviour: Ambient Effective Temperature and Attraction', *Journal of Personality and Social Psychology,* July 1970, pp. 240–4.

10. Auger, Jeanine, *Behavioural Systems and Nursing* (Prentice Hall, Englewood Cliffs, NJ, 1976).
11. Graham, H., *Women, Health and the Family* (Wheatsheaf Books, 1984).
12. See note 10, above.
13. Ibid.
14. Ibid.
15. Ibid.
16. Ibid.
17. Conroy, R.T.W.L. and J. N. Mills *Human Circadian Rhythms* (J. and A. Churchill, London, 1970).
18. *Ibid.*; see also, Turnbull, Eleanor, 'Effect of Basic Preventive Health Practices and Mass Media on the Practice of Breast Self-examination', *Nursing Research*, vol. 27 no. 2 (1978), pp. 98–102.
19. See note 17, above.
20. See note 10, above.
21. Ibid.
22. Langone, John, 'When Hopelessness Kills', *Discover*, October 1980, p. 116.
23. Open University, *Good Health Guide* (Pan, London, 1980).
24. Ibid.
25. Ibid.
26. Ibid.
27. Pender, Nola, *Health Promotion in Nursing Practice* (Appleton-Century-Crofts, Norwalk, CT, 1982).
28. Jarvis, Linda, *Community Health Nursing: Keeping the Public Healthy* (F.A. Davis Co., Philadelphia, 1981).
29. Tromp, S.W., 'Weather, Climate and Man', *Handbook of Physiology: Adaptation to the Environment*, eds. D. Hill, E. Adolph and C. Wilber (American Physiological Society, Washington DC, 1964, pp. 283–93).

# 2

# Therapeutic communication: prerequisite for effective nursing

Study of this chapter will enable you to:

1. Define *communication* and describe the elements in the communication process.

2. Identify the levels of communication and use this knowledge in nursing.

3. List and describe the tools used in communication.

4. Discuss ways to use language of size, time, space and colour, as well as words, effectively.

5. Observe various clients and situations and determine whether your observations meet the criteria and what factors influenced your observations and perceptions.

6. Describe the different types of nonverbal behaviour and how each affects communication.

7. Analyse silent periods to determine the type of silence and its effect on communication.

8. Practise attentive listening and explore its impact on the other person.

9. State the definition and purposes of an interview.

10. Discuss interviewing methods and rationale for steps in the method.

11. Interview a person, well or ill, using the correct methods, and analyse the principles used and the effectiveness of the interview.

12. Describe methods of therapeutic communication and the rationale for each method.

13. Analyse the pattern of communication, using knowledge of rationale, after practice of therapeutic communication with a client.

14. Describe modifications in communication approach that will be effective with a child or adolescent.

15. Discuss ways to modify a communication approach to be effective with clients who have communication disorders.

16. Discuss barriers to and ineffective methods of communication, identify personal use of them, and analyse why they are ineffective.

17. Explore how use of effective communication methods is basic to nursing care and contributes to health and the functioning of systems.

My Spanish friend looked puzzled when I said, 'Let's keep in touch.' I meant, 'Let's talk to each other periodically.'

He heard the literal meaning. Often we don't communicate because we use words symbolically rather than literally, as further illustrated by the following statement:

'I know you believe you understand what you think I said, but I am not sure you realize what you hear is not what I meant.' – Anonymous

The ability to communicate should not be taken for granted; it is not a simple process but rather a complex system by which the world's work gets done.

Communication is the matrix for all thought and relationships between persons and is bound to the learning process. Early sensory experiences shape subsequent learning abilities in speech, cognition, symbol recognition, and in the capacity for maturing communication. Perception of the self, the world, and one's place in it results from communication. Verbal and nonverbal communication is learned in a cultural setting; if the person does not communicate in the way prescribed by the culture, many difficulties arise, for that person cannot conform to the expectations of society. Disordered thinking, feeling, and actions result, along with mental anguish, and perhaps even physical illness.

Communication is the heart of the nursing process, for it is one of the primary methods used to accomplish specific and general goals with many different kinds of people. It is used in assessing and understanding the patient and family as well as in nursing intervention. Communication helps people express thoughts and feelings, clarify problems, receive information, consider alternate ways of coping or adapting, and remain realistic through feedback from the environment. Essentially the client learns

something about the self, how to identify health needs, and if and how he/
she wishes to meet them.

## DEFINITIONS

The word *communication* comes from the Latin verb *communicare*, 'to make
common, share, participate, or impart'. **Communication** *establishes a sense
of commonness with another and permits the sharing of information, signals, or
messages in the form of ideas and feelings.* It is a continuous dynamic process by
which one mind may affect another through written or oral language, gestures, facial expressions, music, painting, sculpture, drama, dance, or other
signs.

**Communication pattern** *refers to the relatively consistent network of messages sent and received in short- or long-term exchanges, the habitual way of interacting with others.* Part of this pattern is the **social amenities pattern,**
*the interaction that uses socially prescribed rules, ceremonies, or customs* according
to the situation and usually results in superficial communications. The social pattern includes **small talk,** *social chitchat that encompasses mundane
topics* and is used to kill time, to test the reactions of others, to avoid involvement, or to serve as a bridge to significant conversation. The **information pattern** differs in that it *involves a request for or giving of information or orders* but it is not likely to establish intimate understandings because
there is little disclosure of self. Neither the social nor the informational pattern is adequate by itself in the nursing process. The communication pattern in the nurse-client-family relationship should be a **dialogue,** involving *purposeful, reciprocal, close expression between the participants* and focusing
on the problems of the one seeking help rather than on those of the helper.

## THE COMMUNICATION PROCESS

Every communication process includes a sender, a transmitting device, signals, a receiver, and feedback, as shown in Fig. 2.1. The sender attempts to
convey a message, idea, or information through the appropriate use of
symbols or signals directed to another specific person or group. That the
message is sent does not guarantee that it will be received at all, let alone by
the person for whom it is intended.

Many factors influence how the message is sent and whether, how, and
by whom it will be received: the needs and condition of both the sender
and the receiver, emotionally, physically and intellectually; the occasion or
setting; and the sender's knowledge about the relationship with the receiv-

er. Other factors include the content of the message or the vocabulary to be decoded; the mood or attitude present in the situation; and the communication experience already in operation.

The receiver, in turn, perceives, interprets, and responds to the message. Through some process, feedback goes to the sender, confirming that the message has been received. The receiver at that point becomes the sender of a message. If the original message does not result in a response or feedback, there is no official interchange.

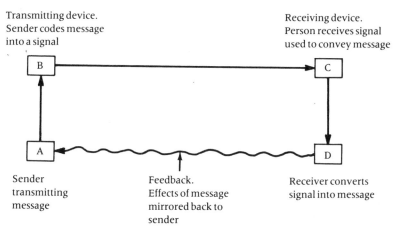

*Fig. 2.1* Elements in the communication process

Communication involves feedback and each message sent, including feedback, affects the next message sent and its feedback. The process is circular; communication from A affects B and B, in turn, affects A.

Communication and related behaviour can be studied only in context. Studying only the information, the command, the question – the words – is not enough. Behaviour and the way of communicating are not static; they vary with the specific situation. In certain situations, seemingly inappropriate responses may be highly appropriate behaviour. The apparently senseless talk of an emotionally ill person, for instance, may be the only feasible reaction in an absurd or untenable family communication context – the only way of achieving family equilibrium.

Or a child's aggressive behaviour may be the only way of maintaining initiative and self when the mother communicates overprotection or 'smothering' nonverbally. Communication is influenced by the family and social systems in which the person lives.

In the strictest sense, all behaviour in the presence of others is communication and all communication affects behaviour. How you gesture, posture, dress, move, speak, behave, or fail to carry out certain behaviours will provide an understandable signal for someone. To illustrate, two persons sitting side by side on a plane may neither speak nor look at one another. Yet there is a communication process present, for the behaviour of each conveys to the other a wish not to engage in an interchange of words, for whatever reason. Contrast this situation with two persons sitting side by side who do not speak but occasionally look at one another and smile. Then a few words are exchanged. The initial nonverbal expressions encourage the eventual verbal exchange. Thus anything perceptibly present or absent can serve as a signal of communication that need only be decoded to be meaningful.

*Levels of communication*

Communication occurs on several levels because of the perceptions of each person involved in the communication, and each level becomes increasingly abstract, as demonstrated in Fig. 2.2. When two persons are communicating, the following levels may occur.

1. This is how I perceive me.
2. This is how I perceive you.
3. This is how I perceive you seeing and hearing me.
4. This is how I think you see me seeing you.

In a nurse-client dialogue, on level 1, you are thinking only of the self while talking to the other person. Self-awareness is important, but awareness must include more than that. Level 1 communication would not be very helpful to the person. On level 2, you are thinking of the self but also observing the client's behaviour and hearing what is being said. This level of dialogue is more appropriate for communication of the other's needs. On level 3, you are aware of how the person might be perceiving you in addition to being aware of what both you and the person are saying, doing and feeling. Thus you can better consider the effect of yourself on the other and his/her behavioural cues, and respond to them. In addition, you may ask for validation of personal perceptions – whether the client is actually perceiving you as you believe. For level 4 communication to occur, you must be very alert, feeling energetic and attuned to the situation.

Now, in addition to the foregoing levels, you consider how the person thinks you are perceiving him/her – your feelings and attitudes toward the person as *he/she* perceives them. Level 4 takes considerable empathy, but it will allow you to be most helpful in communicating with the client. These levels increase in complexity with increasing numbers of people. If you understand the levels of communication, you can anticipate the communication process, hear 'hidden meanings', and recognize your impact on the process.

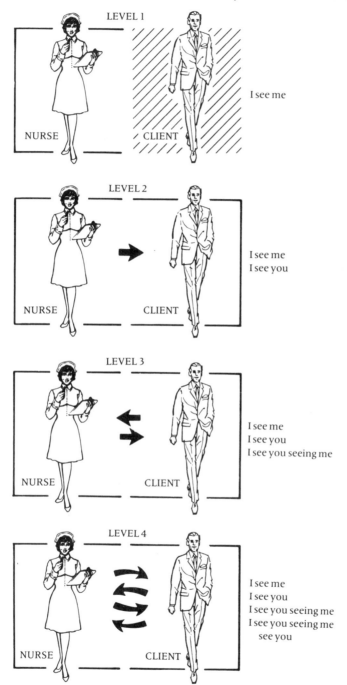

LEVEL 1

NURSE    CLIENT

I see me

LEVEL 2

NURSE    CLIENT

I see me
I see you

LEVEL 3

NURSE    CLIENT

I see me
I see you
I see you seeing me

LEVEL 4

NURSE    CLIENT

I see me
I see you
I see you seeing me
I see you seeing me
    see you

*Fig. 2.2*   Levels of communication

## TOOLS OF COMMUNICATION

The tools of communication – language, observation and perception, non-verbal behaviour, silence, and listening – are closely interrelated and are used simultaneously, although they are discussed separately in the following pages. Knowledge of these tools is essential before appropriately using the nursing process discussed in Chapter 3 and for your effective functioning in any system.

### Language

Language is basic to communication. Without language, the higher order cognitive processes of thinking, reasoning and generalizing could not be attained. Words are tools or symbols used to express ideas and feelings or to indicate objects; they are *not the same as the experience*, although words shape experience, communicate facts, convey interpretations, and influence relationships.

The functions of language can be classified as follows: expressive, arousal and descriptive. A speech act is *expressive* if it informs us of a speaker's state of mind or emotions; it is also likely to serve the function of *arousal*, triggering an emotional response in the receiver of the message. The *descriptive* function serves to inform another person, to convey observations, memories, ideas or inferences.

Visual images are more likely to serve the function of arousal than is language.[1] Viewing a picture can arouse strong emotion, for much of the self can be projected into the image. Yet the visual image is unable to show the many contexts of description or tense of which verbal language is capable, for in listening, the personality of the speaker more easily strikes us.

The same words have different meaning for different people, and you must constantly be prepared to define the meaning of a word or phrase. Also, word meanings change over time in response to new inventions and to developments and changes in travel, mass media and occupations. Thus language is a map of behaviour and communication.

You select, consciously or unconsciously, the part of the world you wish to experience at any time. No two people are in exactly the same spot at exactly the same time; therefore all our experiences are, to some extent, different. Many problems in communication arise because we fail to remember that individual experiences are never identical. When two persons talk with one another, communication is established by determining mutual experience. If the experience being discussed is new to a person, he/she may have difficulty making sense of it. Much difficulty in introducing new ideas and much resistance to change arise from the fact that we must learn *what* to experience in the events we live through.

Words may be used both to express feelings and to avoid expressing them. When a man says he feels 'fine', he may be functioning at optimum level – or he may be physically ill but wish to stop your further enquiry by responding with the word 'fine'. Words may also be used in deliberately obscure ways in order to convey hidden meanings, to test your interest in finding out such meanings, or the degree of your concern for the person, or to express hostility without fear of retaliation.

Nonlinguistic aspects of speech, such as silence, how much of the time and how fast the person talks, how soon the other person stops talking, interruptions, rate of speech errors, hestitations, such pauses as 'ers' and 'ahs', and repetitions also give important signals. Many of these signals indicate anxiety or other feelings, as do loudness, high pitch, rapidity of speech and breathiness. A depressed person talks slowly and at a low pitch and tolerates longer silences. An aggressive, dominating person talks loudly and rapidly, enunciates precisely, interrupts others more often, and may include ridicule, teasing, joking or direct insult in speech.[2]

In addition to the language of words, there is the language of size, time, space and colour.

**The language of size**, both physical and psychological, is related to the impact, influence, or potential for helping what one person has in regard to another. Large physical size conveys dominance, power, authority and control. Large psychological size is perceived when someone is highly knowledgeable, extrovert, aggressive, loud, rapid speaking or moving; also, when someone is stern, distant, holds the body rigidly, places hands on hips, or keeps others at a distance by physical, verbal or emotional stratagems. The psychologically large person may be expected by others to solve problems, to see that all goes well, and to take care of them. Alternately, the psychologically large person may also be seen as someone to avoid, who stifles development and creativity, or who must have the final word. Regardless of the perception, size may interfere with communication. Examples of large psychological size include the business executive, teacher, doctor or nurse as they relate with others in their environment.[3]

The person who is large (psychologically and/or physically) will need to develop insight about and a feeling for others' perceptions and then develop methods to convey accessibility to and acceptance of others. Although changes in interpersonal communication take time and no one principle changes everything, using the principles of therapeutic communication described later in this chapter when interacting with others will be a positive move and help the person seem more empathic and approachable.

**The language of time** conveys feelings not expressed by words and may depend on the culture and one's concept of time. The nurse who frequently looks at her watch, who walks too fast for the patient to stay abreast, or who keeps a person waiting past the hour of an appointment may be conveying rejection, neglect or lack of concern. Sitting at a patient's bedside conveys that you have time to listen.

**The language of space** – the distance between you and another – helps determine the nature of the communication. **Proxemics** *is the term for the study of human use and perception of social and personal space.* Physical distancing varies with the setting and the individual and is culturally learned. Placing a person near the centre of a group is one way of saying that he/she is important. The amount of space given a person – the size of desk or office, the size of the hospital room or ward cubicle – conveys differential importance or status to the person. The distance you maintain between the patient and yourself must be carefully determined, depending on the situation and the needs of the patient, for it may convey feelings to the patient that vary from concern to rejection. You can also use physical space to foster communication and to bring people together. Place chairs in a circular arrangement to foster face-to-face contact, for example.

**Territoriality** *or* **personal space** *refers to an area with invisible boundaries surrounding the person's body.* According to studies by Hall, four distinct zones of interpersonal space exist, primarily in front of us. The intimate zone is reserved for someone who is highly attractive and ranges from 0 to 18 inches; the personal zone is from 18 inches to 4 feet; the social-consultative zone is from 4 to 12 feet; and the public zone from 12 feet and beyond. Different zones are appropriate for different interactions and relationships. The couple, the parent and child, or the nurse and patient, for instance, may interact in the intimate zone. The nurse and doctor may work together on a procedure with a patient in the personal zone but later remain in the social-consultative zone as they discuss the patient's progress. As you teach a class of expectant parents, you would tend to maintain the public zone. Attraction is also indicated by the zone. People who are attracted to each other at a business meeting stand farther apart than they would at a party. Everyone is expected to be closer at a party than at a meeting. Some details of the person's appearance are observable only in the intimate zone, although visual perception of the other may be slightly distorted. Persons talk softly or whisper; body heat and odours are transmitted. Touch is possible in the personal zone and visual perception and loudness of voice are normal. The social zone is used when impersonal business is conducted; sensory involvement is less intense. Distance of the public zone is outside the sphere of personal involvement. Others are perceived as somewhat smaller than life-size and verbal communication is formal.[4]

Knowledge of personal space or proxemics is useful in nursing. Research shows, for instance, that people need more space between them in a public area, such as a waiting room, than in an outdoor area. People tend to tolerate a stranger in their intimate or personal zones for about ten minutes and then they are likely to move to a different location if at all possible. People use chairs or other objects or silence as barriers to protect their personal space. In one study chairs that were lined up in a nursing home corridor for residents and visitors were rearranged to promote corner-to-corner seating or face-to-face seating at a small table. After a two-week period of adaptation interaction among the nursing home residents had doubled. The furniture rearrangement allowed for more eye contact and for more distance between individuals than had been possible in the row of chairs. Close proximity of beds (rows of beds two feet apart) in a recovery room, caused the patients to react with civil inattention to avoid one another's presence. Adjacent patients were not recognized; eyes remained closed; heads were under the covers or toward the wall.

Patients apparently need more personal space in the morning than in the evening. The client's cultural background will influence use and need for personal space. Americans, Canadians and British require the most personal space or territory; Latin Americans and Arabs need the least. People interpret another's spatial behaviour according to their own cultural and personal patterns; friendly actions may be misconstrued as aggressive acts.

In health care, especially hospital admission, where the patient is deprived of most personal possessions, role and social function, where close contact is necessary for many nursing interventions, and the person's body is hardly considered his/her own, it is essential to be mindful of the person's need for territory and privacy whenever possible in order to reduce feelings of threat and anxiety. Knock before entering the patient's room. Don't handle the patient's possessions without permission. Explain what you are going to do before you do it. Keep conversation focused on or with the patient rather than talking about an unrelated topic to another person in the presence of the patient. Raising the head of the bed to a height acceptable to the patient extends the sense of personal boundaries. Arrange furniture to decrease crowding when possible. Screen the patient adequately with curtains, solid dividers, closed doors or other barriers when performing any procedure. Encourage the patient to place personal objects on the locker as a way to stake out his/her territory. Adapt your interventions to promote the person's sense of personal space and preserve personal identity.

**The language of colour** elicits fairly specific responses. In British culture warm colours, such as yellow, red and orange, stimulate creative, happy responses. Cool colours, such as blue, green and grey, tend to encourage meditation and deliberation and have a dampening effect on equality of communication. Colour in the environment can be better planned to be therapeutic and to enhance communication in nursing if you are aware of what is being conveyed to the client through the colours in the surroundings. You should also be aware of what the colour of your uniform (or other dress) and hair means to the person. White clothing for example, may arouse fear in children with past illness experiences. Or the patient may perceive any redheaded nurse as quick-tempered or 'sexy' until learning otherwise through observation.

*Observation and perception*

The second tool of communication is observation and perception. **Observation** *is the act of noting and recording facts and events.* **Perception** *is the personal interpretation of observations.* Rarely do observations exist alone. Frequently the person attaches meaning to or makes judgements about observed events, based on one's knowledge, experience, and/or bias. The observer is part of the observed. What you communicate depends on the quality of your observations and your interpretation of them. Observations are made because of curiosity, a desire to understand others, a need for adequacy, security or self-preservation, or any combination of them. In nursing, each client's needs vary and constantly change. Because you are the one health-team member who has continuous contact with the client and because the diagnosis, treatment and prognosis frequently are determined by your observations, your keen perception will help guide the other team workers in their services.

Factors influencing observation and perception are similar to those influencing the communication process generally and include the following:

1. Physical, mental, emotional, social, and spiritual status, capabilities, limits, goals, and needs of the person.
2. Cultural, social, and philosophical background and values.
3. Number and functioning ability of the senses involved, length of time of contact with or exposure to the stimuli or event.
4. Past experiences associated with the present situation.
5. Meaning of the observed event to the self.
6. Interests, preoccupations, preconceptions, and motivational level.
7. Knowledge of or familiarity with the situation being observed.
8. Practice in purposeful observation; ability to focus on stimuli and maintain concentration.
9. Environmental conditions and distractions.
10. Availability of technical devices.
11. Presence, attitudes, and reactions of others – for if observations and perceptions are accurate but do not agree with group consensus, the person is likely to conform to the group.

One aspect of communication to remember in nursing is that when two sounds are presented simultaneously to both ears, any verbal signals, such as words, nonsense syllables and separate speech sound, are more readily heard and identified by the right ear whereas music and environmental noises are better recognized by the left ear – *if* the person hears equally well with both ears.[5] This information may be critical when you care for people who are depressed, medicated or comatose.

Observations must fulfil certain criteria in nursing. They must be purposeful, planned, objective, accurate, complete and orderly. In *purposeful* observation, you decide what to observe, which are the general and which the specific factors, and why the observation is important. The *planned* observation considers timing, duration, interval between observations, and kind and location of observations. An observation is *objective* when it can be validated directly, indirectly, or through replication by others and is not based on personal bias. *Accuracy* involves use of knowledge, concentration, memory and problem solving. A *complete* observation meets the purposes for which it is made. *Orderly* or systematic observation permits relating parts of data gathered, observing the commonplace and general data, and then focusing on minute details.[6] Whenever you make an interpretation, it should be stated as such.

Perception of the same event varies from person to person and within the same person at different times, depending on personal feelings, preparation, and desires. In addition, the person often simplifies what is not understood, leaving out important facts or substituting others, even if distortion results. Recognize this factor in relation to yourself, the client, the family and co-workers because perception of the event determines action.

Peplau describes four types of relationships between the observer and the observed in nursing:

1. The spectator relationship in which the person is not aware of being observed and the nurse is outside the focus of attention. This situation could occur when you observe the sleeping or critically ill patient.
2. The interviewer relationship in which the person is more or less aware of being studied and that you are taking notes of what he/she is saying in response to a situation or question. This situation could occur during the admission procedure or nursing rounds.
3. The collector relationship in which you use records or reports prepared by other health-care workers to learn what has happened to the client. It occurs in the change-of-shift conference, team conference, or when reading the chart to assist in planning care.
4. The participant-observer relationship in which you engage in ordinary acts connected with nursing, such as morning care, and at the same time observe the relationship between the client and self. The person is aware of receiving care but not necessarily aware that his/her response to a situation and your attitudes about giving care are being observed and studied.[7]

*Action or nonverbal behaviour*

Movement or action is the third tool of communication – for example, finger pointing, head nodding and other gestures; eye contact, a wink, gaze, eyebrow movement, smile and other facial expressions; a touch or a slap on the back, general posture, body movement, and body sounds such as belching, knuckle cracking, and laughing.

Nonverbal communication is powerful and honest and is culturally learned. Signals are often sent without the person's being aware of it. Research findings indicate that nonverbal behaviour conveys 65 per cent of the message.[8] The skin flush, the tiny tremor around the eyes or corners of the mouth, and the brief hestitations in speech indicate stress or agitation in the person. Certain preening behaviour has sexual overtones: stroking the hair, adjusting clothing, or changing position to accentuate maleness or femaleness.[9] Our pupils dilate when we see an attractive person or object or are being presented with an attractive idea or positive line of reasoning, and they constrict whenever something unpleasant is encountered.

Several taboos related to nonverbal behaviour exist in the United Kingdom. Touching, standing close to, or looking directly at a stranger, a person of the same sex, or someone we are not attracted to are all considered impolite and intrusive. As a relationship grows closer, the area open to touch increases, the amount of direct eye contact increases, and the distance between the two people decreases.

*Eye behaviour*

For most people, the eyes are an important part of nonverbal behaviour and body image. The size, shape, and colour of eyes often elicit a response from others as well as from self. Throughout history we have been preoccupied with the eye and its effects on human behaviour, reflected by such phrases as the following:

> She/he looks right through you.
> That was an icy stare.
> He's got shifty eyes.
> She's all eyes.
> Did you see the gleam in his eye?
> Now we're seeing eye to eye.
> He looked like the original Evil Eye.
> His eyes shot daggers across the room.
> She could kill with a glance.
> The eyes are the mirror of the soul.

Literature reveals numerous cases in which the eye is used as a symbol for either male or female sex organs.

Eye behaviour begins at birth. An infant responds positively to its mother's eyes very early. Throughout childhood the person is subtly taught how to use the eyes during interactions, when to gaze and when not to gaze, and at whom and what to look.

Various eye movements and eye behaviours are associated with expression of feelings. Large pupil size may indicate, physiologically, either disease or use of drugs. Large pupil size may also indicate fear, anxiety, or arousal and feeling pleased with visual stimuli or the situation. Eyes opened wide with eyebrows raised are associated with wonder, naiveté, frankness, fear or terror. In anger, eyes fix in a hard, direct stare with the upper lid lowered and eyebrows drawn down (simultaneously, the lips are tightly compressed). A constant stare with immobile facial muscles indicates coldness. Eyes rolled upward may be associated with fatigue, a suggestion that another's behaviour is inappropriate, or efforts at organizing thoughts. With feelings of disgust, eyes narrow (and the upper lip curls upward while the nose moves). During sadness the eyes look down, inner corners of the eyebrows raise (simultaneously, lips turn down and the lower lip may tremble). With embarrassment, modesty, or self-consciousness, the eyes look down and away – surprise is shown by raised eyebrows and direct gaze. Aggressive acts include threatening *gestures*, such as a direct look, a sharp movement of the head towards the other person, a frown, and handraising. Flight or defensive behaviours include closed eyes, bodily evasions, withdrawing chin into chest, and crouching.[10]

Each society establishes eye-related norms. Eye contact in most European countries is considered a sign of positive self-concept, a friendly mood, interest in the other person, persuasiveness, credibility, an obligation to engage in an interaction, monitoring of feedback, and attentiveness to events and communication with another. Decreasing, or brief avoidance of eye gaze means lack of interest, insulation of self against threats, a wish to avoid interaction, impending leave-taking, embarrassment, guilt, humility, deep thinking, talking rather than listening, or that the other person has a turn in the conversation if the person has been talking. Prolonged avoidance of eye contact is interpreted as a negative self-concept or feelings of worthlessness or inferiority, rudeness, or even a sign of mental illness. Yet our society also has norms about not looking too long at strangers in public places and not looking at various body parts under certain conditions.

In Latin America, southern Europe, Arab countries, and the Philippines, the use of eyes and eye contact during conversation is important. Eye contact is minimized in northern European countries. And it is taboo to various degrees in Far Eastern countries, such as Pakistan, India or Vietnam.

Studies of blind children show that their spontaneous nonverbal expressions of feelings are the same as for sighted children. Remarkable similarities have been observed in the eye behaviour of adults, infants, and children, blind persons and nonhuman primates. These observations show the universality of nonverbal behaviour, especially because blind children could not learn these behaviours from visual cues.[11]

*Body language*

Through **body language,** *moving or positioning the body or some portion of it, a person conveys what he/she cannot or will not verbalize,* although this body language may be used simultaneously with verbal activity. Expression of self through movement is learned before speech so that under stress the person often reverts to preverbal communication. Thus an individual may overtly manifest the expression that he/she feels is expected in the existing situation – for example, the smile that is only a façade – rather than show what is really felt. Nevertheless, nonverbal behaviour is more likely to express hidden meanings, although they must be interpreted with extreme care. Laughter is not always a sign of humour or happiness; it may be a device to cover anxiety, show ridicule, or seek attention.

Aggressive, controlling, manipulative acts include threatening gestures, such as a direct look, a sharp movement of the head toward the other person, a frown and handraising. Flight behaviours include retreat, bodily evasions, closed eyes, withdrawing chin into chest, and crouching. These defensive behaviours often occur when a dominant person sits too close to a subordinate. Notice these behaviours, along with other signs of tension, such as rocking, leg swinging, or foot tapping, so that you do not push yourself onto the client.

Posture also indicates feeling. A slightly relaxed, leaning-forward position indicates closeness, interest in, or attraction to a person, object or event. The male indicates attraction by the closed posture: arms in front of body with legs closed. The female indicates attraction with a more open posture: arms down at the side, and sitting with legs apart or not crossed at the knees.

Body language is often a reliable index of the real meaning of what is being said or communicated because the person is generally unable to exert as much conscious control over this aspect of behaviour as over the words used. But knowledge of the person's sociocultural heritage is essential here, for various body parts are used differently in different cultures to enhance conversation. The use of the eyes is all important, for example, in India and Greece, but in Africa the torso is frequently moved. In Britain and America head nodding is common. The amount of movement also varies culturally. Normal distance for conversation is much closer in Latin countries than in western Europe. Touching between same-sexed pairs, including male pairs, is more common among Arabs than Westerners. It may be misinterpreted as homosexual behaviour in Britain and America. Subtle cultural variations in the use of nonverbal signs often lead to serious misunderstandings and resentments. Misinterpretations of nonverbal signals can sometimes be avoided only by verbal validation of their meaning, but speaking of the nonverbal signs may often cause embarrassment because many of these signals are sent without much, if any thought.[12]

Other cultural differences are also seen. Gestures are used by Americans and the English to denote activity and by Italian or Jewish persons to emphasize words. The use of facial expression varies with the culture. Italian, Jewish, black and Spanish-speaking persons smile readily or use facial movements, along with gestures and words, to express feelings – happy, unhappy, or physical pain. Oriental, American, Indian, English, Irish and northern European persons show less facial expression and verbalize less, in response to feelings, particularly with strangers.

In Asia it is customary to conceal emotions and bad news with a smile. Even verbal techniques vary. Americans put commands in the form of queries or suggestions. The English talk with considerable understatement so that they will not be considered boastful. Arab speech contains much emphasis and exaggeration. The Japanese kiss to show deference to superiors, a signal that would be interpreted as an insult and be rejected by the superior in the West.[13] Sentence length and speech forms also vary with the social class of a country. The working class typically uses short, simple sentences and is more direct than the more educated class of people.[14]

You must observe the nonverbal behaviour of the whole person in order to interpret communication correctly, for an isolated gesture or expression may require a completely different interpretation in proper context. In addition, you must also validate your impressions with other health-team members who have observed the person, as well as the person, for the same nonverbal behaviour can be interpreted differently by different people. Also, look for inconsistencies between nonverbal and verbal behaviour. A person's eyes may be cold, for example, even though he smiles and sounds friendly. And the meaning of words may be altered or even contradicted by the way the words are said.

*Touch*

Touch is an important nonverbal tool in communication, for touching another with some part of the body or an extension of it is an outside event that stimulates a response. Touch, like movement, begins *in utero* and precedes speech as a form of communication; thus the relationship between touch and communication begins in infancy and remains throughout life as a means of returning to direct experience. Without tactile stimulation that is gentle and nurturing, the child may not live or may have seriously impaired development. Touching stimulates an infant's chemistry for mental and physical growth.[15]

On reaching school age, the child is touched less and less even by the parents. The British teach their children not to touch themselves unnecessarily and to keep their hands off grownups' objects and others' possessions, in general, thereby dampening the child's natural curiosity and desire to explore.[16]

Americans tend to associate touch or physical contact with sexual connotations. Other cultures also consider touching taboo; the British and Germans carry untouchability even further. On the other hand, highly tactile cultures exist – the Spanish, Mexican, Italian, Greek, French, Jewish, Puerto Rican and South American.[17]

Within our culture differences also exist among socioeconomic classes in the use of and response to touch as a form of nonverbal communication. People in upper and middle socioeconomic levels use touch less in communicating and are generally less responsive to this type of behaviour as a positive reinforcement tool than people in the lower socioeconomic level.[18]

Touch is considered magical and healing in some cultures. In British culture, however, there is still a considerable taboo on casual touching, partly because of residual Victorian sexual prudery. Certain health-care workers, however, are beginning to combine laying on of hands (touch) and prayer with other forms of scientific treatment.

Touch must be used judiciously and not forced on anyone. Yet a great deal of communication, closeness, empathy, mutual encouragement, trust, protection, reality contact, comforting, gentleness and caring can be conveyed between two people in rapport when they touch. Touch may convey a connection, excitement, approval, happiness, competence, or frustration, anger, punishment, physical or psychological assault, and the invasion of personal territory and privacy. Touch can help to reintegrate body image and differentiate self from another. The message conveyed through touch depends on the attitude of the people involved and the meaning of touch both to the person touching and to the person touched. In general, the need for intimacy and touch is so strong that the satisfaction of that need is a greater influence on behaviour than is the fear of closeness of possible rejection.

When another human being reaches out to you, it is hoped that you will be there as a fellow, caring human being. Touch can communicate feelings between people who care about one another, when words would fail. The therapeutic use of touch is indispensable in the healing professions. Thus touch is an important tool in the nurse-patient relationship and in the healing art of communication. The back rub, the hand on the shoulder, the squeeze of a hand, each encourages closeness and communication between you and your patient or client.

*Silence*

Silence is the fourth tool of communication even though silence may also interfere with communication. Because one of your essential tasks is to encourage verbal description, you need to intervene effectively when encountering silence. There are different kinds of silence.

**The blank, empty, or blocked silence** occurs when the client says that there is nothing to say and yet nonverbal behaviour reflects anxiety. In this type of silence you initiate speech and somewhat structure the interchange. You might ask 'What are you thinking?' or 'What is going on with you now?' A comment can be made about the person's daily routine. You may even suggest that the person think of something to say as a way to break the impasse.

**The stubborn, resistive silence** occurs when a feeling of anger is present. The person trying to set up a power struggle to gain control over you, a ploy that can stimulate reciprocal anger unless you understand the basis for the anger. A response of impatience perpetuates the power struggle. Sit out the anger; be undemanding but interested. Ask, 'I wonder what is going on with you?' or 'What are you feeling?' When the person recognizes the anger and understands its possible cause, he/she is more likely to give up resistive silence.

**Fearful silence** occurs when a person's previous experiences in similar or identical situations were excessively intimidating. Perhaps other people or hallucinations were threatening when he/she talked. Stay with the person, recognize efforts to talk, show a kind, positive approach, and accept what is said in order to reduce fears.

**A thoughtful silence**, when the person is resolving difficulties or doing problem solving, is productive. Do not interrupt unless the silence is prolonged. Then suggest that the person share thoughts with you.
   Do not cut off silence prematurely because of your own anxiety. Much can be learned from the silence by examining the data preceding the silence and observing the person during the silence.

*Listening*

Listening is the fifth tool of communication. We have two ears and one mouth, which should give us a clue! Everyone loves a listener, but few persons are skilled listeners.

Because listening gives no chance for self-assertion, instruction, or giving opinion, most people think listening is a passive act requiring no special talent. The evidence is to the contrary. You must learn to listen attentively and curb the desire to speak.

The act of listening consists of more than just hearing. Listening occurs only when the mind is purposefully attentive to what is being said or communicated. The mind is a selective organizer and responder to experience. On average, we receive thousands of exteroceptive and proprioceptive impressions every second. Thus a drastic selective process is necessary to prevent the brain's higher centres from being overwhelmed by irrelevant data. Decisions concerning what is relevant and essential and what is irrelevant vary from person to person and are determined by processes and criteria outside the person's awareness. A person may say something that another does not hear because of the latter's selective response, a selective inattention. Selective hearing and listening are influenced considerably by past experience and associations as well as by the need to decrease anxiety over what is being said in the present situation.

Listening is a faster process than speaking. No matter how fast the speaker's mind is racing, it is not possible to articulate more than about 200 words per minute, but the listener can take in words as quickly as he/she can think. The endings of most sentences can be guessed before they are completed. In fact, a person may hear the end of the sentence inaccurately because of the false sense of security and selective inattention caused by this phenomenon. In the nursing situation you should listen attentively throughout the length of each sentence rather than guess or assume what will be said.

Listening manners are vital and may have a subtle but powerful impact on the other person. Elements of good listening described by many authors,[19] include the following points:

1. Show the person that you are listening by looking at him/her; avoid extraneous or distracting movements. Some clients need continuous eye contact as an indication of your attentiveness; others feel uncomfortable and may prefer that you occasionally shift your gaze.
2. Change facial expression in accordance with the topic and personal reactions. A client benefits from nonverbal expressions of face and body that are congruent with your words and feelings.
3. Put aside personal filters – values, biases, ideas, attitudes and experiences – to the extent possible to avoid missing what the other is saying. Personal filters contribute to moralistic judgements, making assumptions before the other has finished speaking, or formulating an answer or interpreting too soon.
4. Be patient – willing to wait until the person has spoken. Then formulate your response. Silence during the dialogue promotes thoughtfulness.

5. Use multidimensional listening. Try to understand not only the content but also the intent, feelings, inconsistencies and nonverbal behaviour. Attend to all aspects of the communication, not just the obvious words. Some people call this 'listening with the third ear'.
6. Use validation. Restate what you heard and ask 'Did I hear and understand you correctly?'[20]

A message is not a spear of thought thrust into the listener's mind by a speaker or writer. Meaning is transferred only when the listener rearranges his/her mind in accordance with the speaker's voice or printed word signals. Your attitude while listening to another person is an important form of feedback. Realize that you may have no control if a client, because of illness or particular feelings, blocks your efforts at communication. But learn to adapt and to control your own behaviour in order to listen attentively and to stimulate the communication of others.

## INTERVIEWING AS PART OF THE COMMUNICATION PROCESS

All activities in nursing involve communication and verbal communication with patients often involves interviewing.

### Definition and factors involved in interviewing

**An interview** *is a transitory relationship between two persons in which one seeks information from another without gaining personal advantage and the other gives information without suffering disadvantage.* The interview is a conversation directed to a definite purpose other than satisfaction in the meeting itself. Interviewing in the nursing situation involves the following five factors:

1. The interview is usually conducted in connection with other nursing activities in which you do something for the client so that he/she can see and feel the immediate effect of nursing efforts; or you use interviewing to determine how best to give care or to evaluate the effectiveness of care given.
2. Either you or the client can initiate the interview.
3. The situation of the interview is flexible in regard to the setting, interruptions, and availability of time for client and nurse. The setting may be the waiting room, home, office, factory or bedside. Interruptions may occur from other health-team members, other clients or visitors. Time limits may be beyond your control, because of intervening demands, so that you may have to return several times to the person to achieve the purpose of the interview.

4. The client is usually physically and emotionally confined or restricted and is relatively dependent on you and the climate created by you.
5. There is a continuum of people who represent 'the nurse' over a 24-hour period. Each nurse, in the process of continuity of care, participates within the framework of the total plan of care. Thus each nurse may achieve a portion of the purposes of the interview – for example, teaching or gathering information – and the entire nursing team together works toward the total purpose.

*Purposes of the interview*

In nursing the purposes achieved through an interview are as follows:

1. Establishing rapport to convey to the person a sense of worth and the fact that someone cares; developing or maintaining feelings of self-esteem; diminishing feelings of isolation.
2. Establishing and maintaining the nurse-client relationship.
3. Listening in order to provide release of tension or allow expression of feelings.
4. Obtaining information; identifying and clarifying needs.
5. Giving information or teaching.
6. Counselling to clarify a problem; encouraging self-understanding and constructive problem solving in the person.
7. Referring the person to other resources of help as necessary.[21]

*Your role as interviewer*

Yourself – your personality – is the principal tool of the therapeutic interview or communication. Your character structure, values and sensitivity to the feelings of others influence your attitude and helpfulness towards people.

As a beginner, you are more likely to have certain problems in interviewing and therapeutic communication than your more experienced colleagues. Often there is a strong fear that you will do something wrong or be criticized by others. Defence mechanisms used to control your anxiety reduce your sensitivity to the emotional responses of others. Fear of being inadequate can be projected onto the client. You may feel competitive toward professional peers and wish to perform better. You may feel guilty about 'using' or 'practising on' the client. With experience, you will learn to overcome or cope with these feelings and become increasingly aware of relationships and subtleties. Refer again to Table 2.2 for clarification on levels communication.

At first you may bombard the patient with questions. Later you will learn when a person has completed the answer to your question or when encouragement is needed to go on. As competence grows with experience, you will be able to hear the content of words and simultaneously consider how the person feels, deduce what is being inferred or omitted, and gauge your emotional response. In addition, you will be able to intervene actively when necessary rather than sit and passively listen.

In order to gain this competence, take careful notes during or after each interview. And regular sessions should be held with a teacher or supervisor who can guide you and promote self-understanding. Practising in a role-play situation with video feedback can be very helpful in learning these techniques.

*Techniques of interviewing*

Prepare for the interview as much as possible through use of records, by applying general knowledge to the specific situation, and by being alert and observant. Know or define what information is needed to achieve the purpose of the interview. What you ask or say depends on the purpose of the interview. Avoid, however, the 'self-fulfilling prophecy', setting up the interview situation in such a way that the person tells you (or *seems* to tell you) only what you have predetermined will or can be told you. If selective inattention causes you to see or hear only what you wish, much information will be missed or misinterpreted and you will not be fully helpful to the person.

The personality and attitude of the interviewer influence the interviewee's responses. The emotional climate and immediate conditions surrounding the interview also affect you and the other person. The following techniques[22] will help promote productive interviews:

1. Establish rapport. Create a warm, accepting climate and a feeling of security and confidentiality so that the person feels free to talk about whatever seems important.
2. Arrange comfortable positions for both yourself and the person so that full attention can be given to the interview.
3. Control the external environment as much as possible. Doing so is sometimes difficult or impossible, but try to minimize external distractions or noise, regulate ventilation and lighting, and arrange the setting to reduce physical distance.
4. Consider wearing casual clothing without excessive adornment instead of a uniform when working in the school, home or occupational setting. Consider what expectations the interviewee may have of you. In some cases, the person will respond more readily to your casual

dress; at other times your professional dress may be needed as part of the image to help that person talk confidentially.

5. Use a vocabulary on the level of awareness or understanding of the person. Avoid occupational jargon or words too abstract for the interviewee's level of understanding or health condition.

6. Avoid preconceived ideas, prejudices, or biases. Avoid imposing personal values on others.

7. Begin by stating the purpose of the interview. Either you or the interviewee may introduce the theme. You may start the session by expressing friendly interest in the everyday affairs of the person or by discussing events related to the person to establish rapport, but avoid continuing trivial conversation. Maintain the proposed structure.

8. Be precise in what you say so that the meaning is understood. Ask questions that are well-timed, open-ended, and pertinent to the situation. This pattern allows the person to stamp his/her own style, organization and personality on the answers and on the interview. Getting unanticipated data can be as useful in an interview as in giving care. Meaningless questions get meaningless answers. Questions that bombard the person produce unreliable information. Open-ended sentences usually keep the person talking at his/her own pace. Carefully timing your messages, verbal and nonverbal, and allowing time for the interviewee to understand and respond are essential in nursing.

9. Avoid asking questions in ways that induce socially acceptable answers. The interviewee often responds to questions with what he/she thinks the interviewer wants to hear, either to be well thought of, to gain status, or to show that he/she knows what other people do and what is considered socially acceptable.

10. Be diplomatic when asking questions about home life or personal matters. What you consider common information may be considered very private by some. Matters about which it would be tactless to enquire directly can often be arrived at indirectly by peripheral questions. If a subject you suggest meets resistance, change the topic; when the anxiety is reduced, you can return to the matter for further discussion. Remember, what the person does not say is as important as what is said.

11. Be an attentive listener. Show interest by occasionally nodding or responding with 'I see' or 'uh-huh'. Remain silent and control your responses when another's comments evoke a personal meaning and thus trigger an emotional response in you. While the person is talking, find the nonverbal answers to the following: What does this experience mean for him/her? Why is he/she telling me this at this time? What is the meaning of the choice of words, the repetition of key words, the voice inflection, the hesitant or aggressive expression of words, the topic chosen? Listen for feelings, needs, and goals. Recognize the levels of meaning in communication previously discussed. Do not answer too fast or ask a question too soon. If necessary, learn if the

words mean the same to you as to the interviewee. Explore each clue as you let the person tell his/her story.

12. Carefully observe nonverbal messages for signs of anxiety, frustration, anger, loneliness or guilt. Look for feelings of pressure hidden by the person's attempts to be calm. Encourage the free expression of feelings, for feelings often bring facts with them.

13. Encourage spontaneity. Provide movement in the interview by picking up verbal leads, clues, bits of seemingly unrelated information, and nonverbal signals from the client. If the person asks you a personal question, redirect it, for it may be the topic that the interviewee unconsciously (or even consciously) wishes to speak about. Only occasionally will it be pertinent for you to answer personal questions. Brief self-disclosure may help the person feel more comfortable and may elicit additional information for the client's benefit.

14. Ask questions beginning with What, Where, Who, and When to gain factual information. Words connoting moral judgments should be avoided; they are not conducive to a feeling of neutrality, acceptance, or freedom of expression. The How question maybe difficult for the person to answer, for it asks 'In what manner . . .?' or 'For what reason . . .?' and the individual may lack sufficient knowledge to answer. The Why question should also be avoided, for it asks for insights that the person should not be expected to give.

15. Indicate when the interview is terminated and terminate it graciously if the interviewee does not do so first. Make a transition in interviewing or use a natural stopping point if the problem has been resolved, if the information has been obtained or given, or if the person changes the topic. You may say 'There is one more question I'd like to ask . . .', or 'Just two more points I want to clarify . . .', or 'Before I leave, do you have any other questions, comments, or ideas to share?'

16. Keep data obtained in the interview confidential and share it only with the appropriate and necessary health-team members, leaving out personal assumptions. If you are sharing an opinion or interpretation, state it as such rather than have it appear to be what the other person said or did. The person should be told what information will be shared and with whom.

17. Evaluate the interview. Were the purposes accomplished? Recognize that not everyone can successfully interview everyone. Others may see you differently from the way you see yourself, thus preventing you from being helpful or obtaining information. Evaluate yourself in each situation.

You must be sincere, knowledgeable about the purpose of the interview, and skilful in using tools of communication during the interview as well as in establishing and maintaining a climate conducive to successful data collection. The effective interview takes a great deal of energy and attention.

## THERAPEUTIC COMMUNICATION

Analysis of your communication pattern will help you improve your methods. Realize that you cannot become skilled in therapeutic communication without supervised and thoughtful practice. As you talk with another, however, don't get so busy thinking about a list of methods that you forget to focus on the person. Your keen interest in the other person and use of your personal style are essential if you are to be truly effective.

To be effective while communicating with the patient or family, use simple, clear words geared to the person's intelligence and experience. Develop a well-modulated tone of voice, especially with the sick person, for auditory sensitivity is increased during illness. Several authors have described principles, attitudes, and methods essential in therapeutic communication that are useful with individual persons as well as with groups.[23]

*Effective methods*

The following methods are basic for conducting purposeful, helpful communication with a person, well or ill, along with their rationale. Some elaborate on earlier suggestions for interviewing.

**Use thoughtful silence to encourage the person to talk.** Silence gives you and the person time to organize thoughts. It directs the person to the task at hand but allows him/her to set the pace, aids consideration of alternative courses of action and delving into feelings, conserves energy during serious illness, and gives time for contemplation and relaxation. There is a time not to talk. Always focus on the person you are talking to, especially during silence.

**Be accepting.** This is a difficult task at times. Realize that *all* behaviour is motivated and purposeful. Indicate that you are following the person's trend of thought. Encourage the client to continue to talk while you remain nonjudgmental, although not necessarily in agreement.

**Help the person strengthen self-identification in relation to others.** *Always use you, I* and *we* in their proper context. Do not say 'We can take a bath now' but rather 'You can take a bath now'.

**Suggest collaboration and a cooperative relationship.** Offer to share and work together with the person; offer to do things *with* and not *for* or *to* him/her. Encourage participation in identifying and appraising problems and involvement as an active partner in treatment. Tell the person you are available to help. 'I'll stay with you' or 'I'm interested in your comfort' are examples of statements that can help to reassure that you will stay and care regardless of the person's behaviour.

**State open-ended, generalized, leading questions** to encourage the person to take the initiative in introducing topics and to think through problems. Examples include: 'Is there something you'd like to talk about?' 'Tell me about it.' 'Where would you like to begin?' 'Go on.' 'And what else?' 'Would you like to talk about yourself now?' 'After that?' Avoid conventional pleasantries after initial greetings because they constrict the person's expression of feelings and ideas. It is important for the person to talk about his/her mental and emotional distress and turmoil and questions, for often he/she cannot cope with feelings until the feelings are stated.

**State related questions.** Do not let a subject drop until it is adequately explored. Peripheral or side questions help the person work through larger issues and engage in problem solving. Explore by delving further into the subject or idea without seeming to pry. Many clients deal superficially with a topic to test if you are truly interested. Avoid questions that call for a yes or no answer. Explorative questions call for answers that elaborate, thereby helping the person to increase understanding and do further problem solving or clarifying.

**Place events described in time sequence.** In order to clarify relationships associated with a given event, determine how it happened, place it in perspective, determine the extent to which one event led to another, and seek to identify recurrent patterns or difficulty or significant cause-and-effect relationships. Ask such questions as 'What happened then?' or 'What did you do after that?'

**State observations that you perceive about the person.** Statements such as 'You appear . . .', 'It seems to me that . . .', 'I notice that you are . . .', and 'It makes me uncomfortable when you . . .' encourage mutual understanding of behaviour. Such observations offer a basis on which the person can respond without your having to probe, and they call attention to what is happening to help him/her notice or clarify personal behaviour. Using this technique, you and the other person can compare observations and you can encourage a desription of self-awareness. In addition, when you openly acknowledge that another's efforts at a task or behaviour are appropriate to the situation, you reinforce the behaviour and add to the person's self-esteem.

**Encourage description of behaviour or observation** through statements like 'What did you feel?' 'Tell me what you now feel', 'What does the voice seem to be saying?' and 'What is happening?' You can better understand the person when you observe and understand matters as they seem to the client. There is the need to act out impulses and feelings if the person feels free to state them.

**Restate or repeat the main idea expressed** to convey that it was communicated to you effectively, thereby encouraging the person to continue. Restate the idea until the person does clarify. Reformulating certain statements and using different words bring out related aspects of material that might otherwise have escaped the client's (or your) attention.

**Reflect by paraphrasing feelings, questions, ideas and key words** to encourage further talking. Indicate that the person's point of view is important; acknowledge the right to personal opinions and decisions. Encourage the person to accept personal feelings and ideas. Show interest in hearing as much as the person wishes to tell you. Emphasize the word *you* while conversing, as in '*You* feel . . .', in order to reflect what the person has said. (However, do not just mindlessly parrot his/her words.)

**Verbalize the implied** or what the person has hinted at or suggested in order to make the discussion less obscure, to clarify the conversation, to show that you are listening and interested, and that you accept what is said. Questions can be used as a subtle form of suggestion. As an example, you might ask 'Have you ever told your wife how you feel?' or 'Have you ever asked your boss for a rise?' Regardless of the answer, you have indicated that such an act is conceivable, permissible, and perhaps even expected.

**Attempt to translate feelings into words.** Sometimes what the person says seems meaningless when taken literally. Hidden meanings of verbal expressions, as well as their actual content, must be considered and can be explored by describing the implicit feelings.

**Clarify** when necessary through statements like 'I don't understand what is troubling you' or 'Could you explain that again?' The person is usually aware if he/she is not being understood and may withdraw or cease to communicate. It is not necessary to understand everything stated as long as you are honest about it and do not pretend to understand when you do not. Attempting to discover what the person is talking about can help him/her become clearer to self.

**Reintroduce reality** by voicing doubt or by calmly presenting your own perceptions or the facts in the situation when the person is being unrealistic. Indicate an alternate line of thought for consideration; do not attempt to convince him/her of error by arguing. Such action only provokes resistance and a determination to maintain the idea. Encourage the person to recognize that others do not necessarily perceive events as he/she does or draw the same conclusions. Encourage reconsideration and reevaluation (even though it may not change his/her mind) through statements like 'What gives you that impression?' 'Isn't that unusual?' and 'That's hard to believe.' Expressing doubts may reinforce doubts the person already has but has discounted because no one else shared them before. A doubting tone of voice can be as effective as any specific statement.

**Offer information.** Make facts available whenever the person needs or asks for them. Well-timed teaching builds trust, orientates, and gives additional knowledge from which to make decisions or draw realistic conclusions. Inappropriate, excessive, or partial information or advice may cause alarm or needlessly suggest problems to the person. Give the person information about what can be expected and what he/she can do to help self. At times it may be appropriate for you to disclose briefly your own thoughts, feelings or experiences; do not elaborate on yourself.

**Seek consensual validation.** Search for mutual understanding; words should mean the same thing to both of you. Therapeutic communication cannot take place if both you and the other person attach autistic (private) meanings to the words you both use. Always ask yourself if what you heard could have a meaning other than what you think. As a person defines self for the listener, he/she also clarifies what is meant. Avoid words and phrases that are easily misinterpreted or misunderstood and encourage the person to ask whenever there is doubt about what you mean.

**Encourage evaluation of the situation by the person.** Help the client to appraise the quality of the experience, to consider people and events in relation to personal and others' values, and to evaluate the way in which people affect him/her personally as well as understand how he/she affects others. A simple query may help the person understand feelings in connection with what happened and refrain from uncritically adopting the opinions and values of others.

**Encourage formulation of a plan of action** by asking the person to consider examples of behaviour likely to be appropriate in future situations. The client can then plan how to handle future problems or how to carry out necessary self-care.

**Summarize.** Summarize important points of discussion and give particular emphasis to progress towards greater understanding. Summarizing encourages both you and the person to part company with the same ideas in mind, provides a sense of closure at the end of discussion, and promotes a grasp of the significance of what was said.

The quality of any response depends on the degree of mutual trust in the relationship. Techniques can be highly successful or they can misfire or be abused, depending on how they are used, your attitude at the time, and the other's interpretation. There must be a feeling of caring, of safety and security in your company, and a feeling that you want to help the person help himself. The more important or highly personal a feeling or idea is, the more difficult it is to say. This situation causes hesitancy in revealing thoughts, feelings, or intimate needs. By using therapeutic principles, such as those previously listed, you will help the person and his/her family identify you as someone to whom ideas and feelings can be safely and productively revealed.

*Communicating with the client who has communication difficulties*

You will need to gather data from clients with sensory impairments. When you interview a person with hearing impairment, inability to speak the language, or visual impairment, the basic principles still apply, although the specific condition will necessitate some adaptations. The guidelines presented in Tables 2.1 and 2.2 will be helpful. For anyone with a communication disorder, develop rapport and a trust relationship slowly to overcome the reticence or suspicion that might be present. Introduce yourself and your purpose. Use appropriate nonverbal behaviour to convey ideas. Use an intermediary, such as a family member or interpreter, if available and necessary, but *not* to the exclusion of talking with the client.

Table 2.1 summarizes guidelines for communicating with hearing-impaired persons.[24]

Table 2.2 summarizes guidelines for communicating with visually-impaired persons.[25]

*Barriers to effective communication*

Various authors have written about communication patterns to be avoided by persons in the helping professions and the rationale for their avoidance.[26] The following approaches and techniques will interfere with helpful communication with the client and family whether you are conducting an interview or communicating in any other nursing situation. Continually study your personal pattern of communication, verbal and nonverbal, to ensure that you *avoid* these practices.

**Using the wrong vocabulary** – vocabulary that is abstract or intangible, full of jargon, slang or implied status; talking too much; or using unnecessarily long sentences or words out of context can be interpreted by the

*Table 2.1* Communication with the hearing-impaired client

1. When you meet a person who seems inattentive or slow to understand you, consider that hearing, rather than manners or intellect, may be the reason. Some hard-of-hearing persons refuse to wear a hearing aid. Others wear aids so inconspicuous that you may not see them at first glance. Others cannot be helped by a hearing aid.
2. Be sure the person's hearing aid is in place, turned on, and in working order. Batteries need frequent replacement.
3. The hard-of-hearing person may depend to a considerable extent on reading your lips to understand what you are saying even if wearing a hearing aid. No hearing aid can completely restore hearing. Always speak in a good light, face the person and the light as you speak, and do not have objects in or covering your mouth (gum, cigarettes, hand).
4. When you are in a group that includes a hard-of-hearing person, try to carry on your conversation with others in such a way that he/she can watch your lips. Never take advantage of the disability by carrying on a private conversation in his/her presence in low tones that cannot be heard.
5. Speak distinctly but naturally. Shouting does not clarify speech sounds; mouthing or exaggerating your words or speaking too slowly makes you harder to understand. On the other hand, try not to speak too rapidly.
6. Avoid excessive environmental noise, which, when magnified by a hearing aid, is distracting and distressing and overrides normal conversational tones.
7. Do not start to speak to a hard-of-hearing person abruptly. Attract attention first by facing him/her and looking straight into the person's eyes. If necessary, touch the hand or shoulder lightly. Promote understanding by starting with a key word or phrase – for instance, 'Let's plan our weekend now.' 'Speaking of teenagers . . .' If he/she does not understand you, don't repeat the same words. Substitute synonyms: 'It's time to make plans for Saturday.'
8. If the person you are speaking to has one 'good' ear, always stand or sit on that side when you address him/her. Do not be afraid to ask a person with an obvious hearing loss whether he/she has a good ear and, if so, which one it is. The person will be grateful that you care enough to find out.
9. Facial expressions and gestures are important clues to meaning. Remember that an affectionate or amused tone of voice may be lost on a hard-of-hearing person.
10. In conversation with a person who is especially hard of hearing or having difficulty understanding, occasionally jot down key words on paper. The person will be grateful for the courtesy.
11. Many hard-of-hearing persons, especially teenagers, who dislike being different, are unduly sensitive about their handicap and pretend to understand when they do not. When you detect this situation, tactfully repeat your meaning in different words until it gets across.
12. The speech of a person who has been hard of hearing for years may be difficult to understand, for natural pitch and inflection are the result of imitating the speech of others. To catch such a person's meaning more easily, watch the face while he/she talks.
13. If you do not understand the person, ask for a repeat rather than ignore the person.
14. Use common sense and tact in determining which of these suggestions apply to the particular hard-of-hearing person you meet. Some persons with only a slight loss might feel embarrassed by any special attention you pay them. Others, whose loss is greater, will be profoundly grateful for it.

*Table 2.2*    Communication with the visually impaired client

1. Talk to the person in a normal tone of voice. Being visually impaired is no indication that he/she cannot hear well.
2. Accept the normal things that a blind person might do, such as consulting a watch for the correct time, dialling a telephone, or writing a name in longhand, without calling attention to them.
3. When you offer assistance, do so directly. Ask 'May I be of help?' Speak in a normal, friendly tone.
4. Be explicit in giving verbal directions.
5. Advise the person when you are leaving so that he/she will not be embarrassed by talking when no one is listening.
6. There is no need to avoid the use of the word 'see' when talking with a blind person.
7. In guiding the person, permit him/her to take your arm. Never grab the visually impaired person's arm, for he/she cannot anticipate your movements. Proceed at a normal pace. Hesitate slightly before stepping up or down.
8. When assisting the person to a chair, simply place his/her hand on the back or arm of the chair. This is enough to give location.
9. Never leave the person without a way to secure help. Have a call signal available.
10. Never leave a blind person in an open area. Instead lead him/her to the side of a room, to a chair, or some landmark from which direction can be realized.
11. A half-open door, low stools, or loose cords or rugs are dangerous obstacles for the visually impaired person.
12. When serving food to a visually impaired person who is eating without a sighted companion, offer to read the menu. As you place each item on the table, call attention to it. Food locations on a plate should be described according to the face of the clock. If the person wants you to cut food, he/she will tell you.
13. Be sure to tell who else is present in the environment.
14. Encourage use of a magnifying glass if it is helpful.
15. Read mail to the person and assist him/her with business matters if necessary.
16. Describe the environment, people, and events surrounding the person to enrich his/her experience and understanding.

person as your unwillingness to communicate. But words alone do not block. Perhaps even more crucial can be your attitudes and prejudices resulting from personal and cultural background and your failure to understand the receiver's background. Think about what the message will mean to the person, depending on age, sex, personality, socioeconomic status, cultural background, occupation, religion, and degree and nature of illness.

**Conveying your feelings of anxiety, anger, strangeness, denial, isolation, lack of control, or lack of physical health** negatively influences your initial and continued responses to another. Such feelings also interfere with your ability to listen and will certainly cause the other person to withdraw, for rapport cannot be established. The appearance of being too busy, of not having time to listen, of not giving sufficient time for an answer, or apparently not really wanting to hear are equally forceful in 'cutting off' another. Establishing contact on a social rather than a therapeutic basis also limits communication to the superficial issues.

**Failing to realize that the person's reluctance to make a message clear** (resulting from the feeling that what needs to be expressed is socially unacceptable or inappropriate) can prevent therapeutic communication. The client may be afraid to ask questions for fear of getting an obscure answer or of being reprimanded for such questioning. This fearful silence can cause a sense of futility and a closure of communication. Lack of dialogue prohibits evaluating the effectiveness of any message and blocks further attempts at communication. Also avoid interpreting cooperation or passivity as understanding. Sometimes the person answers yes to please you but really does not understand you at all.

**Making inappropriate use of facts, introducing unrelated information, offering premature explanation or counselling, wrong timing, saying something important when the person is upset or not feeling well and thus unable to hear what is really said** – all these provoke anxiety and prohibit problem solving on the part of the person.

**Making glib statements, offering false reassurance** by saying, 'Everything is OK', or unfairly indicating that there is no cause for anxiety – these are dishonest ways of evaluating the client's personal feelings and communicate a lack of understanding and empathy. You cannot foretell the future accurately; therefore you cannot honestly say that there is nothing to worry about. Such verbal behaviour belittles the person who feels he/she has legitimate problems, and it discourages further expression of feelings and trust, although it may relieve your own anxieties.

**Using clichés, stereotyped responses, trite expressions and empty verbalisms** stated without thought, such as 'It's always worse at night', 'I know', 'You'll be OK', or 'Who is to say?' makes the person uncomfortable and prohibits you from maintaining objectivity. Such statements, unfortunately common, do not allow expression of feelings or show understanding. You cannot understand who a person really is if you respond automatically. Also, do not jump to conclusions based on initial impressions.

**Being too strongly opinionated** in any aspect of your conversation with another presents a barrier, for you do not allow for a different response. Neither can you be totally neutral; recognition should be given for accomplishments. Approval or agreement and disapproval or disagreement, however, carry overtones of judgment about the person.

**Expressing unnecessary approval**, stating that something the person does or feels is particularly good, implies that the opposite is bad and limits freedom of the client to think, speak or act in ways that may displease you. Excess praise arouses undue ambition, competition, and a sense of superiority, closing off possible learning experiences because the person may continue to speak and act only in ways that will bring approval. This approach does not allow the person to live up to his/her potential. Similarly, *excessive agreement*, indicating the person is right, can be equally inhibiting, for you leave little opportunity to modify a point of view later without admitting error. Do not take sides with the person, but use the time to help him/her gather data in order to draw personal opinions and conclusions.

**Expressing undue disapproval**, denouncing another's behaviour or ideas, implies that you have the right to pass judgment on the person's thoughts and feelings and that he/she must please you. This moralistic attitude diverts your attention away from another's needs and directs attention to your own. *Excessive disagreement*, opposition to another's beliefs or values, implies that he/she is wrong and you are right and puts the other on the defensive. Disagreement usually results in resistance to change and shows lack of respect. Similarly, *rejection*, refusing to consider, or showing contempt for, the person's idea and behaviour, closes off the topic from exploration and also rejects him/her as an individual. We have all experienced some degree of disapproval, disagreement and rejection in the past; but such responses from others reinforce loneliness, hopelessness, and alienation and may even contribute to illness. This person may then avoid help rather than risk further disapproval, disagreement or rejection.

**Giving advice, stating personal experiences, opinion, or value judgments, giving pep talks, telling another what should be done** – such behaviour emphasizes yourself, elevates your self-esteem and relieves your anxiety, but it implies that you know what is best and that the person is incapable of self-direction. Such behaviour inhibits spontaneity, prevents struggling with and thinking through problems, and may unnecessarily promote a state of prolonged dependency. Certainly talking about yourself is of no interest or relevance to the person or family in need of help. Remember that when asking for your advice, opinion or judgment, a client has frequently already made a decision and is actually seeking a sounding board or validation for ideas. (Instead such queries should be met with questions like 'What have you been told to do?' 'What would you like to do?' 'What do you plan to do?' Then you can facilitate the person's problem solving by using the effective methods of communication previously described.)

**Probing, persistent, pointed, or 'yes-no' questioning** places the person on the defensive and makes him/her feel manipulated and valued only for what he/she can give. Often data obtained will not be accurate because the person will give answers he/she feels you want to hear or, to protect self, will give no answers.

**Requiring explanations, demanding proof, challenging or asking 'why ...?'** – when the person cannot provide a reason for thoughts, feelings and behaviour and for events – forces an invention of reasons, partial answers, expanding delusions or rationalizing, for he/she feels 'on the spot'. Emotionally charged topics should be avoided. If the person knew the 'whys', the reasons, he/she could handle the situation.

**Belittling the person's feelings** (equating intense and overwhelming feelings expressed with those felt by everyone or yourself) implies that his/her feelings are not valid, he/she is bad, or that the discomfort is mild, temporary, unimportant or self-limiting. Such statements indicate a lack of understanding and offer no constructive assistance. When someone is concerned with personal misery, he/she is not concerned about or interested in the misery of others but does expect you to be concerned and interested in his/her feelings and problems. Don't say 'Everyone feels that way.'

**Making only literal responses** or asking question related only to practical matters cuts off exploration of feelings. Persons often cannot state feelings directly or in conventional phrasing but must use symbolism or statements with hidden meanings. If you respond to symbolism on its literal level, you may be showing a lack of understanding. For example, if the person makes a statement such as 'It's a grey day' this may have no reference to the weather.

**Interpreting the person's behaviour or confronting him or her** with analytical meanings of behaviour may cause great anxiety, denial or withdrawal and indicates your limited confidence in his/her capacity to cope with, work through, or understand personal problems. Self-understanding does not come directly from someone else but from assistance from another.

**Interrupting or abruptly changing the subject** takes control of the conversation, often to escape from something anxiety provoking. The new topic may be of no interest or relevance to the client. Such verbal behaviour is rude and shows a lack of empathy. The other's thoughts and spontaneity are interrupted, the flow of ideas is cut off or becomes confused, and you will get inadequate information or be unable to do effective counselling or teaching. The relevance of what is being said may not be immediately apparent, but you should remain hopeful for later understanding.

**Defending or protecting someone or something** (nurses, doctors, hospital) from verbal attack by the client is unnecessary and implies that the person has no right to express impressions, opinions or feelings. Stating that the criticism is unjust or unfounded does not change feelings because his/her feelings are valid to the self. Moreover, what he/she is saying may be true. Genuine acceptance, understanding and competent care of the client make defence unnecessary.

## IMPLICATIONS FOR HEALTH PROMOTION

*Applications to nursing*

The first communication problem that you must control is that of personal emotions in the nurse-client-family relationship. Because the main barrier to communication is emotions, you must develop skill in building bridges over these barriers. The basic bridge to effective communication is feeling. Everyone seeks *warmth, security, assurance* and *appreciation*. When these qualities are present, difficult problems can be taken in stride, especially when commitment is combined with skilful use of the methods described in this chapter.

Study yourself to discover those points at which you could be responsible for blocking communication through your own shortcomings. Know your likes and dislikes; recognize them for what they are; and keep them under control. In order to accept another person, you must first accept yourself. You must be aware of your own needs in order to help another meet personal needs.

Cultivate an understanding of the part played by body language in human interactions and be as aware of what you are saying with your body movements as you are of what others say with theirs. Feelings are frequently expressed by gestures, attitudes, gait and body posture and facial expressions. Refer to the following reference for more information on the science of body language.[27]

In order to make full use of therapeutic communication, the person must feel safe with you, respected by and trusting of you. Revealing one's innermost thoughts and feelings to someone one scarcely knows is difficult for any individual, even when help is needed and expected. Use of communication techniques in counselling makes no attempt to influence the speed or direction of the person's problem-solving efforts; be a facilitator instead of a doer or a teller.

The nurse is in a key position to apply an understanding of the communication process and to carry out therapeutic communication methods in nursing while conducting routine procedures, teaching and counselling or giving support. Thus you can enable the person and family to achieve optimum wellbeing and prevent future health problems. In addition, through communication, you will learn of the effectiveness of care you have given.

*Application to daily living*

Although this chapter has centred around nurse–client–family interaction, the discussions of the communication process, of interviewing, and of techniques and blocks to communication apply equally well to associations with your colleagues and other health-team members. In fact, application of all information in this chapter to your everyday relationships with family and friends will promote an increasingly appropriate, harmonious living pattern. The smoother the communication system, the smoother all other systems will function.

Appropriate, realistic, constructive communication between persons is a basic step towards mental, emotional and, indirectly (but no less significantly), physical health. Communication patterns that block or resist the other person reduce feelings of autonomy and equality and increase feelings of being misunderstood. The resultant emotions – frustration, anger, depression, and the like – will eventually affect the relationship between the persons involved as well as the physiological functioning of the body.

As a nurse, you will find yourself refining your personal pattern of communication practising therapeutic communication with others, and teaching others patterns of communication that promote health individually, within the family, and within community social groups.

## REFERENCES

1. Ekiman, Paul, and Wallace Friesen, *Unmasking the Face* (Prentice Hall Inc. Englewood Cliffs, NJ, 1975).
2. Argyle, Michael, *The Psychology of Interpersonal Behaviour* (Penguin Books Inc., Baltimore, 1967).
3. Murray, Ruth, and M. Marilyn Huelskoetter, *Psychiatric/Mental Health Nursing: Giving Emotional Care* (Prentice Hall Inc., Englewood Cliffs, NJ, 1983).
4. Ibid.
5. Jakobson, Roman, 'Verbal Communication', *Scientific American*, vol. 227 no. 3 (1972), pp. 73–80.
6. Peplau, Hildegarde, *Interpersonal Relations in Nursing* (G.P. Putnam's Sons, New York, 1952).
7. Ibid.
8. Knapp, Mark, *Nonverbal Communication in Human Interaction*, 2nd edition (Rinehart and Winson, New York, 1978).
9. Scheflen, Albert, *Body Language and Social Order* (Prentice Hall Inc., Englewood Cliffs, NJ, 1972).
10. See note 1 and note 8 above. Also, Eibl-Eibesfeldt, I., 'Similarities and Differences Between Cultures in Expressive Movements', *Nonverbal Communication*, ed. R.A. Hinde, Cambridge University Press, Cambridge, 1972, pp. 297–312.
11. See note 8 and note 10, above.

12. Seen note 10, above.
13. See note 2 and note 10, above.
14. See note 2, above.
15. Barnett, Kathryn, 'A Theoretical Construct of the Concepts of Touch as they relate to Nursing', *Nursing Research*, vol. 21 no. 2 (1972) pp. 102–10; Goody-koontz, Lynne, 'Touch: Attitudes and Practice', *Nursing Forum*, vol. 18 no. 1 (1979) pp. 4–17; Montagu, Ashley, *Touching: The Human Significance of Skin* (Columbia University Press, New York, 1971).
16. Montagu, *Touching*.
17. See note 3, above.
18. Montagu, *Touching*; also see note 3, above.
19. See note 3, above; also, Enelow, Allen and Scott Swisher, *Interviewing and Patient Care*, 2nd edition (Oxford University Press, New York, 1979); Mattes, Norman, 'Are You Listening?', *American Journal of Nursing*, vol. 58 no. 6 (1958) pp. 827–8.
20. Goldin P., and B. Russell, 'Therapeutic Communication', *American Journal of Nursing*, vol. 69 no. 9 (1969) pp. 1928–30.
21. See note 19, above; also Bird, Brian, *Talking with Patients* (J.B. Lippincott Company, Philadelphia, 1965).
22. Hays, J., and K. Larson, *Interacting with Patients* (The Macmillan Company, New York, 1963).
23. See notes 6, 20, 21 and 22, above; also, Litwack, Lawrence, Janice Litwack and Mary Ballow, *Health Counseling* (Appleton-Century-Crofts, New York, 1980).
24. See note 3, above.
25. Ibid.
26. See note 13, above.
27. See notes 2, 9, and 10, above; also, Bentall, Jonathan and Ted Polhemus, eds. *The Body as a Medium of Expression* (E.P. Dutton & Co., Inc., New York, 1975); Faust, Julius, Body Language (M. Evans & Co., Inc., New York, 1970).

# 3

# The nursing process: A method to promote health

Study of this chapter will help you to:

1. Discuss major historical events and their impact on nursing.

2. Define the *conceptual approach* and describe some concepts used in nursing practice.

3. Describe *holistic care* and the importance of this approach in nursing.

4. Compare the scientific method with the nursing process.

5. List criteria and discuss essential attributes for professional practice.

6. List the steps of the nursing process and define *assessment, nursing diagnosis, planning, intervention* and *evaluation*.

7. Discuss the purpose of an assessment tool and construct an assessment tool appropriate for patients/clients in each life era with various health problems.

8. Formulate nursing diagnoses from nursing assessments.

9. Differentiate nursing diagnosis and nursing history and write a nursing history on a patient or client.

10. Describe purposes, possible formats and uses of nursing-care plans.

11. Write a nursing-care plan for a patient/client, using guidelines given in this chapter.

12. Explain the importance of scientific rationale and a nursing model for intervention.

13. Relate the step of evaluation to accountability in the nursing process.

14. Use the process recording and analysis of care to evaluate your effectiveness in patient-client care.

15. Differentiate between a social and helpful nurse-client relationship.

16. Describe guidelines for a therapeutic nurse-client relationship.

17. List and describe the phases of the nurse-client relationship and the effect of the nurse's and client's feelings on each phase.

18. Compare problem solving and research and explore the importance of each to nursing.

Most nursing in the past, and even today, was practised on an empirical basis. Care patterns established by early nurses, such as Florence Nightingale and Clara Barton, were chiefly concerned with procedures and aimed at providing an environment of cleanliness, comfort and safety. Nursing's responsibility was to foster solely a reparative process and functions toward this end have accompanied the growth of technology in nursing – a tradition that is almost holy.[1] Today, however, this limited approach has proved inadequate. Thus a conceptual approach to care has emerged, an approach that is essential in order to care for a diverse population in a complex society.

The **conceptual approach** *is the uniting, combining, modifying, and using of many theories or ideas from various disciplines into a new form; it is a holistic, dynamic approach.* Thus for resources or inspiration you might draw on methods or approaches of medicine, religion, education, psychology, sociology or business. Your approach will be refined as you constantly look for ideas from other fields that are applicable to nursing. Learning theories that have been successful in psychotherapy, for example, can be translated to nursing and adapted to client/patient teaching. The conceptual approach does not isolate procedures. Instead it fits these aspects of nursing into a health-promotion emphasis, and it uses whatever knowledge is applicable, such as basic human needs and levels of wellbeing, stress and adaptation. Although the conceptual approach is concerned with repair, it is also concerned with prevention of breakdown; even though it is concerned with practical measures, it is also concerned that sound scientific principles underlie these measures.

## HISTORICAL BACKGROUND

Some discussion of historic events will promote a deeper understanding of the nursing process. Events prior to, during, and after the Second World

War and events of the last two decades have significantly influenced nursing.

### Prior to the Second World War

In the early Christian-Judaic era, the needs of the sick were met by individuals through unselfish caring and love of neighbour augmented by the extensive use of apprentices. During the last centuries of the medieval period, the world experienced vast social and political changes, accompanied by great turmoil and unrest, and the practice of nursing reflected these changes in national and social structures. Religious orders devoted solely to the care of the sick emerged, but it was actually not until Florence Nightingale's time (1820–1910) that nursing began its long climb toward professionalism through efforts to attain a sound pattern of education combined with practice.

Miss Nightingale was an innovator, a feminist before the term became popular, and an independent spirit firmly believing in her goals for nursing care. Defying all traditions, she built the foundation on which nursing rests today. She emphasized a clean environment, good nutrition and use of knowledge; she was concerned that the nurse receive adequate remuneration: and she ardently proclaimed the need for advanced preparation for those in administrative and teaching roles. She was, however, against state registration for nurses and this did not come into effect until 1919 through the unceasing efforts of Mrs Bedford Fenwick. Registration for midwives preceded that of general nurses by 17 years (1902).

Yet from the turn of the century until the Second World War nursing made little progress. Education and practice saw little change in the status quo. In fact, complacency existed in all the professions because of the overall letdown during and following the First World War and the Great Depression of the 1930s.

### During the Second World War

The propelling force of the Second World War with its patriotic spirit and large numbers of casualties, together with the explosion of technology and innovative materials, produced steadily on-going changes in health care. The doctor-nurse-client relationship gave way to the health team and this concept has continued to expand.

Ancillary personnel evolved in the health professions. Military corpsmen and nurses aides became essential to the delivery of care. Clinical medicine moved ahead, marked by such advances as early ambulation, new techniques in burn treatment, the discovery of new drugs, especially the antibiotics, and a whole complex of sophisticated mechanical and elec-tronic devices for prosthetic and life support. These changes directly affected the practice of nursing.

*The postwar years*

The two decades following the war brought more rapid change to nursing than any other era. Everyone – lay public and health professionals alike – looked on the health-care system in a new light. The public began to ques-tion what constitutes good care; the population escalated and the composi-tion and climate of urban areas altered radically.

Scientific inquiry and development literally exploded with new ther-apies, medical discoveries and newly perfected techniques. It became im-portant to strive to keep people well and the whole realm of preventive medical and nursing care was opened to exploration and revelation.

The educational scene witnessed fresh developments. People who had been employed in the services as 'medics' and sick-berth attendants de-cided to pursue careers in nursing. Those who had been auxiliary nursing in hospitals were given status and a badge as State Enrolled Auxiliary Nurses.

With the election of a Labour government at the end of the war, the National Health Service, the dream of Aneurin Bevan came to fruition. The first NHS Act was passed in 1946 enabling the establishment of the NHS in 1948. Nursing now became part of politics with nurses on negotiated national salary scales. Hospitals, community health services and health promotion became the nation's business and enshrined in legislation.

Reorganizations of the NHS in 1974 and 1983 with changes in gov-ernmental control and levels of decision-making have altered nurses' perceptions of accountability and autonomy. Nurses are appointed as members to district and regional health authorities as professional equals to promote the nursing perspective in planning for future health-care needs of the population.

From the late 1950s thought was given to the use of the term 'profession-al' as well as to the expansion of health programmes and the interpersonal relationships between nurse, client and allied health personnel.

During the 1960s various approaches in terms of nursing function were used to establish nursing as a profession. Crucial questions arose. How does the nurse affect the client? How significant are the nurse's decisions and judgments for the welfare of the client? How complex are nursing actions with regard to education and experience? Is there an effective check on nursing actions? What are nursing decisions based on? Does performance improve with experience? With education? How can the consumer judge the nurse's actions?

At the core of these questions is the code of ethics published by the UKCC for nurses, midwives and health visitors. The existence of this code meets one criterion for a profession and it is today the basis on which action by the nurse is founded and the standard against which nursing actions are judged.

Nursing continues as an emerging profession, based on the criteria that describe a profession. Genevieve and Roy Bixler have identified seven characteristics of a profession. A profession:

1. Uses a well-defined and well-organized body of knowledge as the basis for practice.
2. Enlarges its body of knowledge and improves techniques of education and service through the scientific method.
3. Educates its practitioners in institutions of higher education.
4. Applies a body of specialized knowledge in practice services that are vital to human and social welfare.
5. Functions autonomously in the formulation of professional policy and in the control of professional activity.
6. Attracts people with above-average intellectual and personal qualities, who exalt service above personal gain, and who consider their profession as a lifework.
7. Strives to compensate its practitioners by providing autonomy of action while being accountable to the client, opportunity for continuous professional growth, and economic security.[2]

Many leaders in nursing have contributed to nursing becoming a profession. It is impossible to mention all of them. Several nurses who have contributed to the profession through their development of a nursing model are mentioned in the following section.

*The nursing model*

In all fields of practice, regardless of the discipline, certain concepts are used to define the practitioner's role with the client. In nursing, observations, diagnoses, and the plans for action are based on a **nursing model,** *a set of concepts that assist the practitioner to simplify and organize the data into a manageable plan of action.* In discussing the nursing process, it becomes clear that the nurse brings to that process a mental profile of the client, the goals of care, and the role of the nurse in the execution of the plan. Thus the nursing model has become increasingly useful in practice for defining the nurse's role, and in research as a guide for collection and interpretation of data.

Some models that exist in nursing are the Systems Developmental-Stress Model, [3] the Nursing Process Systems Model,[4] Adaptation Models,[5] Hierarchy of Needs Model,[6] and the Interaction Model.[7] Other models have been described by Peplau,[8] Travelbee,[9] Patterson and Zdered,[10] Rogers,[11] Orem[22] and Johnson.[13]

*The nursing process today*

The complex nature of *nursing* is evident in the many approaches that are used to define it. Everyone has a different image of the term. To define it, one can use actions, functions, roles, consumer images, images held by peers, the individual nurse's philosophy, settings in which nursing is performed, the value placed on the client, or in respect for the client as seen from the employer-employee standpoint.

The variety of nurses within the profession today and the diversity of their educational backgrounds further compound the problem. The engulfing proliferation of information and knowledge and the tremendous surge of technology in the health fields have had an overwhelming impact on the thrust of societal changes. The public is more deeply concerned with health and illness and the rights of the individual to attain maximum well-being. The evergrowing need for preventive health care and health maintenance presents a new challenge to nursing.

The rest of this chapter discusses concepts basic to the nursing process, the systematic method of nursing practice, ways to evaluate effectiveness of the nursing process, the use of a helpful nurse-patient relationship as one of the unique functions of nursing, and the changing role of the nurse. As you study this chapter, keep in mind that, in addition to acquiring a mastery of skills and knowledge necessary for your clinical area, you will also need to possess a zeal for continuing your learning and a commitment to the good of people rather than to self-aggrandizement. Moreover, you should view nursing as an art, a systematic but compassionate way of applying knowledge and skill to achieve clearly defined goals.

## BASIC CONCEPTS

*The holistic approach to people and their needs*

A person is a system striving to maintain optimal balance by means of discharging and conserving energy. Your goal is to assist the person in maintaining or restoring this balance, to help him/her remain adaptive; thus you will need an understanding of the nature of the person and his/her needs.

*A person is a part of all that is within and around him – whether it be a cell, organ system, family or society. He/she is more than the sum of all the parts. This view, called* **holistic or total**, will provide a foundation for considering all the areas that affect health.

*A person's* **behaviour,** *observable characteristics and responses,* can help you recognize needs. Although the person usually seeks to meet physical and psychosocial needs simultaneously, preservation of physical integrity is basic. According to Maslow, the human must maintain an optimal level of oxygen-carbon dioxide exchange, fluid and food intake, rest and activity, elimination of waste products, temperature regulation, and participation in procreation in order to guarantee the species' survival. Next in order are needs for safety, belonging and love, self-esteem and self-actualization (realizing the best of one's potential).[14] In nursing, you help the person meet the basic needs that he/she is unable to meet. Knowing priority of needs will help you set your priorities of care. For example, you would not expect a person to concentrate on job safety while suffering from excessive hunger.

*A systematic approach to nursing practice*

You will be systematic in your nursing practice through use of the scientific method, long a part of research in other disciplines. The scientific method must also be an intricate part of nursing if goals of health care are to be effectively met.

As you work with patients/clients, you may not always follow the steps of problem identification, formulation of hypothesis, sampling, data collection, statistical analysis and retesting of the hypothesis in a sophisticated manner. You can, however, readily see the similarity between steps of the scientific methods and the steps of the nursing process.

Indentifying the problem and formulating the hypothesis may be compared to the assessment and nursing diagnosis stages of the nursing process. The third, or planning, stage is analogous to the step in the research process wherein the design of the study is prepared and criteria are selected for dealing with sample population. Intervention, the fourth stage of the nursing process, may be seen as similar to the action stage of a research project in which a procedure is carried out by the investigator to test its effect of the sample. The fifth and final step in the nursing process, evaluation, is comparable to the conclusions about the value of a research study leading to further investigation, thereby producing a circular effect.

## DEFINITIONS OF NURSING AND THE NURSING PROCESS

*Definitions*

Many leaders in nursing have defined nursing. You may want to read various references at the end of this chapter to help you formulate your own definition.

The authors define **nursing** *as an art and science in which verbal, nonverbal, tangible and intangible health-related activities are systematically performed by a specially educated, licensed and compassionate person. The purpose of these activities is to promote, maintain, or restore biopsychosocial and spiritual health of the person, family and group, as well as to comfort, protect, or stabilize the same during life or in the face of death, and to aid in their recovery. These activities, legally defined, involve use of self and may be performed independently or collaboratively with other health-team members but always with the person, family, group, or community as the central focus and as actively as possible in the process.*

    *The five steps of the nursing process are* **assessment** *(identifying needs),* **formulating the nursing diagnosis,** *stating the client's needs as related to impairment of function, structure, or adaptation;* **planning** *(setting priorities and developing the care plan).* **intervention** *(implementing the care plan), and* **evaluation** *(validating the effectiveness of the care).* In this sequence of operations that uses the scientific method, your knowledge, plus available resources, will combine with your personality, compassion and commitment to produce an effective art and science of nurturing. Thus the nursing process is what you do as a nurse. Every decision for action is carried out within the context of one of the five steps, whether it be an instantaneous decision in an emergency or a long-range plan that grows out of a team conference. Only the time factor varies. The process can be as simple as deciding to sit with a lonely elderly client or as complicated as intensive-care nursing. After you engage in a knowledgeable, purposeful series of thoughts and actions, you then evaluate their effectiveness.

*Assessment*

*The first step in the nursing process is* **assessment,** *study of the whole person to establish a baseline of information and determine the person's potential and need for help.* Once established, this baseline is fluid and your assessment is a continuous process. As changes in the person yield new data, nursing problems and objectives may require restatement or may no longer be relevant for care.

    Assessment is accomplished through observation, the use of knowledge and resources, and communication.

**Observation** includes recognizing objective signs in the patient, family or community; watching their interactions with one another; determining the response of the person or family to you; and discerning the way in which the person arranges personal belongings and speaks of self. Observation and perception are closely related and are more fully described in Chapter 2.

**Knowledge** from previous experiences and courses of study must be used in assessment. Knowledge of normal physiology and anatomy and of growth and development provides a basis for understanding pathological states and enables you to predict patient/client responses and plan care accordingly. Sociology, psychology, philosophy and theology are also examples of areas of information you must use to enhance your conceptual approach to care. Both units of this book, as well as other texts, present theory and facts on which to base assessment. Essential to assessment is a sound knowledge of the developing person.[15]

**Other resources** include data gathered from the person's chart and health history. The literature pertinent to the person's condition must be explored, including information about the medical regimen, such as treatments and drugs, and their implications for nursing care must be considered. A word of caution is needed about the use of literature in assessment. Do not attempt to fit the patient/client completely into a textbook pattern. Everyone's adaptational response is unique and any information gathered is to be used only as a guideline.

**Communication** as part of assessment involves a goal-directed approach to the patient, the family or significant others, the physician as your colleague, and other members of the health team. Verbal and nonverbal exchanges take place between you and the patient, ideally leading to the meeting of minds – a sharing of the same meanings as each sees the other's point of view. Clarification of meaning is necessary when any doubt exists so that needs can be met in a way acceptable to patient and family.

Methods of effective communication and interviewing and barriers to communication are discussed in Chapter 2 and must be used for thorough assessment.

Assessment occurs on two levels. **First-level assessment** *is done on initial contact with a person to determine the perceived health threat, the adaptive ability, and priority care measures.* **Second-level assessment** *continues while the person is in your care and adds depth and breadth of understanding about the physical, emotional, mental, spiritual, cultural, social and family characteristics and needs.* This more comprehensive view of the person enables you to plan and give more individualized care.[16]

A district nurse, for example, is asked to visit by a GP. Along with the client's name, address, phone number, age and race, the nurse has the diagnosis of chronic degenerative arthritis and chronic bladder infection. The nurse is to change a No. 20 Silastic in-dwelling urinary catheter every two weeks and when necessary.

On the first visit the nurse finds a person who is essentially bedfast and who is crying because 'my catheter hurts so much. And my stomach is swollen. Oh, I think I'm going to die.'

The nurse will obviously act at the *first level of assessment*. She/he discovers a distended abdomen. The old catheter is removed; its openings are clogged. The pooled urine flows out with the insertion of a new catheter. The person's pain is gone. She stops crying and seems relieved and comfortable as the nurse explains what happened and how to avoid this problem in the future.

The nurse can now proceed to the *second assessment level*. Actually, she/he has been gathering information for this broader assessment while driving through the community by noting the kind of neighbourhood the person lives in. From the moment the nurse walked in the door she/he has been taking mental notes: general home arrangement, family relationships (the manner in which members talk to each other), leisure activities (macramé bag in the making), cognitive state (verbal communication between nurse and client), emotional state (crying and then smiling), obvious physical status (breathing pattern, appearance of skin, body movements and limitations), elimination pattern (urinary catheter and 'Dear, I'm constipated'), safety factors (arrangement of bed, rugs, etc.), sensory status (hearing and visual acuity) and nutritional status (obesity, snacks within reach).

The nurse will need to elaborate on each of these areas in the written report. She/he will also have to elicit health history, financial status, and a more detailed physical assessment.

*Assessment tools*

Each profession has its tools and nursing is no exception. Nursing tools are not the devices with which treatments are carried out but rather the methodology through which assessment of needs is compiled or the vehicle through which *planning*, the third step, is carried out. These tools include the nursing history and a special format for systematic assessment of the patient's/client's functional areas, leading to a clear indentification of *nursing diagnosis*.

*The* **nursing history** *is distinct from a medical history in that it focuses on the meaning of illness and health care to the person and family as a basis for planning nursing care*, whereas the medical history is taken to determine or rule out pathology as a basis for medical care.[17] Instead of recommending a specific format or a list of steps to follow, the following discussion explains the kind of data that a nursing history provides and the ways in which you can make use of this tool.

The initial interview with a person/family on entrance into a health-care agency-hospital, clinic, physician's office or home visits – must be done by the professional nurse if personalized care is to be planned effectively. Systematically collecting data will help you make maximum use of your limited time with the person.

Whether you use a standard form or an unstructured interview will depend on agency policy, your own ability to collect data, the effectiveness of your communication, and the time available. Techniques for this initial gathering of data are the interview, direct observation and inspection. Subjective as well as objective data are collected and recorded. Analytical thinking and the knowledge you bring from the contributing sciences permit you to make judgments and decisions for care.[18]

To be of practical use, a *nursing history should reflect the client's perception of the illness, the need to seek care, and expectations regarding the care he/she hopes to receive. The history must provide clues to personal needs and ability to deal with health problems.* These areas can be covered in an interview guide that includes the following:

1. The meaning of illness and agency care to the person and to the important family members with whom he/she lives; interests; and projected care plans after discharge.
2. The person's specific needs and the extent to which nursing intervention will be required to help satisfy basic needs: hygiene, rest, sleep, relief of pain, safety, nutrition, fluids, elimination, oxygen and sexuality.
3. Additional data that can be labelled 'other,' such as allergies, adverse reactions to medications, language barriers, educational level (prerequisites for successful communication and health teaching), emotional reactions, social situation, and *anything* the person thinks would be helpful to you in caring for him/her.
4. Your impressions and a summary of the initial interview. If a questionnaire is used, this last area could be completed away from the client.

The entire form can be the first nursing entry on the patient's/client's record and serves as a complete admission note.

*Systematic assessment of the functional areas,* using a specific guide, is basic to ongoing understanding of the person and the development of a nursing plan. This assessment tool is distinct from the nursing history, which focuses on relatively unchanging information that identifies potentials, strengths, attitudes, efforts and weaknesses present on admission. The assessment focuses on areas that change, depending on the person's position on the illness – healthiness continuum.

All working guides developed by nursing leaders cover the primary areas of physiological and psychosocial needs. Several typologies are in use and variations are emerging. Well known to nursing are the 21 problems suggested by Abdellah[19] and Henderson's activities of daily living.[20]

Figure 3.1 shows a tool that could be used for a more extensive second-level assessment of biopsychosocial status during the patient's hospitalization or during the client's or family's use of other health-care services.

Another method of assessment uses the Weed problem-oriented record (POR), a series of progress notes in which each problem is listed and numbered by the physician, the nurse, and other members of the health team. Under each listing are four subheadings, the inititals of which form the acronym SOAP. The S stands for subjective data, O for objective data, A for assessments and interpretations, and P for plan of treatment.[21] The following variation of the problem-oriented record is helpful when charting conventional nurses' notes, for it assists you in writing notes that reflect the nursing care plan. Begin each note with the subjective symptoms expressed by the person; add your observations about the person's current situation, and conclude with the intervention or nursing action that you carried out. Staff and students alike have found it useful to visualize this method of charting as follows: 'What does the patient express?' 'What do I see, hear, touch, smell?' 'What did I do about it?'

*Fig. 3.1*   Example of second-level assessment guide

---

*Identifying data*

Name:                                                    Sex:         Age:
Race/Ethnicity:                                          Date of admission:
Referral source, if any:

*Social status*
Environment (neighbourhood, geographic area):
Home arrangement or retirement care:
Occupation:                                              Educational level:
Leisure activities:
Organizational memberships:
Lifestyle usually followed; effect of illness on lifestyle:
Special preferences in care related to lifestyle:
Financial status; insurance; special concerns:

*Family relationships*
Marital status:                                          Number of children:
Other important family members:                          Other significant people:
Role in family:
Patterns of sexual relations:
Effect of illness upon family life:

*Religious practices*
Church affiliation:                                      Clergyman:
Special rituals/preferences in care related to religion:

*Cognitive status*
Level of consciousness:                                  Orientation:
Ability to communicate verbally and nonverbally:
Memory recall:                                           Attention span:
Ability to grasp ideas, to think logically:
Apparent insight into health problem:
Special values related to health:

*Emotional status*
Feelings about present illness/hospitalization:

Feelings about past experiences with health-care agencies/staff:
Stressful event(s) prior to this illness:
Perceptual abilities (vision, hearing, touch, etc.):
Special awareness of any body part or function:
Feelings about self:
Prefer being alone:                                    With others:
Attitude towards life:
Goals or aspirations:
Sources of pleasure:                                   Displeasure:
Situations causing upset feelings:
Ability to cope with stress:
General behaviour:

*Health history*
Usual health status:
Usual activity level, hours of work:
Pattern of biological rhythms:
Usual eating habits; fluid intake:
Usual sleep habits:
Use of beverages, alcoholic beverages, tobacco, drugs (prescribed, nonprescribed,
legal, illegal):
Present illness and its onset:
Past illness(es), hospitalization(s):
Usual health-care practices:
Usual source of health care:
Special home-care needs/discharge plans:
Family illness(es):

*Physical status*
Height:                                                Weight:
Posture:

Position of comfort:                                   Body movements:
Appearance of head:                                    Face:
    Eyes:                    Ears:                    Nose:
    Mouth:                   Teeth:                   Throat:
Appearance of skin:                                    Temperature:
    Circulatory status:                            Blood pressure:
Muscular build, tone:
Condition of chest (size, shape, movements, cough):
    Heartbeat:                Pulses:               Respirations:
Condition of abdomen (soft, distended, rigid, painful, other symptoms):
Appearance of back:
Appearance of extremities:
    Arms and hands:
    Legs and feet:
    Fingers and toes:
    Range of motion:
Elimination pattern:
Body excretions/secretions:
Reproductive status; appearance of external genitalia:
Presence of pain:
Other signs or symptoms:

Assessment of specific patient/client needs or problems can also be done. The medication history described by Parker, for example, can help you obtain detailed information about medications taken, both prescription and nonprescription, potential drug interactions, and effects of medications on the person.[22] Forms can also be devised to obtain a nutrition history.[23] Joyce Snyder and Margo Wilson describe the following factors to be included in the psychological assessment:

1. Response to stress and coping and defence mechanisms.
2. Interpersonal relationships.
3. Motivation and lifestyle.
4. Thought processes and verbal behaviour.
5. Nonverbal behaviour.
6. Awareness and handling of feelings.
7. Support systems.
8. Talents, strengths and assets.
9. Physical health.
10. Nurse's impression of the interview and interaction.

Janis Reynolds and Jann Logsdon describe a tool for assessing mental status that includes information about identifying data; responses based on the nurse's judgment, such as appearance, motor movement and level of consciousness; and responses based on the person's self-description about illness, family, living arrangements and life patterns.[24]

In assessing a community, consider the following items:

1. Geographical area or neighbourhood, including distribution of residences, industry, commercial establishments or service facilities, and ecological factors such as natural resources or presence of pollutants.
2. Sources of income, income stratification, and the amount of interaction between various income levels.
3. Educational facilities, educational levels, and occupations of the population.
4. Cultural and ethnic background of the community and its residents.
5. Number, age, sex, and family-size distribution of the population.
6. Health facilities, their accessibility, and care available.
7. Other facilities, such as churches, leisure and recreational facilities.
8. Service people in the community, such as health-care workers, police, clergy, social-welfare workers, and their use by the population.
9. Designated and informal community leaders and their roles.
10. Means of communication in the community, such as face-to-face interchange, directives, and nonverbal messages, as well as the formal communication systems and presence of media.
11. The decision-making process and enforcement of decisions in the community, including informal and governmental.

12. Acceptance and integration of new residents into the community.
13. Level of trust in the community between residents, between leaders and residents, and between leaders and service providers.
14. Changes that have occurred in the last several years, as well as rapidity of change, cause of change, and acceptance of change by the community.
15. Degree of cohesion in the community.
16. Acceptance of members who do not conform to the cultural norm.
17. History of the community.[25]
18. Local health authority policies for provision of care.
19. Political influences in resourcing care.

*Nursing diagnosis*

The nursing diagnosis is formulated as a result of judgments made after the assessment. The word diagnosis means to *state a decision of opinion or make a judgment after careful examination and analysis of facts*, and it is not limited to medical conditions.[26]

**Nursing diagnosis** is a *'statement of a potential or actual altered health status of a client which is derived from nursing assessment and which requires intervention from the domain of nursing'*. It includes a statement of the etiology or possible causes and manifestations of signs and symptoms. Nursing diagnoses are distinct from pathological states identified as being responsive to the physician's treatment. The area in which nursing diagnoses are made involve potential or current disturbances in life patterns, body functions, emotional states, spiritual aspects or developmental level, including those occurring secondary to disease. The nursing diagnostic category suggests the status of the person, primary elements of the care plan, treatment and potential outcome. This framework tends to describe the client rather than the nursing activity. Instead of using functional concepts, such as 'provide adequate oxygenation', for instance, you should shift the emphasis by evaluating why the person needs suctioning or any other nursing activity. The answer is found in a description of the client's state: potential respiratory dysfunction resulting from (*condition*) as noted by (*signs and symptoms*). This approach forces the nurse to use knowledge of anatomy and physiology. Nursing diagnosis may be indicative of the medical diagnosis and, conversely, the medical diagnosis may indicate the nursing diagnosis. Thus a nursing diagnosis of respiratory dysfunction might be related to the medical diagnosis of pulmonary embolus. Similarly, the medical diagnosis of fracture might suggest the nursing diagnosis of impaired mobility. But the medical diagnosis remains the same, even during rehabilitation. The nursing diagnosis changes as the person's condition or reaction to the condition changes.

Other examples of nursing diagnosis include ineffective breathing pattern, alteration in bowel elimination, alteration in cardiac output, impaired mobility, alteration in nutrition, ineffective family coping, impaired verbal communication, ineffective individual coping, deficit in diversional activity, fear, anticipatory grieving, dysfunctional grieving, potential for injury, disturbance in self-concept, impairment of skin integrity (actual or potential), sexual dysfunction, spiritual distress, social isolation. The list could go on; it is still being added to, based on research.

The nursing diagnoses emerge quite naturally from the assessment of the client. These statements may express needs or concerns in any or all five areas of human experience and awareness: the biological, physical-environmental, sociocultural, psychological, and spiritual-humanistic realms and are applicable to health promotion as well as acute or chronic illness.

There are times when a specific diagnosis may be stated by several members of the health team – for instance, physician, social worker and nurse. The physician's diagnosis of 'anxiety' in a patient who has undergone a colon resection for cancer may refer to the patient's fear of a recurrence. The social worker may make the same observation of anxiety and be referring to the patients's worry over the cost of special clothing and diet. The nurse may diagnose anxiety and be referring to the patient's difficulty in caring for his colostomy. Each will subsequently intervene in a different manner. The physician may prescribe a tranquilizer, the social worker arrange for financial assistance, and the nurse intervene by teaching and giving support to the patient as he learns colostomy care.

Given a general idea as to the meaning of a nursing diagnosis, the next step is to understand how it can be used in a practical sense. It will be helpful to think of it in terms of a specific, common situation that frequently confronts the nurse: that of a patient admitted to the hospital with a medical diagnosis of diabetes. This patient has not been adhering to his prescribed diet, has neglected his food care, and has been careless about taking his oral hypoglycemics. After a comprehensive assessment, the nurse will have formed some judgments regarding the patient's needs. How can they be expressed in writing? The answer lies in the ability to relate the patient's needs to something that is amenable to nursing care. When stated in these terms, which reflect the definition of nursing diagnosis, it will be helpful to all who care for this patient.

The following examples of a nursing diagnosis might be used for the preceding patient:

1. Nonadherence to prescribed drug therapy *related to lack of understanding of the disease process*, manifested by _____.
   (behaviour, signs, symptoms)
2. Nonadherence to prescribed diet therapy *related to lack of knowledge of diet restriction*, manifested by _____.
   (behaviour, signs, symptoms)

In each statement the cause of the problem is within the ability of nursing to alleviate, either directly by patient teaching or by referral to another health discipline.

Other examples that may serve to clarify the use of a nursing diagnosis might be as follows:

1. Potential skin breakdown over coccyx related to impairment of circulation, manifested by ____.
2. Urinary frequency related to bladder infection, manifested by ____.
3. Dehydration related to elevated temperature, manifested by ____.
4. Withdrawal related to embarrassment over odour, manifested by ____.
5. Impaired mobility related to necessity for continuous traction, manifested by ____.
6. Anxiety related to concern about surgical outcome, manifested by ____.

The accepted use of the term 'related to' is necessary for clarity. It is useful in that it ties the need or problem directly to the area most apt to be responsive to nursing actions; at the same time it allows for other factors that may impinge on the problem and so is less confining in its meaning than the phrase 'due to' might be.

The nursing diagnosis sets the stage for the fourth step in the nursing process – planning the care.

*Formulating nursing-care goals and a plan of care*

On the basis of your systematic study of the patient, decide which functional area is in most need of your help. The problems of care must be determined before you can set priorities. Then you will be able to state **goals,** *a positive statement of what is to be accomplished or the objectives for the person's return to health – the priorities for today, this week, and for eventual discharge to his/ her usual life with optimum health for the individual.* Thus you formulate a **nursing care plan,** *a record summarizing all information required to carry out appropriate nursing care for an individual, family, or group at a given time. The plan is built on the nursing assessment and diagnosis of health needs and indicates specific goals to be reached with the client through designated nursing actions.* The goals and plan are established with the patient/client and family.

Essential to planning care is setting priorities. Once the nursing diagnoses are made, they are ranked in order of priority for care. This step is often a stumbling block for the beginning nurse. Here Maslow's Hierarchy of Needs model may be helpful; priorities can be set according to the Hierarchy.

Consider Mr Denton, age 62, who sustained a cerebral vascular accident and has been in the hospital 24 hours prior to your being assigned to care for him. He has a right hemiplegia and is on complete bedrest. What are the immediate priorities of care? You might select his bath or the monitoring of his intravenous fluids. These steps are important but not ends in themselves; instead they are ways of meeting the needs of those functional states that are in varying degrees of maladaption.

Assuming that you know Mr Denton's age, occupation, social-cultural background, and general response through a nursing history, you can decide what you hope to accomplish. Immediate priorities may be to establish rapport and guide his understanding of the situation, preserve musculoskeletal function, prevent skin breakdown, assist the family in the crisis situation, and establish adequate elimination and nutrition. Long-range goals may include rehabilitation to optimum physical function, a return to work, or help with the acceptance of a disability.

The nursing diagnoses on which you base Mr Denton's care might be:

1. anxiety related to unfamiliar surroundings and personnel;
2. immobility related to right hemiplegia;
3. family apprehension related to concerns for Mr Denton's care and comfort;
4. dehydration related to his inability to help himself to fluids;
5. erratic bowel pattern related to immobility;
6. weight loss related to inadequate food intake;
7. lack of communication related to aphasic speech.

It is not difficult to see from this list how priorities can be set and a plan formulated for Mr Denton's care.

The *purpose of the nursing-care goals and an established plan* is to improve care and minimize wasted efforts. Care plans can be very effective. However, if the plan is not kept up to date, the wrong care may be given.

Remember, too, that a diagnosis may be initially incorrect through faulty writing, misspelling, or incorrect transcribing by the admitting clerk or unit ward clerk.

On the other hand, care plans make the difference between poor care and adequate care. Consider the patient who is almost totally deaf but who is used to nodding and saying 'Fine', to any comment. She was being taught how to irrigate her new colostomy. Although she kept smiling and saying 'Fine', she never seemed to learn how to manage the procedure. Finally, a worker perceived that she was deaf (a rather late perception). This information, along with explicit instructions on how to teach under these circumstances, was incorporated into the care plan. Within several days the woman was managing the procedure adequately.

Not only are care plans useful for people with physiological problems, but people with communication barriers, as in the preceding examples, or those with psychological problems are also in need of an ongoing, up-to-date plan that each health worker can follow. The format used for the written care plan will vary from agency to agency, but in any situation the plan must be simple to use and capable of being readily understood by all workers. A nursing care plan or card usually contains spaces for basic information: diagnosis, age, activity, type of bath, diet, directions regarding intake, output and vital signs, and space to note communication barriers (such as visual or hearing impairment, aphasia, or speaks a foreign language). Diagnostic tests, treatments and medications, as well as a space for special instructions in administering them, are also noted. For example, the size and number of dressings to be used, any special way equipment should be arranged, and difficulties to be anticipated and avoided can be noted in a space under 'Special Instructions'.

Table 3.1 illustrates some of the entries that might appear on a nursing care plan for an elderly man with diabetes and arteriosclerotic-heart disease. Notice that the nursing diagnoses are stated in the context of a dysfunction in an area to which nursing care can be addressed for the necessary help or support.

Teaching begins at the time of the patient's admission and should appear in your care plan from the beginning. It may appear as a part of intervention aimed at a current need, such as explaining the importance of elevating the legs or of using foam pads. Or it may be geared to discharge arrangements, as is the plan for teaching a diabetic. Whatever the need, include it in your plan in such a way as to ensure teaching that can be carried out easily and consistently by everyone. Writing instructions is not enough. Conference discussions and individual help to team members in interpreting the need for teaching are necessary if instruction is to be productive.

In writing your care plan, be sure to use precise action verbs, such as raise, turn, move, place, direct or apply. Put the nursing action in the most descriptive verb form: what is to be done or how it is to be done. Use

*Table 3.1*    Example of Entries for Nursing Care Plan

| Nursing diagnosis | Nursing actions |
| --- | --- |
| 1. Shortness of breath, related to respiratory dysfunction. | 1. Head of bed 45°. Check position frequently. Keep footboard in place. |
| 2. Mouth dry, related to constant mouth breathing. | 2. Oral care T.D.S. Keep lips lubricated with Chapstick. |
| 3. Generalized edema, related to cardiovascular insufficiency. | 3. Monitor IV flow carefully – 15 drops/min. Keep legs elevated when sitting in chair. Discourage sitting on edge of bed. |
| 4. Reddened areas on back and extremities, related to pressure of bed on edematous areas. | 4. Change position 2 hourly. Skin care 2x each shift. Use protective boots on feet. |
| 5. Inadequate self-management of diabetes related to lack of knowledge of disease processes. | 5. Set up teaching programme for diabetic management with dietician and nurse specialist. |

modifiers for precision: gently, slowly, firmly, and so on. The which, what and where are important: which joint, what position, where is it located. The time and frequency elements need to be stated: when, how often, how long. For example, 'turn q.2h' may need to be stated so as to consider individual patterns: sleep habits, right- or left-handedness, sleep position most favoured, time at which visitors may be expected, or time at which the patient may desire to read or watch television.[27]

Because one tends to think of care plans in terms of a hospital setting, the example in Table 3.2 has been offered. It is important to note that planning for health maintenance and health promotion for the more than 70 per cent of persons with chronic illnesses who are not in hospitals is an urgent need in our society today. Table 3.2 shows a care plan used for a female client with hypertension.

A nursing care plan is the nurse's responsibility. When she admits the patient, taking vital signs, weighing the person and writing the results, she/he can also write other information: 'says he often feels faint' . . . 'has an artificial leg' . . . 'likes to sleep with the window open' . . . 'requires kosher food'. These observations can then be sorted out and used by the professional nurse to formulate care goals with the patient and family and to begin the written nursing care plan in a more formal sense. Much of the potential success of written plans lies in the ability of the professional nurse to involve team members on all levels in the task of keeping the plan current. If ancillary personnel are never consulted about the plan or coached in its use, it will never become a viable part of the scheme of care.

Although each member of the nursing team (including all three shifts) is to be involved in the task of updating the plan and keeping it current, the nursing orders must be one person's (head nurse, team leader, or primary nurse) overall responsibility and authority. Nursing strategies cannot change daily or at random if consistent care to meet established goals is to be given. There may be several approaches to a given problem, each one good in itself; when combined, however, they are likely to be less effective than each would be if used alone.

*Discharge planning* is an integral part of the nursing goal and care plan in any setting. Discharge planning must begin the day of admission and involve the patient and family unit. Because the entire plan of hospital care is geared toward discharge, it is only logical to consider the nurse as being primarily responsible for plans for continuity of care at home or for referral to a hospital-based home-care department, a home-health-care agency, or other agencies. Other health-team members who may contribute to discharge plans are the physician, social worker, dietitian and physiotherapist. The degree to which these people collaborate with the nurse depends on the patient's specific needs and the conditions of life to which the patient will return.

When a patient enters the hospital for a colostomy, for example, the postoperative progress will be followed by the nurse each day, often in conjunction with an ostomy therapist. Together they will do patient teaching, note how well the patient adapts to his colostomy, and evaluate the learning of self-care. The nurse is responsible for investigating the need for home care and any necessary agency referrals, involving the family in all of this planning. How well the family members are coping with the patient's condition; their abilities, strengths, and limits; and the physical setting in the home all need to be explored. Similarly, the diabetic, the patient who has a stroke, and all patients in need of continuity of care will need this kind of planning.

Nurses are the best qualified members of the health-care delivery team for discharge planning because they are familiar with all aspects of their patient's/client's care, they are able to interpret medical as well as nursing information, and they are in a position to transmit this information to those who will render follow-up care.

*Table 3.2*   Example of entries for nursing care plan

| Nursing diagnosis | Nursing actions |
| --- | --- |
| *Need for patient teaching*<br>Lacks knowledge of hypertension. | Encourage questions and discussion. Supply literature and explain same. |
| 25 lbs. overweight. | Discuss effects of obesity on hypertension. Explore eating habits and suggest modifications in keeping with lifestyle and preferences. |
| Leads a sedentary life at age 70. | Supply literature on simple exercises to promote weight loss and strengthen muscle tone. Encourage walking. |
| Lacks understanding of medications. | Review purpose of medications, explain their action in lay person's terms and importance of consistency in dosages. Teach an awareness of possible side effects. |
| Lacks knowledge of high-salt food products. | Provide lists of salt content in various foods. Assist in planning a compatible diet regimen low in salt. Suggest ways of enhancing flavour of foods without the use of salt. |
| *Need for emotional support*<br>Lost husband 2 months ago after a long illness. | Allow opportunity to express feelings and assist her in moving through the steps of grieving. Recommend Widows' Support Group or bereavement counselling. |
| Difficulty in adapting to lifestyle change due to bereavement and subsequent feeling of having 'time on her hands'. | Encourage to participate in activities in or near the village where she lives, thereby establishing a new routine with other people. Suggest various volunteer activities to help others. |

*Nursing intervention*

*All actions that you carry out to promote the patient's/client's adaptation constitute* **intervention**, the fourth step in the nursing process. You **intervene** (from the Latin meaning 'come between') *when you modify, settle, or hinder some action* in order to prevent harm or further dysfunction.

'Ministering' to people, carrying out 'comfort' measures, or 'caring' for the sick are terms often equated by lay people with conserving the ill person's energy by waiting on him/her. But your interpretation of *care* and *comfort* should encompass the overall goal of professional nursing: to assist the person to function as effectively and efficiently as the limits of illness permit and to encourage him/her to react to the situation in a unique way. Care that is limited to energy-conserving measures on the person's behalf may be very detrimental to his/her progress. You need a comprehensive data base, including a nursing history and assessment that encompasses all functional areas, a list of nursing diagnoses, and a plan that is based on goals so that your nursing actions are pertinent for the individual. In addition, you must know the **scientific rationale,** *the reasons, either physiological or psychosocial, for performing any action.* For example, do you bathe the patient because of a rigid schedule or because of physiological and psychological principles involving (a) increased circulation and aeration; (b) care of the integument; (c) preservation of musculoskeletal function, and (d) opportunity for communication, further assessment and health teaching?

Nursing actions may consist of either dependent or independent functions: those depending on the medical regimen as outlined by the physician or those derived from nursing judgments. Through nursing intervention, you execute all those ministrations that help meet needs that the individual is not able to meet. Intervention includes all comfort and hygiene measures; safe and efficient use of medical techniques and skills; planning and creating an environment conducive to wholeness, including protection from risk and injury; and health teaching, formal and informal. It also includes the offering of oneself for strength and courage in coping with problems through counselling, listening and socializing; and using information for referrals wherever indicated, either for in-patient care or as discharge planning.

The concept of rehabilitation could be considered almost synonymous with intervention, for from the very beginning of your relationship with the client/family intervention must be geared to restoration of the person's potential for optimum functioning. It is unquestionably tied in with teaching and discharge planning, discussed under the section on nursing goals and plan of care.

The importance of the written care plan to organize nursing intervention cannot be overemphasized. It is a powerful instrument that can be used in a variety of ways. The data base is invaluable as the groundwork for later evaluation and judgment regarding patient progress.

Nursing intervention occurs in many settings: hospital, local health department, doctor's surgery, neighbourhood health centre, and patient's own home. Nurses also carry out intervention from other bases, such as the Red Cross, insurance companies, health-maintenance organisations and private nursing agencies.

Because the nursing process is a problem-solving mode of action using the scientific method, your nursing actions are hypotheses to be tested in practice. When they are shown to be effective and can be validated, specific actions or ways in which needs are best met become a part of the ongoing individualized nursing care plan. The fifth step of the nursing process, evaluation, is used to determine the validity of nursing actions, to decide to what degree goals have been met, to redefine nursing diagnoses, and to lay the foundation for a further plan of care.

## Evaluation

Evaluation, *determining immediate outcomes and predicting long-range results*, cannot be entirely separated from the first four steps in the nursing process. A circular effect implies constant reassessment of the patient/client situation, redefining of nursing diagnoses, stating nursing goals, and updating of the nursing care plan for action. Interventions will then be modified or expanded and reevaluation will occur. Criteria for evaluating the care as to its effectiveness will evolve from the goals inherent in the nursing diagnoses: for instance, if the nursing diagnosis was 'erratic bowel pattern related to immobility', the gain or lack of a consistent bowel pattern will be evidence to support the success or failure of the nursing actions taken to accomplish the goal. Validation must include feedback from the recipients of care – patient or family – and from members of the health team who are objective observers. Subjective symptoms, such as pain, and results of intervention are best evaluated by the patient. Observable signs may be evaluated best by the health team.

The goal of your chosen action within the nursing process is always to minimize objectively the negative consequences to the greatest degree possible and to capitalize on those outcomes that are positive. In evaluating results of intervention, you will seek to duplicate the positive effects and to determine the cause of unexpected outcomes, whether positive or negative. In a negative outcome, attempt to control or help the person control the events responsible so that the outcome does not recur.

Recognizing that an act may have more than one consequence, you must evaluate who will be affected by the act, what results can be anticipated, and the value of the consequences to those involved. Being aware of this evaluation process will help you appreciate that even the simplest activity is a means of achieving the goals you have set for the patient in striving towards health. Emptying a bedpan then becomes not an isolated menial task but a part of your intervention for carrying out some priorities of care, such as provision of needed rest and maintenance of elimination and fluid balance.

Evaluation of care is directly related to what is termed **accountability,** *the state of being responsible for one's acts and being able to explain, define, or measure in some way the results of decision making.* Accountability involves evaluating the effectiveness of care on the basis of 'how', 'what', and 'to whom'. Just believing that your care makes a difference is not enough. You must have criteria that justify both the need for and the effectiveness of your nursing actions.

The 'how' is measuring your effectiveness against a set of criteria – a predetermined outcome to be observed. Noting that an immobile patient who has been given daily prune juice is now able to have a normal stool at reasonable intervals without requiring enemas or cathartics is one example of observing a predetermined outcome. You can evaluate the care of an individual patient, care given within a nursing unit, or care delivered by an entire community health agency or clinic.

The 'what' of accountibility involves intervention measures and intangibles, such as attitudes and subtle nuances. The nursing measures you carry out are important, but equally important is the meaning of care to the person.

In order to decide 'to whom' you are accountable, you must first clarify for yourself the nature and the purpose of your care. You will be accountable to the patient/client, family, group, doctor, nursing staff, agency administration and community.

One way in which nurses can contribute to improvement of care is by developing within their own agency a quality control system that applies specifically to nursing. This system must be one in which desired nursing criteria are identified and it must incorporate a way in which nursing practice can be compared to the established criteria. Process standards rather than structure standards must be used. (The difference between process and structure standards can be illustrated by examples: *Structure* – Are written care plans used? *Process* – Is the written care plan appropriate to the patient. Does it consider personal needs, disease-related needs and therapy-related needs? *Outcome* – What is the outcome in terms of mortality, morbidity and social functioning?)

The scope of the system may be determined by the objectives and specific needs of the agency. It may be limited to patient care or may include administrative functions; it may be used for a particular department exclusively; or it may apply to a specific group of patients – for example, those with respiratory diseases. Once it has been determined, a form can be prepared, one with a format that is simple, easy to use, and readily interpretable by all who use it. Because the design will influence the way in which the standards are worded, the evaluation form must be prepared first.

Basic to any quality-control system, or as it is sometimes called, a nursing audit, is a plan for recording accurate and objective observations of patients in their clinical record or chart. Without written data relevant to patient progress, patient response to therapy, and completion of physician's orders, the nursing process would be incomplete. *The nurse's charting must reflect the nursing care plan.* Only by validation of nursing actions can the profession hope to demonstrate its commitment to quality care.

Whatever system of charting is used – narrative nurses' notes, a problem-oriented record in which progress is noted by using the SOAP format, or a goal-oriented record – it must be capable of being analysed in terms of the quality of care given. Such analysis includes both technical aspects and the 'art of care'. The 'art of care' includes rules, manner, and behaviour of care providers, and their communication with clients. This responsibility rests on the nurse and requires accountability to the patient, profession, other members of the health team, the institution and, not least, oneself.

An essential part of the nurse's accountability is a personal commitment to continuing education that is related directly to the practice of nursing. The current explosion of knowledge, advances in technology, and public demand for more effective health care make it essential that nurses continue their learning beyond their basic education.

Lately there has been a move toward mandatory continuing education for nurses with arguments pro and con. Whether mandatory continuing education for registration as a registered nurse becomes widespread, the responsibility for improvement of practice through education will always rest with the individual nurse.

TOOLS FOR EVALUATING YOUR EFFECTIVENESS

*The process recording*

Communication is essential to the nursing process and thus is repeatedly emphasized throughout the book. One tool for analysing your communication pattern with patients is the process recording.

The **process recording** *is a written account of the responses of client and nurse and the analysis of these responses* providing for the reconstruction of a nursing incident in order to identify and examine the elements in it. It may be written during the time the conversation or interview is occurring or from recollection. You should obtain the person's consent if you plan to take notes during an interview.

The reconstruction of an interview or conversation is valuable for picking out clues to behaviour and for determining inconsistencies in your response to the person. The process recording allows you to evaluate your responses in relation to communication principles and methods, improve communication, focus more accurately on the person's needs, and make predictions about nursing intervention. In addition, you provide the person a seldom available opportunity to express self to someone who listens in a nonjudgmental way. Thus you help him/her to sort out thoughts and feelings. The process recording is also a teaching tool. When you share with other team members what you have told the person and his/her reaction to the illness, they can use this information as a guide in further therapeutic communication.

You will build on the foundation of interviewing and therapeutic communication studied in Chapter 2. The person must be able to sense your regard and interest in his/her ideas, hopes and fears. You nonjudgmental attitude is essential to help the person sort out ideas and reach the solution that seems most feasible.

As soon as possible after the interview, reconstruct it from your brief notes and make an analysis of the verbal and nonverbal dialogue. This expansion can help you gain insight into yourself and the client and provide data for planning care. If your approach to the person seems unproductive, a process recording in which incidents are reconstructed may help identify the problem. Clues can be analysed for their meaning by writing out what preceded certain of your or the client's responses. You can better realize ways in which you could have intervened in a more direct or helpful manner, perhaps by rephrasing or refocusing your portion of the dialogue.

*Written analysis of nursing care*

Another tool for evaluating your effectiveness in the nursing process and nurse-client relationship is a **written analysis** *of nursing care*. The written analysis provides a way of looking at your assessment of needs, your intervention as a result of planning, the scientific rationale on which your intervention was based, and of evaluating the care you gave.

**Assessments and nursing diagnoses** may be put down in a sequential order if your wish or they may be sorted out according to functional areas.

**Intervention, together with the reason for your action**, is placed in a second column and shows the results of your planning. A stumbling block in this portion of your analysis is often the confusion of medical intervention with that of nursing. If the patient has an intravenous pyelogram done in X-ray, for example, that is medical intervention. If you explain the test to the patient, allay fears through communication and teaching, and prepare him/her for the test by administering prescribed medication or treatments, these are nursing interventions.

You should justify or give the rationale for action on the patient's behalf, validating your rationale with the literature. Therefore familiarity with the current nursing literature, as well as an ability to use the literature of related disciplines, the natural and behavioural sciences and humanities, will be a necessary part of your continued independent study as you practise nursing.

**Evaluation** is the step often overlooked or given minimal attention. Yet it is the basis for reassessment and improvement of care and should be included in your written analysis. You may not always write an analysis, but you should have the same information firmly in mind and be able to describe it to others. You may be able to incorporate some of the process recording in your evaluation. Your reassessment is then based on a more complete data base and can be done with a number of interrelated facts, some of which, if missing, would considerably change your approach to the improvement of the patient's care. You may see, for instance, that the outcome of the bath you have given is increased relaxation for the patient, including a restful nap before lunch, but fail to evaluate the feeling of dependence and loss of self-actualization expressed by the person verbally and nonverbally. Rehabilitation may then be seriously impaired through inadequate evaluation.

## THE NURSE-CLIENT RELATIONSHIP IN THE NURSING PROCESS

*Differences between a social and a helpful relationship*

Establishing a helpful relationship is one of the unique functions separating nursing from other health services.

The **nurse-client relationship** *is a helpful, purposeful interaction over time between an authority in health care, the nurse, and a person or group with health-care needs, with the nurse focusing on needs of the client while being empathic and using knowledge.* Through this relationship the nursing process is put to use, and it must be differentiated from mere association. Social contact with another individual, verbal or nonverbal, may exert some influence on one of the participants and needs may be met. But inconsistency, nonpredictability, or partial fulfilment of expectations often results. Characteristics of social relationship are as follows:

1. The contact is primarily for pleasure and companionship.
2. Neither person is in a position of responsibility for helping the other.
3. No specific skill or knowledge is required.

4. The interaction is between peers, often of the same social status.
5. The people involved can, and often do, pursue an encounter for the satisfaction of personal or selfish interests.
6. There is no explicit formulation of goals.
7. There is no sense of accountability for the other person.
8. Evaluation of interactions does not concern personal effectiveness in the interaction.[28]

A nurse-client relationship is established *when the person's or family's needs are met consistently and unconditionally.*

A working nurse-client relationship is, by definition, good, helpful, therapeutic. There is no such thing as a poor nurse-client relationship; there are only poor or unsatisfactory experiences that prevent establishing the relationship. Interactions moving toward a relationship occur whenever direct patient care, health teaching, listening, or counselling are done, or when the person's/family's activities are being directed or modified in some way.

The following interactions are *not* helpful to the patient because needs are met inconsistently or conditionally:

1. Automatic, in which there is no meaning to either person.
2. Impersonally helpful, in which a service is expertly given but no personal interest or empathy is displayed.
3. Involuntary, in which 'carrying out orders' is done as a duty, often the result of the nurse's perception of work as just a job to be done.
4. Inconsistent (that which is conditional in nature) assisting the patient only when the situation is interesting or when it fulfils the nurse's needs.

The nurse-client relationship is one in which the person's real complaint is uncovered. The focus is on the client's needs rather than on your own. The person is not a social chum. There is a giving of self in an objective way to the person and family; yet you do not identify with (feel the same as), pity, or reject the one seeking help. Neither do you feel you are the only person who can help the client. You use the resources that a team can offer whenever doing so is beneficial to the person or family.

### The effect of feelings on the relationship

Only through mutual striving for self-awareness and appreciation of the other person's reactions can a nurse-client relationship grow to maturity. Knowing that each person has needs to be met gives meaning to this relationship. You must expect both positive and negative feelings in yourself and in the other, and you must realize that both can be expressed either overtly or covertly.

The client's positive feelings may be those relating to a sincere desire to cooperate in his/her own care and may include a polite manner toward others. The feelings may be a result of educational, religious or cultural background, or a combination of these factors. In any event, you are in a position to capitalize on such positive feelings in order to establish rapport and a sense of trust as a foundation for the nurse-client relationship. Additionally, make every effort to learn the person's negative feelings. Insecurity; distrust of unfamiliar persons, routines and treatments; or helplessness or hostility because of a lack of control over his/her own responses – all may be present.

Unfortunately, when either positive or negative overt feelings dominate a patient's behaviour, the person may be labelled 'good' or 'bad' by the staff. The 'good' patient is the one who never complains, who accepts illness no matter how distressing or painful, and who receives the care given without question. The characteristics of the 'bad' patient are usually described by staff as demanding, complaining and displeasing physically and conversationally. Such a person is seen as not helping himself/herself, unappreciative and uncooperative. Nurses often become upset or judgmental with the intransigent patient as well. He/she does not understand the rules in the same way that you do and interferes with the established routine. Yet the interference may be an expression of the very self-determination necessary for rehabilitation.[29] Often the behaviour of the person from a different culture, social class or ethnic group is misinterpreted. When the person's behaviour does not match your expectations, do not label it. Instead try to understand why the behaviour might be different.

The positive feelings that you may have towards the client are strongly bound to your commitment to nursing as a way of life. They cannot develop if you are merely doing a job because the negative feelings we all possess can overpower the positive and interfere with the nurse-client relationship. Negative feelings, which may at times be expressed in your reactions, will provoke inappropriate behaviour. Talking out your negative feelings with the staff is better than unloading them on the client or family.

*The effect of behaviour on the relationship*

To develop an awareness of the feelings that you take with you to the client, examine your behaviour to determine whether it is modified for some people in a helping way and for others in a manner that hinders your effectiveness. Modification of your behaviour with, or approach to, different persons is a valuable tool. Surely you would behave differently towards the child than towards the aged person. But behaving differently because a person is rich or poor, black or white, quiet or boisterous, grateful or ungrateful, in agreement or disagreement with your value system may prevent you from meeting that person's needs.

Remembering that all behaviour has meaning will help you to sharpen and improve those qualities you possess that produce a positive response in others. When inappropriate reactions do occur, analyse them in terms of what preceded them and of what happened after the incident. Search for clues to establish the meaning of feelings. Using the process recording format, you might record the event by writing the conversation and the non-verbal responses of both you and client for closer analysis. Discussing the incident with objective persons may help, perhaps in team conference. Become familiar with your own coping mechanisms; seek to understand their relative value and the ways in which you use them in your approach to nursing care. Take sufficient care of your personal needs outside the nursing setting so that you can give your best professional care to the person or family or group.

Although the relationship with a client is a reciprocal experience, the responsibility for establishing it and for making appropriate changes in it rests with you, not with the client. The relationship is based on each person's perceiving the other as a unique individual without stereo-typing. Help the person *not* to see you as the command officer or the 'angel in white' and avoid seeing the patient as a 'gallbladder' or a room number.

You may unconsciously exhibit a middle-class tea-and-cakes niceness combined with Puritan morality that insists on uncompromising obedience on the part of nursing student, nurse, patient and family alike. You may represent a punitive social system, and the person may sense your moral indignation toward health problems that some regard as stemming from 'indiscretions': alcoholism, drug addition, unwed motherhood, obesity, venereal disease, or even diabetes uncontrolled because of dietary carelessness. Superimposed on this attitude may be the ethic of cleanliness in which you loom as a threat to the other, judging the person in terms of how clean he/she is, internally as well as externally.

Hospital administrations sometimes contribute to stereotyping by commending the nurse as 'good' if she/he gets the beds and baths finished, the pills passed, the treatments done. Because these things are tangible, they do not require time for involvement with patients' reactions, behaviour, or qualitative responses of nurse to patient or patient to nurse. Tasks must be done and are vital to nursing care, but over-emphasis on tasks leaves little time for exploring the meaning of the person's health status and health goals.

Carrying out the person's planned regimen for health maintenance or restoration will be accomplished more easily because of the nurse-client relationship, for it will naturally foster the tangible as well as the intangible aspects of your care. Above all, keep expectations mutual and remember that the major characteristic of the nurse-client relationship is that *the nursing needs of the individual or family are met in an emotional climate of warmth, support and mutual trust.*

*Guidelines for the nurse-client relationship*

If you consider your behaviour an influence on the person's or family's behaviour, you will be in a better position to advise specific approaches for bringing about change. You will want to develop characteristics of a helping, humanistic relationship. These characterisitics include being:

1. *respectful* – feeling and communicating an attitude of seeing the client as a unique human being, filled with dignity, worth and strengths, regardless of outward appearance or behaviour; being willing to *work* at communicating with and understanding the client because he/she is in need of emotional care;
2. *genuine* – communicating spontaneously, yet tactfully, what is felt and thought, with proper timing and without disturbing the client, rather than using professional jargon, façade, or rigid counsellor or nurse role behaviours;
3. *attentive* – conveying rapport and an active listening to verbal and non-verbal messages and an attitude of working with the person;
4. *accepting* – conveying that the person does not have to put on a façade and that the person will not shock you with his/her statements; enabling the client to change at his/her own pace; acknowledging personal and client's feelings aroused in the encounter; to 'be for' the client in a nonsentimental, caring way;
5. *positive* – showing warmth, caring, respect, and agape (love); being able to reinforce the client for what he/she does well;
6. *strong* – maintaining separate identity from the client; withstanding the testing behaviour of the client;
7. *secure* – permitting the client to remain separate and unique; respecting his/her needs and your own; feeling safe as the client moves emotionally close; feeling no need to exploit the other person;
8. *knowledgeable* – having an expertise based on study, experience, and supervision; being able to assist the client in formulating goals;
9. *sensitive* – being perceptive to feelings; avoiding threatening behaviour, responding to cultural values, customs, norms as they affect behaviour; using knowledge that is pertinent to the client's situation;
10. *empathic* – looking at the client's world from his/her point of view; being open to his/her values, feelings, beliefs, and verbal statements; stating your understanding of his/her verbal or nonverbal expressions of feelings and experiences;
11. *nonjudgmental* – refraining from evaluating the client moralistically or telling the client what to do;
12. *congruent* – being natural, relaxed, trustworthy and dependable, and demonstrating consistency in behaviour and between verbal and nonverbal messages;

13. *unambiguous* – avoiding contradictory messages; using purposeful communication;
14. *creative* – viewing the client as a person in the process of becoming, not being bound by the past, and viewing yourself in the process of becoming or maturing as well.[30]

Other features that correlate highly with being effective in a helping relationship are being open instead of closed in interaction with others, perceiving others as friendly and capable instead of unfriendly and incapable, and perceiving a relationship as freeing instead of controlling another.[31]

Establishing and maintaining a relationship or counselling another does not involve putting on a façade of behaviour to match a list of characteristics. Rather, both you and the client will change and continue to mature. As the helper, you are present as a total person, blending potentials, talents and skills while assisting the client to come to grips with needs, conflicts and self.[32]

Working with another in a helping relationship is challenging and rewarding. You will not always have all the characteristics just described; at times you will be handling personal stresses that will lower your energy and sense of involvement. You may become irritated and impatient while working with the client. Accept the fact that you are not perfect; remain as aware as possible of your needs and behaviour and your effect on the other. Remember that the most important thing you can share with a client is your own uniqueness as a person. As you give of yourself to the client, you will in return be given to – rewarded with warmth and sharing from the client.

*Phases of the nurse-client relationship*

Unless the encounter is brief, the feelings between you and the client and the family and the work jointly done evolve through a sequence of phases. The phases are not sharply demarcated and they vary in duration. They can be compared to human developmental stages because of the degree of dependency-independency and feelings of trust involved: the orientation phase is comparable to infancy, identification to childhood, the working phase to adolescence, and termination to adulthood.[33]

**The initial or orientation phase** of the relationship begins when you first meet the person or family. You might carry out intervention measures shortly thereafter, as you function in the role of technical expert, counsellor, teacher, referral person, or substitute mother. Your main tasks during this phase, however, are to become orientated to the other's expectations, health needs and goals through assessment while simultaneously orientating the person to your role and health-care goals and his/her role in the health-care system. You formulate a tentative care plan. Establishing rapport and showing acceptance are vital for assessing and orientating the other person. Be aware of how you are affecting the person and how he/she is affecting you. During this period the person clarifies the health status and its meaning through your exploration of the many factors affecting him/her. Essential to this phase is caring for the person or family in such a way that a sense of trust and confidence in you is established.

**The second phase, called the identification phase**, marks the time when the person has become better acquainted with you, places trust in your decisions and actions, works closely with you, follows your suggestions, and at times imitates your behaviour. He/she sees you as 'his/her nurse'. You continue the nursing process, actively guiding him/her but also providing opportunities for participation in self-care. You accept dependency without fostering it excessively.

**The third, the working phase**, is the time when the client is becoming more independent, actively using all services and resources offered by the health team. He/she becomes more assertive and no longer relies so heavily on you. By now he/she is usually regaining physical and emotional health – optimal function – so that the behaviour begins to change as he/she becomes more involved in decision making about certain aspects of the situation. Although the person seems more independent and even self-centred, you can now work as equal partners in meeting health goals. The client is preparing for convalescence and discharge from your services.

**The maintenance phase**. Often the nurse who works in an acute-care setting does not really experience the rewards of a relationship with the patient. The short stay typical of hospitalization or even the few visits given by a district nurse allow nothing more than establishing rapport, if that.

The maintenance phase in the relationship is only possible in the setting in which a client is followed by the same nurse over a period of time – for example, in a rehabilitation centre, nursing home, old people's home or psychiatric/mental-health agency. Also the district nurse or health visitor may visit the same clients over a period of years.

In this phase, termination does not occur for a long time. Often termination only comes with the death of the person. The active, working, therapeutic stage goes on until the person has reached his/her potential. In this situation, the client has reached a plateau where support and maintenance are essential for daily living. The client may live at home, following your directions for health-promotion measures, and may call on you for assistance only when chronic illness becomes uncontrolled or when a new condition of pathology or aging arises. Or the client may be in an institution and need maximal or minimal assistance with daily physical care. What characterizes this phase is that you must actively pursue interventions in order to maintain emotional and social well-being. The reward will be the gratification of seeing a person reassert his/her will to live, to become creative in coping with problems or making 'ends meet', and to remain independent.

**The last phase, termination**, is marked by the person's becoming as fully independent as possible, leaving the health-care system to return to the community. Together you plan the management of the health situation after discharge, especially if the client requires any special life-style modifications, such as in exercise, hygiene or diet. This is a time of separation and both you and the person must work through feelings about separation – sometimes past as well as present situations. Mutual attachment develops between you and someone you take care of for a long time and either one or both of you may feel uncertain about the person's ability to manage without you. Together you need to talk about feelings about separation and your confidence in the ability to be independent and remain healthy. Avoid increasing dependency on you at this time to meet your needs. When the client leaves the health-care system, each of you should feel no regret about the termination. On the other hand, if there is need for follow-up visits after discharge, your interest and concern in the person or family extend to this ongoing care.

Without the nurse-client relationship, the person's needs are not met and the nursing process is not in force. Mechanical tasks become an end in themselves and the person is not helped to prevent or adapt to his/her illness.

There may be people with whom you cannot form a helpful relationship. There may be situations in which it would be best for the client if someone else were to work with him/her. You need to be aware of your own feelings of discomfort with a client and you should be able to accept the fact that you cannot work with certain people. Often the reasons will be obscure; you may want to work through the reasons with an instructor or supervisor of your own personal growth. For more information on barriers to an effective nurse-client relationship, see the list of references at the end of the chapter.[34]

*Problem solving versus research in the nursing process*

In nursing you will do problem solving and research; both use the scientific method discussed in this chapter. Although problem solving and research are frequently thought of as synonymous, a fundamental difference in purpose exists between them.

The purpose of problem solving is to solve an immediate problem in a specific setting. The solution is not necessarily new knowledge and cannot be generalized to a larger population. Consequently, the precision of study is not so exacting, and statistical analyses are seldom done.

The purpose of research is to reveal new knowledge. All elements of the scientific method are precisely followed. The results of a research study cannot be expected to produce information to solve a specific problem.

Knowledge obtained through research may contribute to the solution of an immediate problem and problem solving may reveal new knowledge applicable beyond the immediate situation. But the basic difference remains. Problem solving as a health-teaching method is discussed in the next chapter.

*Research in nursing*

Historically nursing research has been scarce, although Florence Nightingale reportedly valued astute observation and gathering of evidence and indicated their importance for nursing. Research has been considered the exclusive domain of academicians, nurse-scientists, doctoral candidates – or worse, researchers from other disciplines who have found nurses a rich source of data for study in the behavioural sciences. Study of the nursing profession by behavioural scientists has resulted in certain benefits. Many pertinent facts have emerged that have given insight to nurses concerning their responses to patients and to each other. However, nursing cannot justify its worth as a separate discipline unless clinical research is performed by its own practitioners.

Staff nurses are extremely valuable resources for ideas that nurse researchers can use. At the bedside or in a one-to-one patient-client relationship in any setting, nurses can observe and report those areas of nursing care that need to be studied. Nurses can start listing ideas or problems that require further investigation and these items can be brought to the attention of someone interested in developing the idea. Staff nurses are invaluable in the collection of data. They know the patient's individual characteristics, limitations and availability and thus can facilitate the researcher's work.

Although the Ph.D is usually considered the research degree, many Master's level programmes prepare nurses to do beginning-level research. All nurses are taught the problem-solving process, which is the basis of all research. The nurse without a doctorate who wishes to do research would be wise to consult a qualified researcher for assistance in developing the methodology of the project.

Most research in nursing is not funded. Countless small projects are carried out by individual nurses or groups of nurses with little or no financial help. Many faculty members in universities are able to do research with small amounts of money through some plan of the institution that encourages pilot studies. Larger studies may be supported by private foundations. Most large research grants come from the government or commercial funds and are difficult to obtain.

To qualify, one must have completed one or more pilot studies and have published the results of the research. In rare instances, organizations or institutions will support nursing research by providing released time for the nurse so that proposals may be developed and data collected and analysed.

Nursing research begins with a **discrepancy,** *a perceived difference between two states of affairs,* or an uncomfortable feeling about the status quo. A difference is felt between what is occurring now and things as they could, ought, should or might be. A gap might exist between what is known and what needs to be known to take action. Or there might be a discrepancy between sets of facts.

In the final analysis, the curiosity of the individual nurse and the belief in the value of nursing practice will determine whether significant research is done in nursing. Each nurse must be responsible for noting if certain situations or sets of circumstances produce specific patient responses. Collecting such data over a period of time can obviously result in increased knowledge for nursing. More importantly, if carefully analysed and reported, the data can result in improved care for patients, families and communities.

## REFERENCES

1. Riehl, Joan, and Sister Callista Roy, eds., *Conceptual Models for Nursing Practice,* 2nd edition (Appleton-Century-Crofts, New York, 1980).
2. Bixler, Genevieve, and Roy Bixler, 'The Professional Status of Nursing', in *Conceptual Models for Nursing Practice,* 2nd edition (Appleton-Century-Crofts, New York, 1980), pp. 53–9.
3. See note 1, above.
4. Brown, Sally Jo, 'The Nursing Process Systems Model', *Journal of Nursing Education,* vol. 20 no. 6 (1981) pp. 36–40.
5. Roy, Sister Callista, *Introduction to Nursing: An Adaptation Model* (Prentice Hall Inc., Englewood Cliffs, NJ, 1976).
6. Maslow, A.H., *Motivation and Personality* (Harper & Row, Publishers, New York, 1954).
7. Brodish, Mary, 'Nursing Practice Conceptualized: An Interaction Model', *Image,* vol. 14 no. 1 (1982) pp. 5–7.
8. See note 32, below; also, Blade, Mary, 'The Peplau Developmental Model for Nursing Practice', in *Conceptual Models for Nursing Practice.*
9. Travelbee, Joyce, *Interpersonal Aspects of Nursing* (F.A. Davis Company, Philadelphia, 1967).
10. Patterson, Josephine, and Loretta Zderad, *Humanistic Nursing* (John Wiley & Sons, Inc., New York, 1976).

11. Rogers, Martha, *The Theoretical Basis for Nursing* (F.A. Davis Company, Philadelphia, 1970).

12. Orem, Dorothea, *Nursing: Concepts of Practice* (McGraw-Hill Book Company, New York, 1971).

13. Johnson, Dorothy, 'The Behavioural System Model for Nursing', in *Conceptual Models for Nursing Practice*.

14. See note 6, above.

15. Murray, Ruth and Judith Zentner, *Nursing Assessment and Health Promotion Through the Life Span*, 3rd edition (Prentice Hall, Inc., Englewood Cliffs, NJ, 1985).

16. See note 1, above; also, Bower, Fay, *The Process of Planning Nursing Care: A Theoretical Model* (The C.V. Mosby Company, St Louis, 1972); Saxton, Dolores, and Patricia Hyland, *Planning and Implementing Nursing Intervention* (The C.V. Mosby Company, St Louis, 1975).

17. Little, Dolores E., and Doris L. Carnevali, *Nursing Care Planning*, 2nd edition (J.B. Lippincott Company, Philadelphia, 1976).

18. See note 10, above.

19. Abdellah, Fay, *et al.*, *Patient-centered Approach to Nursing* (The Macmillan Company, New York, 1960).

20. Henderson, Virginia, *Nature of Nursing* (The Macmillan Company, New York, 1966).

21. Weed, Lyle L., *Medical Records, Medical Education, and Patient Care: The Problem-Orientated Record as a Basic Tool* (The Press of Case Western Reserve University, Cleveland, 1969).

22. See note 6, above.

23. Butterworth, Charles, and George Blackburn, 'Hospital Malnutrition and How to Assess the Nutritional Status of a Patient', *Nutrition Today*, vol. 10 no. 2.

24. Reynolds, Janis, and Jann Logsdon, 'Assessing Your Patient's Mental Status', *Nursing '79*, vol. 9 no. 8 (1979) pp. 26–33.

25. Murray, Ruth, and M. Marilyn Juelskoetter, *Psychiatric/Mental Health Nursing: Giving Emotional Care* (Prentice Hall, Inc., Englewood Cliffs, NJ, 1983).

26. See note 13, above.

27. Ibid.

28. See note 25, above; also, Hopson, B., and M. Scally, *Life Skills Teaching* (McGraw-Hill Book Company, New York, 1981).

29. See note 9, above.

30. Rogers, Carl, *Client-Centered Therapy* (Houghton Mifflin Company, Boston, 1951).

31. See note 25, above.

32. Ibid.; also, Peplau, Hildegard, *Interpersonal Relations in Nursing* (G.P. Putnam's Sons, New York, 1952).

33. Ibid.

34. See note 25, above.

# 4

# Health Teaching: a basic nursing intervention

Study this chapter will enable you to:

1. Discuss why teaching is a major nursing responsibility in all settings.

2. Differentiate the traditional and simple definitions of *teaching*, *learning* and *education* from the nontraditional and complex.

3. Define *health education* and *self-care*.

4. Describe changing educational trends with an emphasis on the future.

5. Identify the varied opportunities for teaching health promotion.

6. List the fundamentals of teaching.

7. Explore and apply the many facets of creativity in teaching-learning.

8. Discuss and translate into practical examples various teaching-learning theories, including how they are affected by language, culture and other factors.

9. Compare methods of teaching with various ages, including individual and group approaches, and predict when each might be appropriate.

10. Discuss how teaching may differ from institution to home setting.

11. Sharpen your ability to identify significant teaching-learning opportunities through analysis of case studies.

12. Teach patients, families, and co-workers in the nursing setting when appropriate.

On entering nursing you may not have understood that to nurse is to teach. Teaching provides a major way to help another adapt. This chapter does not attempt to review the many teaching-learning theories. Instead it presents various theories and methods that seem applicable to nursing and that you can begin to use.

The authors have not attempted to emulate educational jargon, but they, too, are imprisoned in words. You must take the words and phrases and apply them to people, yourself included, making the ideas alive and active. Only then will you experience the teaching-learning process.


DEFINITIONS

**Learning** *is the process of acquiring wisdom, knowledge or skill; an overt change in behaviour may be observed.* **Teaching** *is the process of sharing knowledge and insight, of facilitating another to learn knowledge, insight and skills.* These definitions are deceptively simple. Popular magazines, textbooks and library shelves are full of theories and explanations about how these processes take place. Yet no one can say learning *will always* take place under certain conditions or teaching *will never* take place under certain conditions. In spite of quantities of information, people with their unique minds and personalities are always modifying the existing theories.

In actuality, teaching and learning cannot be separated, for while a person is teaching, learning is also taking place, or at least should be. Perhaps the substandard use of *learn*, as in the sentence 'I'm going to learn you something' has more accuracy than people have thought. Both terms connote a lifelong process, an internalization (learning) of thoughts, attitudes, facts, and a consequent externalization (teaching) of those thoughts, attitudes and facts. Teaching and learning can be conscious and formal, as in the announced situation 'Today we are going to learn about the digestive system.' Or they can be unconscious and informal, as when a mother frowns and says with a certain tonal emphasis, 'What is *that* smell?' The listening and watching child combines a certain smell with a negative mental attitude.

One word that connotes a chilly, stiff learning process is *pedagogy.* Originally the word meant teaching children, but today it refers generally to teaching. Unfortunately, most knowledge about learning has come from studies of children and animals and most knowledge about teaching has come from teaching children who are in compulsory attendance. Thus adults are often taught as though they were children. To combat this erring process, Knowles has coined a new word, **andragogy:** *helping adults learn.*[1] Consequently, he turns from traditional pedagogical methods. His and others' ideas will be more thoroughly considered later in this chapter, for they are useful in patient teaching.

The word *education* has traditionally meant a process that transmits the culture. But the word originally came from a Latin word meaning 'to draw out'. Although we are more familiar with education as a cramming full of facts and information, the other side of the definition is to draw out the mysterious hidden qualities within a person. The amount of education a person has gained and retained has long been measured by IQ (intelligence quotient) tests. But many qualities cannot be measured this way. The IQ test cannot measure how much creative imagination a person has, how much ambition, perseverance, or willingness to cooperate. And these qualities are significant, although previously not often considered or given priority. Thus a balanced definition of **education** is the *continuing process of using immeasurable inner resources to gain external information.*

**Health education** *specifically transmits information, motivates the inner resource of the person, and helps people adopt and maintain health practices and lifestyles.* It is also concerned with the environment, professional training, and research to maintain and evaluate the process. Traditionally health education focuses on what the professional thinks is good for the patient/client.

**Self-care**, increasingly popular in recent years, *focuses on what the learner perceives as needs and goals to maintain or enhance health and wellbeing.* It is generally undertaken prior to illness rather than in response to disease.

## THE NURSE AS TEACHER-LEARNER

As a professional nurse, you may be more of a teacher than someone actually called a 'teacher'. A history instructor may teach secondary school students from 9.00 a.m. to 3.00 p.m. 5 days a week. But you can spend nearly every waking moment in teaching health promotion. You teach through example: through health precautions and personal hygiene as well as by words.

If you have a family, either children of your own or brothers, sisters and parents, you constantly do health teaching. You may lock the medicine and caustic material in a cabinet, explaining the dire results of taking too much internally. You may notice early diabetic symptoms in your father and direct him to a doctor for tests. You may quickly take the proper first-aid action when your sister fractures a bone. You will additionally be a teacher to your neighbours and friends.

Teaching those near you takes on unprecedented magnitude when you analyse the barrage of so-called health information directed at us daily through communication-advertising media: natural or organic foods are superior to processed foods; certain vitamins and minerals will provide pep and sexual vigour; certain exercises will promote breast development. Or again, certain procedures will grow hair on a bald male head or remove hair from a female face; a particular cream will slow down the aging process; a certain diet will cause drastic weight reduction; certain medications will wake you up, put you to sleep, or remove all your aches in moments.

Obviously Westerners are concerned with staying slim and appropriately masculine or feminine, with looking young and retaining their vigour. They have a fear about their own and their loved ones' health. You can supply sound information on the essentials of good nutrition, exercise and rest, while pointing out that people must accept periods of strain, fatigue, lesser energy, and the aging process. You won't always teach with words alone. Your standards of cleanliness – for example, how frequently you wash your hands – will be imitated by your children and observed by your patients.

You will teach no matter what professional position you hold. The nurse can teach while giving a bath. The nurse in the health centre or clinic can do spot teaching while preparing a patient for examination. The health visitor or district nurse can teach while working with specific situations in the home. The industrial nurse can teach while taking down worker information. Of course, the nurse is also a teacher while instructing students, but teaching is more basic than a professional job. Also, your teaching is not limited to the task at hand. Often occupational-health nurses will encounter problems offered by the employees that are unrelated to their treatments. Most problems will concern health needs of family members.

In trying to help each individual reach the maximum health potential, you must consider the total person. The particular culture, social class, religion, environment, definition of health and illness, developmental stage, whether the person is in a crisis, and what kind of communication he/she responds to will affect understanding and your consequent teaching.

You might ask yourself: What does the person want to learn? How can he/she best be taught? Can I help the person project a positive image of what he/she will be in the future? For example, can I help the person who is a diabetic think of self as slim, healthy, and enjoying the proper foods rather than as a deprived person who will moan and reminisce about delicious sugary desserts? Can I help the person understand that he/she must continue to learn about the disease and possible new treatments as medical research probes now-unknown possibilities? Can I improve my skills, and the person's skills, in the four crucial areas of learning, relating, choosing and problem solving?

Practising health teaching is part of holistic health care – care that encompasses the whole person.

## FUNDAMENTALS OF TEACHING

Although no set rules can be laid down as absolute standards for effective teaching, the following suggestions are recommended:

1. Be trustworthy and consistent.
2. Have self-esteem and enthusiasm. Generate a sense that what you are teaching will benefit the learner.
3. Don't discuss your personal problems with a client.
4. Think through your teaching image. What do patients learn from your cleanliness (or lack of it), dress, posture, tone of voice, gestures, yawns and facial expressions?
5. Determine what the client *wants* and *needs* to learn before you begin your instruction.
6. Know your teaching area. Organize and present your material so that patients feel you know what you are doing.
7. Utilize available teaching methods, resources, various emotional climates, and referral systems when appropriate. Encourage practice of skills and use repetition if it is needed.
8. Respect the client as more important than a procedure, a potential disease process, or a research project.
9. Involve the client actively in the learning process in order to enhance learning.
10. If you ask the client to do something, explain why. Be sure that what you ask is realistic.
11. Distinguish between lack of intelligence and misunderstanding caused by cultural, ethnic or religious differences, and do not equate intelligence level with educational level.
12. Strive for learning from inner motivation through recognition of need, not from outward pressure.
13. Practise sensing the moment of learning. A sense of appropriate timing is essential in teaching, based on assessment of the learner's interest, knowledge, motivation, and values.
14. If you write instructions, write legibly.
15. Plan for interruption.
16. Don't overwhelm with technicalities or excessive, complex facts.
17. Reinforce progress. Give positive feedback when appropriate.
18. Accept errors in the learning process without harsh judgment but with correct information.
19. Don't allow your racial bias to control your attitude about another's ability to learn.
20. Don't reinforce destructive thinking. When a client says 'My mother

died of this disease', don't reply 'It's a real killer. My two aunts died from it, too.'

21. Record your teaching experience and share these notes with other staff members (or teachers from other disciplines) who may instruct the patient.

22. Be realistic about teaching and learning. Accept good days and bad days. Sometimes you will be elated, sometimes depressed, about results.

## CREATIVITY

Assume that your best teaching device is you. You may be open to new knowledge and you may agree with the fundamentals of teaching but not always know how to implement them. Thus you will benefit from the following investigation of creativity and its application to teaching and learning.

What is *creativity*? The word has been used freely. It has been defined as a process, a product, a personality, and an environmental condition. **Creativity** *is the ability to sense gaps or problems with known information, forming ideas or hypotheses about what should be done, testing and modifying those ideas, communicating those ideas, and taking appropriate action in a unique way.* From this process you will obtain ideas to carry out activities that are new, unique and useful to you even though they may not be new, unique or useful to other people.

An appropriate question might be 'How do you sense gaps and problems?' Without this essential tension in thinking, the rest of the process will not follow. One answer is to improve your observation. People can look at a slowly changing object for years and not notice the change, as the surveyor proves who points to a foundation beam largely destroyed by rot. The astonished homeowner says 'I've gone past here every day for a year but didn't notice the change.' Or less dramatic, can you describe in detail from memory the tree outside your kitchen window?

These are two examples (or at least one, if you can describe that tree in detail) of lack of sight perception. Other senses that need sharpening are sound, touch, sensation of movement, taste and smell. Recreate in your mind the following sensations: the voice of your mother or father when you were little and being reprimanded, the feel of the hair on your pet dog, the sensation of your body as you hiked the last 100 feet of the mountain last summer, the taste of lemon juice, the smell of cooking broccoli. Practising this kind of observation exercise of your sensory memory will improve your teaching because you will have a broader sensitivity base from which to sense gaps and problems.

Observing emotional reactions is also significant as you work with patients. Can you recreate the emotion of despair you felt when, after working hard and counting on a certain achievement, you failed the test, were disqualified in the race, or didn't get the job or school position you wished? How did you feel when you lost the love and understanding of someone you were counting on? You really can't walk a mile in the patient's shoes, but your helpful understanding of his/her emotions, through understanding your own, can increase the value of your teaching.

Lowenfeld lists this quality of sensitivity in observation among his criteria for creativity, along with fluency of ideas, flexibility, originality, and the ability to redefine or rearrange, analyse, synthesize, and coherently organize problems.[2] You might display fluency of ideas as you think of the various ways you could apply a bandage, form recipes, or adjust meals in a particular situation. You might show flexibility as you quickly incorporate changing circumstances into a situation. For instance, a procedure doesn't work because a previously unknown factor has been introduced. Instead of saying 'It won't work', you take the factor into account and get desirable results.

Originality is variously defined. Some say there are no new ideas and hence no true originality. Others say that every time you associate or combine two or more ideas that you already have and come up with a new perspective, you have been original.

The rest of Lowenfeld's criteria work into a systematic process. You redefine a disease process with new research results or you rearrange a procedure with the new knowledge that the patient is left-handed instead of right-handed. You analyse, or take apart, the significant factors involved in an unwed mother's situation. You synthesize, or put the parts back together, when you help a senior citizen create a new way of life. You exhibit coherence or organization when you arrange all the aspects of any teaching plan to form a unified working unit.

Creativity, then, conjures up visions of curiosity, imagination, discovery, innovation and invention. It is a number of abilities rather than a single characteristic. The creative person often has a high degree of psychologic health, is persistent, self-assertive, energetic, dominant, individualistic and playful. The creative person can see many relationships among elements, relationships that baffle the conformer, the person who does only what is expected and does not ruffle the system. The creative person isn't always accepted by the traditional teacher because he/she has to be dealt with uniquely and can't be treated in the ordinary way. Can you tolerate creativity in your patients? Will you help them learn through exploring, manipulating, questioning, experimenting, testing and modifying rather than by accepting your word as final authority?

No one knows if creativity has a genetic link or if it is totally a function of the environment. But sex differences do exist in the human brain. Female infants show a somewhat larger area of visual cortex in the right hemisphere of the brain than do male infants. According to J. Wada of The University of British Columbia, this fact implies a possible anatomical basis for the female advantage in nonverbal ideation.

The two cerebral hemispheres differ in function. The left hemisphere is almost always dominant for language, logical reasoning and mathematical calculation. The right hemisphere is nonverbal and processes spatial and visual abstractions, recognition of faces, a sense of one's body image, music, and it may be closer to intuitive or preconscious processes and fantasy.[3]

In a 10-year-study of creative people Getzels and Csikszentmihaly found that some definite factors in a child's environment can encourage the child to become a problem finder (one who is creative) before he/she becomes a problem solver. These factors are (a) being the oldest or only child; (b) having a working mother who delegates responsibility; (c) having parents who support creativity; and (d) going to schools that encourage problem finding.

During their children's elementary years, the British tend to stress conformity to the peer group, use punitive discipline, orientate their children to success, equate divergency with abnormality or delinquency, and make a sharp distinction between work and play. In their secondary school years, the young are frequently pressured into striving for popularity, achieving high grades, getting work done on time, and making conventional occupational choices. In college students are sometimes forced to overemphasize the acquisition of categorized knowledge, memorization of facts, and standard testing. Thus covering subject matter rather than seeing the interrelationships is often the result. You may recognize this pattern in your own experience.

Suggestions to foster creative learning as you teach patients/clients are to:

1. allow opportunity for creative behaviour, such as providing for independent learning through the study of appropriate literature or asking questions that require more than recall;
2. develop your own skills in creative learning according to methods described later in the chapter;
3. reward creative achievements by respecting unusual solutions and by not threatening with immediate evaluation before an idea is completely tested;
4. develop a constructive rather than critical attitude toward information gleaned;
5. establish creative relationships, especially with children; permit one

thing to lead to another and embark on the unknown, yet provide adequate guidance;
6. provide for continuity of creative development in problem finding and solution finding.

*Creativity* is *not* synonymous with *permissiveness* or *chaos*. You are the re-source, the organiser. Often you will be authoritative. You will say 'Sugar elimination will modify your diabetic condition. Omitting egg yolk may help lower your cholesterol. Chewing sugarless gum will cut down on dental caries. Adequate exercise will strengthen those muscles.' But how you then help the client work with those facts in the situation will reveal either your authoritarian or your creative teaching manner.


SOME IDEAS TO CONSIDER

In addition to developing a creative teaching manner, you may want to ponder the following ideas concerning the nature of teaching and learning. These ideas originated in various disciplines: psychoanalysis, adult education, language and communication studies, anthropology and nursing.


*Significant learning*

Carl Rogers defines *significant learning* as learning that makes a difference – that affects all parts of a person and influences behaviour, course of action, attitude and personality.[4] Rogers substantiates his claim that such learning does take place by citing his experience with psychotherapy. He assumes that it can also take place in an educational setting under certain ideal con-ditions:

1. The person must clearly perceive the problems and issues that are to be resolved.
2. You, the nurse-teacher, must be openly aware of the attitudes you hold and accept your own feelings.
3. You must accept the person as he/she is and understand his/her feel-ings.
4. Resources (such as literature about health promotion, crutches, cook-books, yourself) should be given if they are useful to the person and not an imposition.
5. Evaluation should be conceived as knowing that the client is adequately prepared to solve the problem if he/she so desires, but leaving the per-son free to choose whether to put forth the required effort.[5]

*Pedagogy versus andragogy*

The saying from the Talmud, 'Much have I learned from my teachers, even more from my classmates, but most of all from my students', has special significance in Knowles's theory of adult education. As a person matures, he/she:

1. Moves from dependency to a self-directing position.
2. Accumulates experiences that become an increasing resource for learning.
3. Moves in the direction of learning that harmonizes with current developmental tasks.
4. Changes from subject-centred, postponed applications characteristic of children's education to problem-centred, immediate applications of knowledge.[6]

Others have also emphasized these guidelines for adult learning.

As a nurse-teacher you may be working with a variety of age groups. Some will be self-directing adults. You can apply these crucial assumptions as you teach adult patients and their family members if you let them help plan and conduct their own learning programmes to some extent. Build on and make use of their life experiences to gain greater learning, and be sure learning is appropriate to their developmental tasks. (For example, don't try to get the 40-year-old heart patient to plan his retirement if he still has realistic aspirations for becoming managing director.) Teach what is significant to their particular life problems, not what you think is a good subject. You may need to help them in organizing material, refocusing thinking, reassuring by pointing out what they already know, giving authoritative answers when needed, and giving individual attention to those who do not learn well alone. Keep in mind that the adult learner has many priorities other than learning. Other life responsibilities will greatly affect the ability to learn and the time he or she can spend. The adult learner, however, may use a small portion of time effectively because of having learned how to integrate previous experiences with new learning.

Other factors must be considered for the learner in later maturity. Probably this person will need the reassurance that he/she isn't too old to learn. The person will also need such features as large print and excellent lighting for diminished eyesight; clear, distinct speaking for less acute hearing; and frequent summaries and slower presentation because it may take a little longer to synthesize the material.

Similarly, you must adjust to the children and young adults you teach, to their dependency needs, lack of experience, developmental tasks, and lack of sophistication in problem solving. Children lack the seasoned habits of adults and may respond more quickly to a change in pattern. Use a developmental approach.[7] You have a special responsibility to children as a teacher of health promotion because eating, exercise and health practices become routinized early in life. The child who comes to you may have had little health teaching at home or in school.

The child may be inspired to learn through playing games, reading appropriate books or cartoons, or using puppets. Simple drawings, with explanations in the appropriate age-level language, may help explain a body part, a procedure, or what a medicine will do in the body. Children also enjoy arts and crafts, cooking, planting and drama (such as simple role playing). Incorporating any of these activities into health teaching may enhance learning.

There are a range of specific materials available developed for use in primary and secondary schools by the teacher. For example, the 'MY BODY' project from HEA. The nurse is the advisor and supporter here, leaving the teaching to the schoolteacher.

*Language: prohibitor in teaching-learning*

Language, our primary tool for education, can open up new worlds to people or leave them in a state of confusion. Nonverbal behaviour is also significant. Communication developed first through the physical movements of people or objects; then through drawings, which represented objects or needs of people; next through giving spoken names to important ideas, concepts and objects; and finally through establishing written signs to correspond to these names.

We sometimes forget that written signs have no physical resemblance to their referents. Two people must have a mutual understanding about the meaning of a word or communication does not occur. We also do not have distinct and separate signs for each observed occurrence. Thus although dwellings can be generally subdivided into houses, apartments, bungalows and mobile homes, even these words cannot give a unique description of your dwelling. Because we cannot keep producing exact sounds for all different experiences, we have words that have many different meanings, such as *fast*, which can mean a speed, a dye that remains in place, or a certain type of friend. *High* can mean a physical elevation, a degree of alcohol or drug intoxication, a musical pitch, or a kind of religious ceremony; it can mean 'grave' or 'serious' (as in *high treason*), or 'expensive' or 'costly'. *Reading* a skin test is not the same as *reading* an essay. Furthermore, the mind seems to decode messages in relationship to its own background situation, prejudices, and moods. For example, a person can hear and repeat exactly what you have said without believing a word of it.

Given such possibilities of faulty language communication, even if technical language is adjusted to the client's level and explanations are logically coherent and complete, the patient should have additional understandable experiences about the new concepts to be learned. Comprehension must not be evaluated totally on the basis of language or reading response. Because motion pictures, television images, photographic slides, and pictures look like their referent, and the first two also sound like their referent, these and other (audio) visual aids should be strongly considered as adjuncts to verbal explanations.

## *Culture: prohibitor in teaching-learning*

The preceding ideas on adult education may work in European majority culture but fail in a culture where authority is unquestioned and where concepts of self-help and audience participation are not valued. For instance, if a married woman from a strict patriarchal system is a patient, you should teach the husband what must be done in order to be effective.

Evidence is lacking to support the claim that more health education alone will improve health.[8] The nation's major health problems – alcoholism, heart disease, obesity, certain cancers and accidents – stem from ignorance or irresponsibility on the part of individuals rather than from inadequacies on the part of health providers.

Culture is often the prohibiting factor when people cannot seem to change lifestyles and attitudes that are responsible for illness, disability and death.

Cultural and subcultural expectations have a powerful effect on behaviour – yours, the patient's and the family's. Accepting what the group believes to be true on the main issues of life is beneficial to all members of society. When one is relieved of the need to make choices, peace of mind and security result. Thus health education to change habits is likely to fail unless social pressures to maintain the old customs are overcome. At the same time, the new proposed behaviour cannot cause too much insecurity, uncertainty or mental stress.

People conform to the expectations of prestigious members of society and prestige may have little to do with money. Thus important persons need to be consulted and given an opportunity to maintain prestige by having a major part in the changing of health habits. Programmes are accepted only to the extent that local representatives – priests, teachers, grandparents, shop stewards, doctors, businesspeople, or the mass media – take part in planning and conducting them.

Ritualistic customs or behaviours are usually tied to elementary functions of life – menstruation, feeding, gestation, defecation. Sometimes the ritual is harmful to health, but attempts to change it may cause resistance because time has sanctified the custom. Examples are female circumcision, defecation in open places, and food taboos for pregnant women.

Every culture accepts and absorbs new ideas, provided that they do not conflict with its own fundamental tenets. All new ideas are at first judged according to existing customs and beliefs and then gradually accepted if they mesh sufficiently with what already exists.

Consider the following suggestions in promoting health education and changes in health practices in any culture:

1. Get intimately detailed knowledge of beliefs, attitudes, knowledge, and behaviour of the cultural group and evaluate their psychological and social functions. Try to share the feeling of the culture. Avoid being culture-bound: do not automatically reject concepts and patterns different from personal ones.
2. Identify numerous subcultures, for programmes based on premises valid for one group may not be successful with another group.
3. Determine leadership patterns within a community or group. Define the decision makers in the family and larger social institutions, the status of various groups within the community, as well as the status of the health worker in comparison to these groups.
4. Remember that every culture is layered: each has certain characteristics that are manifest and others that are latent – certain components that constitute the stated ideal pattern of behaviour but that are seldom practised. Consider and study both levels. Least visible are the values that give direction and meaning to life.
5. Don't make direct attacks on the fundamental beliefs of the group: instead patiently and gradually change ideas by appealing to the group's desire for health and normality. Avoid abrupt change. Use **linkage ideas,** *ideas consistent with both public health and the cultural belief system.* If no common ground exists, you should add on your ideas to the cultural ideas.
6. Consider unanticipated consequences of the health education programme and estimate how permanent the introduced changes are expected to be. Consider the untoward consequences of the programme. Positive results from your teaching in one situation may be considered negative in another situation.
7. Beware of the aspiration gap. Expectations of better living or health conditions, once aroused, are likely to rise more rapidly than improvements in the actual life situation. Supplying help and hope runs the risk of intensifying rather than satisfying felt needs, as rising aspirations outrace material gain, causing discontent and disillusionment. Programmes of preventive health measures are the most difficult to establish because of the low value on health, the lack of understanding of cause and effect or the reasons for preventive measures, and the existence in local cultures of competitive preventive measures.

*Other prohibitors in teaching-learning*

A nursing student, somewhat dissatisfied with her nursing education, used an analogy to make a point. She compared some of her nursing instructors to delicate flowers who wilted as teachers. She declared that when she taught, she would be like a dandelion – tough, common, almost indestructible, and with functional component parts.[9]

The idea is commendable, but caution is needed. Although armed with the best of theory and methods and with respect for the person, you will at times fail to impart positive health habits through teaching knowledge based on scientific information.

You will be dealing in health education with many myths and forms of unconscious resistance. Some people try to undermine their own health as a means of attracting attention or avoiding a hated job. Others, out of desire to belong, will cling to a false diet theory. Some believe the whole body is a mobile dirt factory with a constant need for cleaning. Even health educators, although highly trained formally, are subject to these devices and beliefs. You may need to teach other teachers.

Occasionally situations arise in which significant learning simply cannot occur. Perhaps you remind the patient of her employer, whom she detests. Or if you are a black female heterosexual health teacher working with a Caucasian male homosexual patient, you may not succeed in teaching him because of prejudice (his or yours).

In a hospital setting the question of who shall teach, and when, may be impossible to answer. Health professionals cannot decide who should teach about diagnosis – nurse or physician. And if both, how? Aiming primarily for efficiency runs counter to allowing teaching time. The physician suddenly writes the discharge order. No teaching time is available. In some hospitals and health-care agencies a health educator is employed. However, most nurses believe that teaching is an integral part of nursing and that no one person should be hired for that role.

Teaching can be harmful if goals are unaccepted, inappropriate, misunderstood, or not broken down into manageable steps. If teaching materials are not appropriate, if teaching is not thorough, or if evaluation is not adequate, the patient may be confused, lose self-confidence, and be unable to adapt to his/her health problem.[10]

Obviously the hardest look you take must be at yourself. Communication is often easiest with a person of one's own class or status group because each shares similar premises. But what happens when basic premises are dissimilar? Sometimes you fail.

Failure need not be permanently defeating. Sometimes it escalates the maturing process. Thus you should evaluate and revise working principles from your varied experiences in an attempt to produce better results (and to realize when you can't). This is analogous to the step of evaluation in the nursing process.


METHODS OF TEACHING

*Techniques of teaching*

Methods or techniques of teaching are nearly as varied as people. A given technique can be effective in one setting and totally inappropriate in another. The key is in planning the technique for the specific situation.

Basically a climate for teaching-learning must be set. All involved must want teaching and learning to occur and anticipate an improved self-image as a result of learning. Time must be set aside for in-service teaching preparation and patient/client teaching. General team or individual goals must be set. Teaching guidelines and audiovisual materials must be available. The actual setting for the teaching-learning must be conducive. For example, learning is difficult in an overcrowded, poorly ventilated room where people are looking at each others' backs or are uncomfortably seated.

Your responsibility is to know your patient/client and the situation. You might write individual teaching guides on your patients that include such items as:

1. The nature of the person's disease, including the person's normal functions, pathological changes, and results of the changes.
2. Hospitalization and nursing care measures, such as diagnostic procedures, treatments, medications, fluids, diet and rehabilitation.
3. Discharge and home care, including diet, fluids, medications, activity, dressings, rest, general hygiene, prophylaxis, special equipment, and suggestions for improvisations.
4. Community agencies and resources.
5. Helpful bibliography.

Obviously age, mental and emotional attitudes, family status, and other factors affecting the person's learning should also be included in this guide. With this ongoing information, you can construct a design for teaching that is based on a priority system.

The priority system may be developed by identifying *acute educational needs* when a lack of understanding causes psychosocial anguish or physical danger; *preventive educational needs* when a person is threatened with a condition and doesn't know how to handle it; and *maintenance educational needs* when an alteration in normal functioning demands an ongoing understanding and skill.

Use of the nursing care plan as an integral part of teaching is discussed in

Chapter 3. Just as a work of art calls for unity, continuity, and a certain sense of pace and movement, so does teaching. Your presentation, behaviour, knowledge and concern will each add components to your effectiveness.

Although certain techniques generally work better than others in specific situations, there are no definite rules. *A teaching method represents a way of thinking.* You must choose a method that you can use effectively and that is beneficial to patients/clients.

Table 4.1 depicts some techniques for producing desired behavioural outcomes.[11] You can use your creativity to adapt these methods to your specific situations.

Note that you can build skills without imparting a lot of underlying knowledge. Through demonstration and return demonstration, for instance, you can teach a 10-year old how to take and report a blood-pressure reading accurately without having to explain all the underlying physiology

*Table 4.1*  Some techniques for producing desired behavioural outcomes

| *Rationale* | *Teaching methods* |
|---|---|
| *If you wish to:* <br> impart generalizations about experience. | *Use:* <br> lecture, symposium, panel, reading, audiovisual aids, a book- or pamphlet-based discussion. |
| apply information to experience through insight and *understanding.* | feedback devices, problem-solving dicussions, laboratory experimentation, group participation, case problems. |
| build *skills.* | role playing, drill, coaching, demonstration, and return demonstration. |
| *create new* attitudes. <br> (Attitudes are learned through repeated reinforcement of a response to a stimulus. If a response different from the original one is given and reinforced over a period of time, a change in attitude occurs, evidenced by a change in behaviour in a particular set of circumstances. Eventually the attitude may become a value.) | reverse role playing, experience-sharing discussion, counselling-consultation, environmental support, games designed to produce certain attitudes, and nonverbal exercises which draw out certain attitudes through gesture, posture, and facial expression, positive and negative reinforcement. |
| change *values* through the rearrangement of the priority of beliefs. | speakers who have adjusted satisfactorily to a certain condition now facing the patient, biographical or autobiographical reading, drama, philosophical or direct-value-placement discussion with provision for reflection. |
| promote new *interests.* | field trips, audiovisual aids, reading, creative expriences. |

of the heart and all the technicalities of the equipment involved. If, however, through role playing followed by group discussion, you are trying to teach someone how to get along in his/her family, you will need to teach the underlying principles of group dynamics and how to use them in a situation that is ever changing.

*Individual and group teaching*

Some techniques are best suited for teaching on an individual basis whereas others are best for large groups or several subgroups.

**Individual teaching** can be provided through programmed learning, reading material, audiovisual aids, and one-to-one instruction. **Programmed learning** *provides material in carefully planned sequential steps that leads the person to a mastery of the subject.* The material is presented through programme instruction books or a **teaching machine,** *a simple manually operated machine or a complex computer.* One frame of information is presented at a time. The learner then tests his/her grasp of the information in the frame by writing a response to a question, usually a multiple-choice type. The book or machine then gives the correct response. If the learner's response was incorrect, the programme then presents (or, in the case of a book, directs him/her to turn to) a repetition of the information or a more detailed explanation, depending on the programme and his/her response. The advantages of programmed learning include logical presentation, active learner participation, immediate disclosure of correct response, reinforcement of material, and individual pacing.

Another method of giving individual instruction is by providing factual material. The health organizations discussed later in this chapter provide preventative health-teaching literature as part of their programmes. Evaluating the benefits gained from these materials is difficult because people who receive the material often do not respond to the organization's request for feedback, even when given a stamped answer form. One study tried to determine the effectiveness of a breast self-examination by seeking the reactions of 383 women one year after they received teaching kits with filmstrip, teaching notes and commentary; only 41 per cent responded. Women in the upper half of the social scale reacted more favourably: 48 per cent of them had established an examination pattern (though not necessarily monthly, as the material suggested).[12] The tendency of upper-class persons to read better and to respond more readily to scientific health teaching than lower-class persons seems evident here.

Other factual reading materials include autobiographies of persons with certain disease processes and 'how-to' books by persons who have experienced certain health problems directly or indirectly and want to pass along suggestions to others. Fiction also provides valuable insights into physical and mental illness.

With the constant introduction of more sophisticated audiovisual equipment into the teaching-learning area, you can get and adapt these devices to individual learning. A recorder and cassettes explaining preventive measures, disease processes, or specific instructions can be loaned to the client. He/she can stop the cassette at any point and replay necessary portions until satisfied with the learning. 'Talking Books' is a programme that records information for the visually impaired. Closed-circuit television or videotape set-ups allow the person to hear and view material. You can be involved in producing teaching cassettes and television or videotape programmes.

These methods of individual instruction are only individual to a certain point. Only when the client can check learning with a resource person, ask further questions as necessary, and have help in making personal applications, will learning become significant. That process involves you. The person doesn't learn from a machine alone. These discussions with patients need not be long. The important point is to be available when they do have questions and to convey that any question or problem is worthy of your consideration.

**Group teaching** can meet the person's need to achieve status or security through being a group member. Client groups provide a channel through which feelings and needs can be expressed and met, especially if the people have similar problems, such as colostomy or diabetes. Thus you can use the group process to enhance health teaching or for therapy to aid coping with problems. You may also have an opportunity to work with a group that has formed to accomplish some specific goal, such as losing weight, promoting research to find a cure for cancer, or providing guidance to parents with mentally retarded children. In some cases, information is not enough. Social support is also necessary, especially when engaging in a lesser-valued activity – like not eating sugar when society says that dessert is the best part of the meal. One study of hospitalized diabetics, some taught individually and some taught in a group by a nurse specialist, showed that the group demonstrated as much or more knowledge and skill in urine testing as the former.

In another study 25 experimental patients participated in a small group session the night before surgery. They discussed their concerns and fears and learned what to expect and how to aid in their convalescence. A randomly selected matched control group of 25 patients who underwent similar surgery but who received only routine care were compared, after surgery, with the first group. Results showed that extra preparation increased patient participation, decreased tension and anxiety, and led to more rapid postoperative recoveries.[13]

One minister who had visited hundreds of patients on the night before surgery said, 'Fear of the unknown is what I continually find. I don't necessarily mean about the outcome of the surgery, although that is involved. I mean they don't even know about the recovery room process. Instead of giving spiritual help, I find myself telling them many details which the nursing staff should have taught. With these important details at their command, I can see their anxiety lessen.' Small group sessions could reduce these fears.

Not only should the rather complicated procedures such as surgery and its accompanying routines be explained; positive results have also been obtained with minor procedures. One group, for example, was told what sensations to expect and then had blood pressure cuffs placed on their arms and the pressure pumped up to 250 mm Hg. Another group was told only of the procedure – that is, 'Your blood pressure will be taken.' The conclusion was that accurate expectations about sensations do reduce stress, but that patients should be told only about sensations usually experienced, not those rarely experienced.[14] Excessively detailed explanations can raise rather than lower anxiety.

If you work with a group, you should initially set a working social climate. People do not automatically start revealing their problems and supporting and helping each other. You must use some introduction technique that focuses on the individual, his/her personality strengths and resources, rather than on a disease or problem. (The person already knows why he/she is there.) Each person can introduce himself if the group is small. If the group is large (25 or more), you can break it up into subgroups of 5 each and allow each subgroup at least 20 minutes to plan a presentation using one of the following creative techniques. In *the enquiring reporter*, one person in each group (or subgroup) is chosen to compose a feature story about the personalities and resources of group members. The person then presents the story to the total group in 3 minutes. In *the living newspaper*, each group picks a type of newspaper feature – a news story, column, book review or editorial, for example – and presents a 3-minute group description through that format. In *the television variety programme*, each group has a 3-minute segment to present its members through interview, skit, song or comedy. These methods produce immediate ego-involvement, create an atmosphere conducive to participative learning and sharing of problems and resources, and start the spirit of creative enquiry.[15] You can think of other introductory techniques for your particular group situation.

Whatever your reasons for teaching the group, you must assess needs and interests, define purposes and objectives, construct a design and evaluate success. As you teach, rely on many approaches to accomplish your purpose.

A sample of group approaches that you could use follows:

1. *Support groups.* The total group breaks up into subgroups of three or four

people. The purpose is for subgroup members to support one another. If one person misses a session or doesn't understand a procedure, the other members of the subgroup are responsible for getting the missing information to that person. Each has a feeling of being active and of being responsible to one another and each can clarify his/her own understanding while teaching someone else.

2. The *whip group*. This is a variation of the support group. One person in each subgroup is designated to interpret the concepts being taught. Misunderstandings can be caught early, for periodic times are designated for interpretation and discussion.

3. *Directive note taking*. The entire group listens to a lecture for 2 or 3 minutes. Then all stop and write notes on what was said. The teacher checks sample summaries to see how well the ideas are getting across. This procedure is repeated until the end of the session.

*Problem solving*

Another approach to teaching-learning is the problem-solving technique, which is useful with either individuals or groups and is essentially the creative process discussed earlier. Parnes outlines a seven-step creative problem-solving process that can be written out to clarify thinking.[16] The person starts with *confronting 'the mess'*, acknowledging the predicament and the resultant dissatisfied feelings. Creative efficiency is increased if people understand the psychological process by which they operate. The emotional and irrational factors in peoples' thinking are more urgent than the intellectual and rational. People are free to go on more effectively after acknowledging this first step.

The second step is *clarifying the 'fuzzy problem'*, writing a factual rather than an emotional explanation of the situation by answering such questions as who, what, when, where and how. The third step is *fact finding*, writing information the patient would like to have related to the situation described. The fourth step is *problem finding*, listing all the creative-type questions or challenges suggested by the preceding two steps, such as 'How might I . . .?' and 'In what ways might I . . .?' The fifth step is *idea finding*, or deferred judgment, selecting the most likely ways of solution finding. The sixth step is *solution finding*, in which the best approaches are evaluated; and the seventh step is *acceptance finding*, or adoption of solution. These steps are merely guides to be adapted to personal and group characteristics (see Fig. 4.1.).

Some persons are capable of going through these seven steps relying only on their insight. Others can work through the steps themselves but will need you to present the plan to them. And still others will be so engulfed in 'the mess' that they will need your careful guidance to move them toward a solution.

*Fig. 4.1*    Seven-step creative problem-solving process

| | (Monologue of a 55-year-old woman who has just learned, after routine bloodwork in a clinic, that she appears to be a borderline diabetic. She leaves without getting an adequate explanation.) |
|---|---|
| 1. Acknowledging *the mess* (emotional aspects) | 1. I can't possibly change my ways. I love desserts. I can't cook without sugar. My husband and friends won't accept me. I'll never go to another party. I can't stand to have diabetes. |
| 2. Identifying the *fuzzy problem* (known facts) | 2. Yes, I have been awfully thirsty lately. And that cut on my foot healed so slowly. I have been too tired to carry on my usual work. |
| 3. Looking for *additional helpful facts* | 3. Maybe there is a diet I can follow. Maybe I can find a cookbook which will teach me to cook without sugar. Maybe I will have more energy and be a better companion to my husband if I look into the management of diabetes. |
| 4. Asking *creative questions* to help deal with steps 2 and 3 | 4. Where can I get this cookbook? Where can I get more literature on diabetes? How can I test my urine myself? Who can help me? |
| 5. Selecting *tentative solutions* | 5. Let's see, I could call Jane's family doctor. I think she said he works with diabetics. Or maybe I can find a doctor who specializes in diabetes. I can look in the phone book to see if a diabetic association exists. I can talk to Mrs Jones; she has had diabetes for 10 years and seems to handle herself well. |
| 6. Evaluating tentative solutions and selecting a *solution* | 6. Well, I think I'd better find a specialist. If I have diabetes, I want to get all the facts. I'll also call Mrs Jones; she can probably give me lots of hints from her everyday life. |
| 7. Accepting the findings through *adopting a plan* of action | 7. I'm glad I found out while I'm borderline. Lots worse things could happen. I will follow the regimen. It should help me live longer. |

## Other approaches

*Appropriate visual aids* should be used with whatever method is used. Letting people work with their hands as well as their minds is often effective. Groups may make a collage from magazine pictures of, for example, foods acceptable to a diabetic versus unacceptable foods; good hygiene versus poor hygiene; elements of health versus elements of illness. Children in an elementary classroom went through numerous magazines, cutting out pictures of people who appeared to be in good health and people who appeared to be in poor health. When all the pictures of unhealthy people were arranged on one poster and all the pictures of healthy people were arranged on another poster, the contrast was startling. This visual confrontation enabled the teacher and students to begin to discuss why these differences existed and to apply the principles to the children's lives.

The *HEA Graphic Handbook* (1986) and *Video Handbook* both present factual 'how to' information in an easily assimilated form.

Clients are also eager to get *handouts*, appropriate visual or written materials that they can keep. Ideally, they will use this material and even pass it on to a relative or friend. You must know each patient's reading ability (or lack of it) and select materials accordingly. Not being able to read is a source of embarrassment to patients. Go over the handout with the person; do not just hand it to him/her.

The *local library* is a useful centre for setting up health teaching courses, and it is committed to presenting a variety of programmes based on community needs. Additionally, you can use the library's books in your teaching, especially on such subjects as childhood illnesses or sex education. You may even want to use books in the children's library for an elementary presentation of some subjects.

Use the health promotion department in your local District Health Authority. You, as a nurse-teacher, can also make use of the local college library to keep up to date on educational insights and teaching methods. Do not limit yourself to nursing literature exclusively.

Teaching *patient/client rights* uses a direct approach either with individual persons or with groups. Although people may have vast resources within themselves, they sometimes do not use them because they have been taught to respect the doctor: 'Do not question the doctor's judgment. He/she is too busy to explain.' While you and the patient should respect the doctor, the doctor should also respect you and the patient. We question the plumber about the new parts he/she is putting in our sink, ask their cost, and refuse to pay if the work is ineffective but often we fail to question the doctor about medications we take, their effects, or the side-effects.

One study questioned 60 patients in a teaching hospital about the drugs they were taking and concluded that (a) patients have little information about their medications; (b) younger patients know more about their drugs than older ones; and (c) patients who would like more information do not ask.[17] Another study confirmed that patients want specifiic information about their condition.[18]

Table 4.2, based on suggestions from a medical physician, indicates how patients can get specific information from their doctor.

*Evaluation*

Evaluation is judging how effective teaching has been. Evaluation is sometimes difficult because clients cannot always be followed long enough to

*Table 4.2*    Teaching guide for client's rights

| *Five do's* | *Five don'ts* |
|---|---|
| 1. When you call the nurse or secretary for an appointment, state your request or problem so the appropriate appointment time can be scheduled. | 1. Unless an emergency arises, don't take up extra, unplanned-for time. For example, don't say, 'Oh, while I'm here for my ear infection, why don't you do my complete physical.' |
| 2. Organize thoughts about your present health status or illness and write them down so you can present pertinent facts to the doctor. These will aid him/her in giving a thorough examination or in making a diagnosis. | 2. Don't lie to yourself or to the doctor. Don't let fear cause you to ignore a situation that may need immediate but minimal treatment. |
| 3. Cooperate during the physical examination and allow the doctor to be complete. Don't tell the doctor to skip certain procedures. | 3. Don't tell the doctor to give you pills. Don't feel cheated if you don't get medication; many illnesses are minor and self-limiting. Your own observance of a health-promotion regimen may be all you need. |
| 4. Ask your doctor about proper diet, work load, exercise, and rest to help you maintain maximum health. Ask about realistic limitations. If ill, ask your doctor questions about availability of treatment, medication, diagnosis, causes of condition, chances for recovery, or whatever you want to know related to situation. If you have more questions after you leave, write them down and call back for answers. If hospitalized, continue to ask questions about drugs and ongoing treatment. | 4. Don't ask for unnecessary hospitalization for X-rays or tests because its your right or because grandma is burdensome. Talk with your doctor about alternate plans that will promote long-range health for everyone involved. |
| 5. Follow instructions after health promotion plan is established. After time, effort, and money are spent, you are the only loser if you refuse to follow suggestions or directions. | 5. Don't leave the doctor's office dissatisfied. At least express and explain your feelings. The doctor needs to understand your point of view. Maybe a change can be made or perhaps you need additional information to understand a suggestion or decision. |

see the results of teaching, and human behaviour is so complicated that true changes are hard to measure.

Evaluation can be informal or formal. Informal judgments are made constantly. A patient/client compliments or complains. You react to these judgements. You observe how well a client dresses a wound, irrigates a catheter, or cooks a meal after your demonstration. You may write evaluation notes on the learning ability. By questioning the person's understanding, you are evaluating your teaching. If he/she has learned appropriately – can give explanations and can perform the activities that were taught – the teaching has been adequate. Patients/clients can evaluate their own learning, whether goals were met, and your teaching by using a rating scale or checklist, which further assists your evaluation process.

Every person connected with a teaching–learning programme should be involved in evaluating the programme. Depending on the specific situation and programme, these people might include the participants (patients and teachers); the programme director and staff, who can see the programme as a whole; the directing committee, who establish objectives and policy; and outside experts who can be totally objective. Community representatives can supply valuable evaluative information when the teaching is aimed at serving the general public.[19]

## HOME TEACHING

So often there is no continuity in teaching from health-care agency to home. Ideally, all teaching should include the patient's family and its particular circumstances in the plan, but in a setting other than the home the true circumstances often cannot be discerned. When a mother returns to the clinic for the third time with a child who has pneumonia, the doctor and nurses may reprimand her for not taking better care of her child. She may be too proud to say she can only afford to keep one room partially warm, that she doesn't have enough quilts, and that their diet consists mostly of rice.

Sometimes lower-class persons give up before ever starting on a health-promotion plan because they know they cannot afford the fancy equipment or the expensive nutritional supplements recommended by the hospital staff.

The nurse who goes into the home can, in one half-hour, make observations that could never be made under any other circumstances, certainly not in a hospital room. When you enter the home, you see, smell, hear and feel how the people think and live. Peeling plaster, unpainted walls, holes in the floors, spilled old food underfoot, the smell of urine, piles of dirty clothes, oppressive heat or pervasive cold all give information regarding health (or lack of it). A row of shined shoes, religious articles, a certain painting, photos of children and relatives, framed certificates, rows of books or of store-bought medicine also give valuable information. These are extensions of the personalities. From these observations you can begin realistic health teaching as part of your nursing intervention.

One visiting nurse said her goal was to teach health promotion under existing conditions, to make patients both comfortable and as healthy as possible in their own circumstances. She said that if a patient needed a diet change for heart disease or diabetes, she would ask him to keep a record of everything he ate for three days. Then she would plan an adequate diet ıd that information. She felt it was futile to change the existing plan ıically, or take away all his favourite foods and add new ones that he aıu.ı't like or didn't want to try.

## AGENCY TEACHING

Effective teaching often involves making a pertinent referral. Once you understand the health status of the person and of the family and home situation, you can refer the person to the agency that can give the most help. In fact, you should not attempt to provide services in areas where you are not fully trained, especially if expert service is simply a matter of proper referral.

Survey your local community for health-teaching agencies. You should know which services you can expect from these agencies. Larger cities sometimes have community-service directories that give this information. Keep abreast of newly added programmes. Don't overlook church and club groups that sponsor or help with health education.

## CURRENT CHALLENGES

Teaching–learning is important at any stage of the healthiness-illness continuum, but more emphasis now is given to teaching health promotion and early prevention. You have a brigade of definitions, theories, methods and agencies to assist you in teaching. But before you can teach effectively in the health care or social systems, you must have good health rather than a pathological orientation. Health educators should shift their emphasis from pathology that has never been experienced to things the person has done and enjoyed and will be unable to continue to do if health behaviour is not implemented.

**Health behaviour** *is any activity undertaken by a person who believes self to be well.* Health behaviour and self-care have come to be synonymous.

Practising health behaviour or teaching health behaviour is not dramatic. One nurse said that teaching proper diet, weight control, the need for rest and sleep, stress reduction, the importance of exercise, cleanliness, periodic health examination and immunization is so humdrum. Yet these areas of teaching can eliminate much time, effort and money spent on teaching in later disease stages as well as eliminate suffering for the person.

For example, on a routine blood pressure check, a 33–year-old black male learned that the reading was 170/110 mm Hg. Blood testing showed high cholesterol and triglyceride levels. He was also 50 pounds overweight.

With teaching and monitoring over a period of a year, he avoided high sugar and salt intake, started regular exercise, and subsequently lost 30 pounds. His blood pressure returned to normal limits so that medication was unnecessary.

According to the often-quoted studies of Breslow and Bellac, persons who followed seven common health habits were not only healthier than those who did not but also lived longer. The practices are:

1. Sleep 7 to 8 hours a night.
2. Eat breakfast.
3. Do not eat between meals.
4. Get exercise regularly.
5. Do not drink alcoholic beverages to excess.
6. Do not smoke.
7. Stay within 10 per cent of your proper weight.

In a following study several years after the original one, only the third practice – do not eat between meals – seemed less significant than the other six.

Providing you have a good health orientation, you still must deal with the client where he/she is – culturally, socially and developmentally. Previously the average layperson did not place health in the same level as did the health worker. The lay person generally takes health action only when he/she believes there is susceptibility to a health threat that could have serious effects on the person's life, when he/she knows what actions to take to reduce the health threat, and when the health threat is greater than the action threat.

Besides teaching health promotion and prevention measures to lay people, you may need to direct your teaching toward health educators who continue to focus only on the curative process. You may also establish courses to teach schoolteachers, fire fighters, police officers, ambulance attendants or health-agency workers – those who are in a direct position to aid in illness or injury prevention and control.

Health promotion/education forms part of the audited plans of each regional health authority. Each district health authority has a health promotion department which often works closely with schools of nursing as well as the local education authorities.

The UKCC curriculum guidelines place much emphasis on health promotion activities in its competencies.

REFERENCES

1. Knowles, Malcom. S., 'Teaching-Learning Teams in Adult Education', in *The Changing College Classroom*, eds. P. Runkel, R. Harrison and M. Runkel (Jossey-Bass Inc., Publishers, San Francisco, 1969).

2. Lowenfeld, Viktor, 'Creativity: Education's Stepchild', in *A Source Book for Creative Thinking*, eds. Sidney J. Parnes and Harold F. Harding (Charles Scribner's Sons, New York, 1962) pp. 9–17.

3. Hughes, Helen, 'Creativity in Women', *AAUW Journal*, vol. 70 no. 3 (1976) pp. 6–9.

4. Rogers, Carl, *On Becoming a Person* (Houghton Mifflin Company, Boston, 1961).

5. Parnes, Sidney J., *Creative Behavior Workbook* (Charles Scribner's Sons, New York, 1967).

6. See note 1, above.

7. Murray, Ruth, and Judith Zentner, *Nursing Assessment and Health Promotion Through the Life Span*, 3rd edition (Prentice Hall Inc., Englewood Cliffs, NJ, 1985).

8. Bayer, Mary, 'The Red Dandelion', *Nursing Outlook*, vol. 21 no. 1. (1973) p. 32.

9. Ibid.

10. See note 5, above.

11. Knowles Malcom S., *The Modern Practice of Adult Education* (Association Press, New York, 1970) pp. 37, 39–40, 225, 271, 294.

12. Hobbs, Patricia, 'Evaluation of a Teaching Programme of Breast Self-Examination', *International Journal of Health Education*, vol. 14 (1971) pp. 189–95.

13. Hayward, Jack, *Information – A Prescription Against Pain* (Royal College of Nursing, 1975); Schmitt, Florence E., and Powhatan J. Wooldridge, 'Psychological Preparation of Surgical Patients', *Nursing Research*, vol. 22. no. 2 (1973) pp. 108–15.

14. See note 5, above.

15. See note 1, above.

16. See note 5, above.

17. See note 5, above and note 18, below.

18. Fahrer, Lois, and Ronnie Berstein, 'Making Patient Education Work', *American Journal of Nursing*, vol. 76 no. 11 (1976) pp. 1798–9.

19. See note 11, above.

# 5

# Application of adaptation theory to nursing

Study of this chapter will help you to:

1. Define *adaptation, adjustment,* and key concepts related to adaptation.

2. Discuss the application of adaptation theory and related concepts to nursing.

3. Differentiate between stress and anxiety and describe physiological, cognitive, emotional and behavioural reactions to stress responses in each stage of the General Adaptation Syndrome.

4. Discuss examples of physiological processes and physical defence mechanisms in the body that are adaptive and factors that influence these adaptive processes.

5. Describe psychological adaptive processes and factors that influence these processes.

6. Differentiate levels of anxiety and physical, cognitive, emotional and behavioural manifestations at each level.

7. Discuss examples of and factors influencing cultural and social adaptation.

8. Identify adaptive behaviours used in family interaction.

9. List examples of situations or behaviours that interfere with adaptation.

10. Discuss nursing measures that will assist the person or family to adapt to or cope with internal or external changes (physical, emotional, social, cultural).

A concept that is easily applied to the science and art of nursing is **adaptation.** *Through this process people, either individually or in groups, constructively* *ms imposed internally or externally in order to meet their needs.* .erent, or threatening conditions – stimuli, forces, stressors, .nay be entirely beyond a person's control or may result from *.o* choose alternatives. The term **adjustment** *refers to minor* *tomary behaviour to meet life's problems more effectively.*

*m* and life are synonymous; each involves the whole organism. All systen.s previously described must be adaptive in order to function. Adaptation permits forward movement by reducing or negating the effects of discord, deviance or adverse forces accompanying change. No adaptation is permanent or static because change is constant. Change or adaptation should be accomplished without excess physical illness, loss of long-range goals or values, psychological disintegration, or disruption of the person's or system's overall social functioning.

The definition of *health* and its related concepts outlined in the first chapter of this book introduced you to the concept of adaptation. Although adaptation as a concept is not emphasized in other chapters, its implications permeate the book. An appropriate teaching method promotes adaptation. Carrying out the nursing process aids adaptation. Behaviour in the phases of crisis is the person's way of adapting. Environmental, cultural, religious, social-class, and family influences are integral factors in adaptation. In each development era the person undergoes adaptive changes.[1] This chapter explores the application of adaptation to nursing practice.

ADAPTIVE PROCESSES

Although adaptive processes may seem to be strictly physiological, they affect the whole person. Thus the key concepts discussed here regarding these processes in general should be considered in relation to psychological, sociocultural and family adaptations as well. Nursing implications are related throughout.

*Homeokinesis*

**Homeokinesis** *refers to the ability of the organism to preserve its integrity* *through change and the element of motion* that is characteristic of physiological adaptation. Dynamic, self-regulating processes work to maintain or restore the internal environment to normal. Homeokinesis involves **negative** **feedback** *in which a deviation in one direction results in a reaction in the opposite* *direction.* The classic example is the maintenance of a relatively constant environment in the home by means of a control device, a thermostat.

*The body as an open system*

Physiological adaptation may be considered by viewing the body as a complex open system in which a dynamic balance is maintained with the surrounding environment. Each interrelated subsystem (organs, tissues) of the body is an open system made up of additional subsystems (cells). Levels of organization within and among systems include the cellular, structural, organ-system, and physiological-process aspects. To illustrate, the regulation of body temperature involves skin, respiratory, circulatory and neurological structures. Variations in the degree of adaptation may also occur. Changes in function of one body part mediate change elsewhere. Examples include the carotid sinus reflex that slows the heart rate, thereby reducing blood pressure through decreased vasoconstriction, and eye adaptation to light and dark through pupil dilation and changes in the rods and cones. Increased production of antibodies occurs in response to the presence of foreign protein in the form of a bacterium. And decreased oxygen tension at higher altitudes increases blood hemoglobin content.[2]

Basic adaptive responses are sufficiently known to permit prediction of outcomes that relate directly to many aspects of nursing care. Detection of **hyperpyrexia**, an *increased body temperature*, in the patient, for example, will permit you to plan for increased perspiration, resultant dehydration, increased cardiac and respiratory rates, increased surface heat loss, and eventual decreased metabolism, leading to a decreased heat production.[3] Plans for fluid replacement, rest, conservation of body heat, and monitoring of vital signs will be some basic components of the febrile patient's care plan. Special skin care will promote adaptation of the integumental system, preventing skin breakdown caused by deprivation of moisture and nutrition to the skin during hyperpyrexia.

*Maintaining a steady state*

A person's functioning as an integrated behavioural unit can be viewed on a continuum: at times he/she is operating as a stable integrated unit with consistent, orderly behaviours and at other times as an unstable, ineffective nonintegrated unit in coping with stimuli. The human is remarkably adaptive.

In the **stable** or **steady state** *there is an optimal energy balance between utilization and conservation.* Any disturbance in a system stimulates return to a steady state or **equifinality,** *a characteristic or original state that the organism strives by nature to assume through self-regulatory processes.*[4]

All people have a potential for energy imbalance and inappropriate energy allocation. One of the best ways to assess imbalance is to note inconsistency between behaviours: the person says one thing and does another.

The apparently calm, friendly patient, for instance, may actually be feeling great anxiety, undergoing great energy utilization, and experiencing covert behavioural and physiological instability. Illness is also likely to cause energy imbalance, which indicates that the body's responses are inadequate to its special needs. Illness may be regarded as a life process that is regulating or striving toward normality following a disturbance to the system. Recovery is an adaptive response to maintain the body's integrity, a reestablishment of equifinality, the steady or stable state. Chronic disease or disability represents an altered state between usable energy and the steady state. When a person's regulatory processes are all properly functioning, he/she is in a steady adaptive state and can then deal most effectively with whatever situations are presented.

*The adaptation syndrome*

**Stress** *is a physical and emotional state always present in the person, one influenced by various environmental, psychological and social factors but uniquely perceived by the person, and intensified in response when environmental change or threat occurs internally or externally and the person must respond.* The manifestations of stress are both overt and covert, purposeful, initially protective, maintaining equilibrium, productivity, and satisfaction to the extent possible.[5]

The person's survival depends on constant mediation between environmental demands and adaptive capacities. Various self-regulatory physical and emotional mechanisms are in constant operation, adjusting the body to a changing number and nature of internal and external stressors, agents or factors causing intensification of the stress state. **Stressors** *(stress agents)* include cold, heat, radiation, infectious organisms, disease processes, mechanical trauma, fever, pain, imagined events, and intense emotional involvement. A moderate amount of stress, when regulatory mechanisms act within limits and few symptoms are observable, is constructive. The exaggerated stress state occurs when stressors are excessive or intense, limits of the steady state are exceeded, and the person cannot cope with the stressor's demands. **Distress** *is negative, noxious, unpleasant, damaging stress.*

Responses to stress are both local and general. The **Local Adaptation Syndrome**, typified by the inflammatory response, *is the method used to ward off and control effects of physical stressors locally.* When the stressor cannot be handled locally, *the whole body responds to protect itself and ensure survival in the best way possible through the* **General Adaptation Syndrome.** The general body response augments bodily functions that protect the organism from injury, psychological and physical, and suppresses those functions nonessential to life. The General Adaptation Syndrome is characterized by Alarm and Resistance stages and, when body resistance is not maintained, an end stage, Exhaustion.

*The General Adaptation Syndrome*

The **Alarm Stage** *is an instantaneous, short-term, life-preserving, and total sympathetic-nervous-system response* when the person consciously or unconsciously perceives a stressor and feels helpless, insecure, or biologically uncomfortable. This stage is typified by a 'fight-or-flight' reaction. Perception of the stressor – the alarm reaction – stimulates the anterior pituitary to increase production of adrenocorticotropic hormone (ACTH). The adrenal cortex is stimulated by ACTH to increase production of glucocorticoids, primarily hydrocortisone, or cortisol, and mineralocorticoids, primarily aldosterone. Catecholamine release triggers increased sympathetic nervous system activity, which stimulates production of adrenaline and noradrenaline by the adrenal medulla and release at the adrenergic nerve endings. The alarm reaction also stimulates the posterior pituitary to release increased anti-diuretic hormone. Generally the person is prepared to act, is more alert, and is able to adapt.

Physiologically, the responses that occur when the sympathetic nervous system is stimulated are shown in Fig. 5.1.[6]

To complicate assessment, there are times when *parts* of the parasympathetic division of the autonomic nervous system are inadvertently stimulated during a stressful state because of proximity of sympathetic and parasympathetic nerve fibres.[7] With intensification of stress, opposite behaviours are then observed. They are shown in Fig. 5.2.[8]

The **Stage of Resistance** *is the body's way of adapting, through an adrenocortical response, to the disequilibrium caused by the stressors of life.* Because of the adrenocortical response, increased use of body resources, endurance and strength, tissue anabolism, antibody production, hormonal secretion, and changes in blood-sugar levels and blood volume sustain the body's fight for preservation. Body response eventually returns to normal.

If biological, psychological, or social stresses, single or in combination, occur over a long period without adequate relief, the stage of resistance is maintained. With continued stressors, the person becomes distressed and manifests objective and subjective emotional, intellectual and physiological responses, as shown in Fig. 5.3.

Be aware of these signs and symptoms (shown in Figure 5.3) in yourself as well as in patients. You will encounter considerable stress in the work of nursing. Identify stressors, especially in situations in which your sense of self is threatened or in which you are made to feel incompetent. Share your feelings and talk about your work experiences with someone whom you trust and who will offer feedback about your coping skills. You will need someone who values you as a person, not just as a worker, who sees you as more than nurse, job, position or nurturer, and who can help you put stressful work situations into perspective. Strive to develop a sense of being master of your own life and circumstances, a feeling that you can exert some control over what happens to you by the way you view yourself and

Headache from tense neck & shoulder muscles.

Anti-inflammatory responses increase from glucocorticoid production. Defences against inflammation/infection high for short time.

Respiratory rate/depth increased as bronchi dilate, due to increased epinephrine; allows adequate oxygenation.

Hyperglycemia from glucagon secretion in pancreas causing glycogenolysis; for energy demands after initial hypoglycemia. Increased glucocorticoid production results in gluconeogenesis in liver; body cells have sufficient glucose for stress response. Protein catabolism due to conversion of protein to glucose.

Gastric glandular acid and volume secretion reduced: less essential functions such as digestion and excretion reduced. Intestinal smooth muscles relax, reducing motility. Sphincters contract. Anorexia, constipation, or flatulence may occur.

Salt and water retained by kidneys bolster intravascular blood volume due to increased antidiuretic hormone and aldosterone production and peripheral vasoconstriction; fuller blood pressure, less urinary output, and hemoconcentration result. Sodium chloride in extracellular fluid reduced; potassium levels rise.

Pupils dilate; use maximum light for vision. Vision initially sharp, later blurred.

Myocardial rate, strength, and output increased by greater epinephrine production; more blood available throughout body as pulse rate and strength increase. Palpitations or arrhythmias may occur.

Blood pressure rises when increased norepinephrine produces peripheral vasoconstriction.

Increased blood clotting due to catecholamine stimulation of increased production of clotting factors. Increased blood viscosity may result in stasis and thrombosis if Alarm Stage persists.

In urinary bladder, detrusor muscle relaxes and trigone sphincter contracts; micturition inhibited. Or person voids only small amounts but feels urgency.

Blood supply shunted to brain, heart and skeletal muscles rather than to periphery due to peripheral vasoconstriction. Skin pale, ashen, cool. Vasoconstriction stimulated by increased secretion of renin by kidney with reduced blood supply to kidney. Renin secretion stimulates production of plasma angiotensinogen; in turn, production of angiotension I and II causes vasoconstriction and increased blood pressure in vital organs.

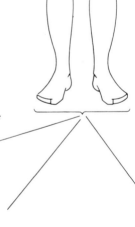

Muscle tonus increased by epinephrine production; activities may be better coordinated, or rigidity and tremors may occur. Metabolic alterations in muscles with glycogenolysis and reduced use of glucose. Blood lactate and glucose increase.

Metabolic changes in adipose tissue; lipolysis and release of free fatty acids for use by mucles. Glycerol converted to glucose.

Metabolism increased up to 150%, providing immediate energy and producing more heat due to catecholamine release. Body temperature may rise. Perspiration. Mild dehydration from increased insensible fluid loss. (Dry lips and mouth occur.) If metabolism remains high, tissue catabolism, insomnia, fatigue, and signs of dehydration such as dry skin, weight loss, and decreased urinary output occur.

*Fig. 5.1*    Response to stressor – adaptive

Alarm phase, General Adaptation Syndrome: physiological responses to sympathetic nervous system stimulation. (From Murray, Ruth, and M. Marilyn Huelskoetter, *Psychiatric/Mental Health Nursing: Giving Emotional Care* (Prentice Hall, Inc., 1983), p. 377. © Prentice Hall Inc. 1983. Used with permission.

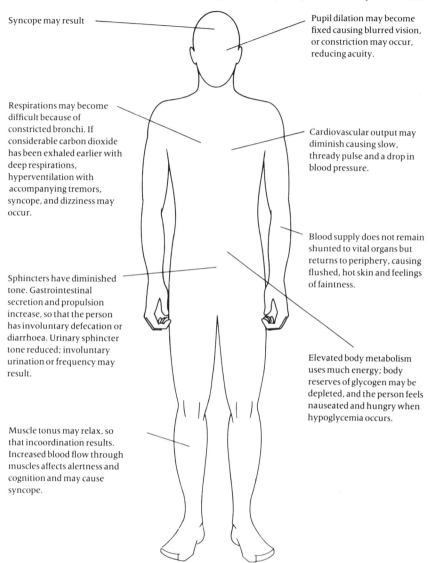

Syncope may result

Pupil dilation may become fixed causing blurred vision, or constriction may occur, reducing acuity.

Respirations may become difficult because of constricted bronchi. If considerable carbon dioxide has been exhaled earlier with deep respirations, hyperventilation with accompanying tremors, syncope, and dizziness may occur.

Cardiovascular output may diminish causing slow, thready pulse and a drop in blood pressure.

Blood supply does not remain shunted to vital organs but returns to periphery, causing flushed, hot skin and feelings of faintness.

Sphincters have diminished tone. Gastrointestinal secretion and propulsion increase, so that the person has involuntary defecation or diarrhoea. Urinary sphincter tone reduced; involuntary urination or frequency may result.

Elevated body metabolism uses much energy; body reserves of glycogen may be depleted, and the person feels nauseated and hungry when hypoglycemia occurs.

Muscle tonus may relax, so that incoordination results. Increased blood flow through muscles affects alertness and cognition and may cause syncope.

*Fig. 5.2* Shock – enhanced response to stressor

adjust your behaviour. When you can cope with your own work-related and other stressors, then you can help patients and their families to be adaptive.

Stress is additive. The repeated or chronic exposure to stress, even when the stressors are of widely differing kinds, including other people and their feelings, ultimately takes a toll on the individual. Reserves of adaptability

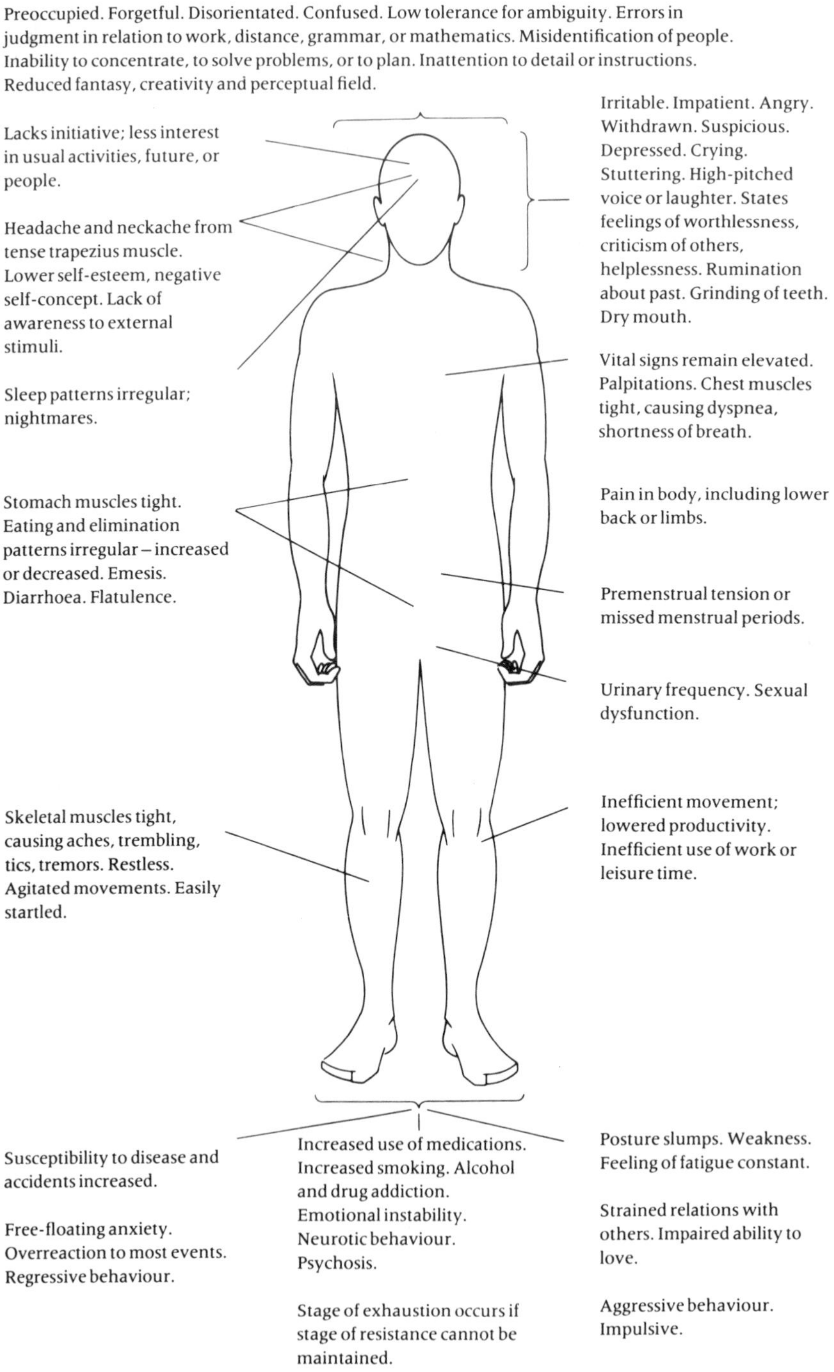

Preoccupied. Forgetful. Disorientated. Confused. Low tolerance for ambiguity. Errors in judgment in relation to work, distance, grammar, or mathematics. Misidentification of people. Inability to concentrate, to solve problems, or to plan. Inattention to detail or instructions. Reduced fantasy, creativity and perceptual field.

Lacks initiative; less interest in usual activities, future, or people.

Headache and neckache from tense trapezius muscle. Lower self-esteem, negative self-concept. Lack of awareness to external stimuli.

Sleep patterns irregular; nightmares.

Stomach muscles tight. Eating and elimination patterns irregular – increased or decreased. Emesis. Diarrhoea. Flatulence.

Skeletal muscles tight, causing aches, trembling, tics, tremors. Restless. Agitated movements. Easily startled.

Irritable. Impatient. Angry. Withdrawn. Suspicious. Depressed. Crying. Stuttering. High-pitched voice or laughter. States feelings of worthlessness, criticism of others, helplessness. Rumination about past. Grinding of teeth. Dry mouth.

Vital signs remain elevated. Palpitations. Chest muscles tight, causing dyspnea, shortness of breath.

Pain in body, including lower back or limbs.

Premenstrual tension or missed menstrual periods.

Urinary frequency. Sexual dysfunction.

Inefficient movement; lowered productivity. Inefficient use of work or leisure time.

Susceptibility to disease and accidents increased.

Free-floating anxiety. Overreaction to most events. Regressive behaviour.

Increased use of medications. Increased smoking. Alcohol and drug addiction. Emotional instability. Neurotic behaviour. Psychosis.

Stage of exhaustion occurs if stage of resistance cannot be maintained.

Posture slumps. Weakness. Feeling of fatigue constant.

Strained relations with others. Impaired ability to love.

Aggressive behaviour. Impulsive.

*Fig. 5.3*    Adaptation – blocking of stressor

are used that can't be replaced. Some experience with stressors may aid coping with stress and be protective against stress-induced disease. Certain coping methods, feeling in command of the situation, and strong family and social ties can help a person to suffer less deleterious effects of stress. Breaking ties by separating from the group or a loved one, divorce, mobility or death, and the resultant sense of loss, rejection and loneliness predispose to disease and death.[9]

The **Stage of Exhaustion** *occurs when the person is unable to continue to adapt to internal and external environmental demands.* Physical or psychic disease or death results because the body can no longer compensate for or correct homeostatic imbalances. Manifestations of this stage are similar to those of the Alarm Stage except that all reactions first intensify and then diminish in response and show no ability to return to an effective level of function. Frequent or prolonged General Adaptation Syndrome response triggers disease through adrenocortical hypertrophy, thymolymphatic atrophy, elevated blood glucose, ulceration of the gastrointestinal tract, reduced tone and fibrosis of tissues, and vasoconstriction.

Health-care workers are concerned with promoting the Resistance Stage and preventing or reversing the Exhaustion Stage, whether through drugs, bedrest, medical treatments, crisis intervention, psychotherapy or social action. Ideally, you should identify potential stressors that the person might encounter and determine how to alter the stressors or best support the person's adaptive mechanisms and resources physically, emotionally and socially, for the person will respond as an entity to the stressors. The relationship of stress to life crisis or changes is discussed in Chapter 6 and must be considered whenever you are doing health-promotion measures or intervening with the ill person.

## PHYSIOLOGICAL ADAPTATION

The processes of homeokinesis, maintenance of a steady state, and the General Adaptation Syndrome just described all affect physiological adaptation.

### Adaptation to the environment

Adaptation enables living organisms to respond to changes in their environment in such a manner that injury or disease is prevented, damage is repaired, or a comfort level for coping with the altered environment is attained. Adaptation assists a person to function within a normal range.

*Regulation of body core temperature*

Regulation of a relatively constant internal temperature is one of the physiological processes that demonstrates the principle of adaptation.[10] Generally the nude body is capable of maintaining the normal body core temperature between 98°F (36.6°C) and 100°F (37.7°C) indefinitely when exposed to dry air temperatures ranging from 60°F (21°C) to 130°F (54.4°C). Certain feedback mechanisms in the nervous system provide the regulatory processes necessary to stabilize core temperature and most operate through the temperature-regulating centre of the hypothalamus.

The preoptic receptors in the hypothalamus are primarily responsible for detection and response when core temperature is above normal; the peripheral receptors are more important when core temperature is below normal. Signals from the peripheral receptors are transmitted to the hypothalamus, where they are integrated with signals from the preoptic area to provide the final efferent message for control of heat gain and loss. This control centre is called the *hypothalamic thermostat*.

Sweating begins at 37°C (98.6°F) and increases rapidly as the core temperature rises; it ceases if the temperature falls below that level. Heat production is similarly adaptive, for at any temperature below 37°C (98.6°F) mechanisms that produce heat are activated, notably muscle activity culminating in shivering. Increased heat loss occurs in two ways in response to overheating: (a) by stimulation of sweat glands to increase evaporation and (b) by inhibition of certain sympathetic centres in the posterior hypothalamus, permitting vasodilation of skin vessels.

Adaptation to cold is equally efficient. Vasoconstriction in the skin is the first change and it occurs over the entire body, closing off conduction from internal structures and conserving body heat. Sweating is completely checked at 37°C (98.6°F) and evaporative cooling ceases.

*Heat production* occurs through shivering and sympathetic excitation. The primary motor centre for shivering is situated in the posterior hypothalamus. It is activated by severe body cooling that sends impulses down the brain stem to the cord to the anterior motor neurons. Skeletal muscle tone is intensified throughout the body; muscle metabolism speeds up, and the rate of heat production is increased as much as 50 per cent. Once the muscle tone reaches a crucial point, shivering begins as the result of feedback oscillations of the muscle spindle stretch reflex mechanism. Maximum shivering can raise heat production as much as five times normal.

Sympathetic stimulation of circulating norepinephrine and epinephrine in the blood can trigger an immediate rise in the rate of cellular metabolism by requiring greater oxidation of foodstuffs to produce the amount of high-energy phosphates required for normal body functions. This adaptive mechanism for increased heat production is called *chemical thermogenesis*. Although not nearly as effective in adults as in infants, it can increase heat production in infants by as much as 100 per cent, a crucial factor for maintaining normal body temperature in the neonate.

The comfort we experience at 72° with a relative humidity of 50 per cent on a calm day could not be enjoyed if our core temperature of 98.6° fluctuated. When a change in weather occurs, our hypothalamic thermostats signal immediately to hold temperature and other vital functions constant. If our bodies could not cool themselves in an environment of 105° during a summer heat wave, permanent brain damage would transpire within minutes; similarly, a drop of but nine degrees on a zero day could mean death.

Research shows that weather affects humans. Body chemistry changes with the seasons; for example, certain individuals burn extra fats in cold weather. Although the body's overall metabolism conserves and endures, surface capillaries close down, resistance to disease lessens, cardiovascular illnesses occur frequently, and the death rate peaks world-wide in winter.

The transitional seasons impose the most stress, especially spring. Switching from winter to summer may trigger such an explosive change in the organism as to almost match the about-face in the weather. Blood acidity rises, cholesterol and sugars climb to high levels, hormones surge. A burst of energy may be felt: the housewife feels impelled to get busy with new tasks and the young man's fancy may indeed turn to thoughts of love (his hair and beard double their rate of growth).

## Mechanisms of defence

The human body is equipped with various defensive physiologic mechanisms. They help to reduce injury and prevent the invasion of pathogenic microorganisms, thus promoting and maintaining a healthy status. When these mechanisms fail, various disease states result: neoplastic, infectious, viral, toxic or traumatic.

Some *defensive mechanisms are of a general nature and serve to protect against many types of harmful agents; they are the basis of* **nonspecific resistance.** Other *defensive mechanisms are specific against a certain harmful agent and no other; they are spoken of as* **specific resistance** or **specific immunity.**

**Nonspecific resistance.** Some principal nonspecific forms of body resistance are the skin, mucous membranes and their secretions, the skull, reflex movements, phagocytosis, inflammation and interferons.

The first line of defence is the unbroken *skin* and *mucous membranes* that protect the deeper tissues from mechanical and chemical injury and that provide a barrier against the penetration of bacteria. The skin and mucous membranes are constantly in contact with microorganisms. Certain microorganisms that are regularly present on these coverings constitute their normal flora of resident bacteria. When the person's resistance is lowered by injury to the tissues or by a disease process that reduces general resistance, these resident microorganisms, as well as pathogenic microorganisms, flourish.[11] Pathogenic microorganisms may gain entry through broken skin or mucous membranes, the respiratory or gastrointestinal tracts, the vagina, or blood vessels, especially the veins. Microorganisms are spread through direct contact, droplet infection (organisms that are sneezed or coughed), food and water, insect and animal bites, or contaminated equipment, such as in intravenous or intramuscular administration of medications.

Reproduction of resident skin flora and the growth of pathogenic microorganisms are minimized by lack of sufficient moisture and the presence of specific antibacterial and antifungal organic acids. A surface film on the skin, which consists of secretions from sebaceous glands and sudoriferous (sweat) glands and of products of *cornification* (the process whereby the epidermis hardens), provides an acid environment and has antibacterial and antifungal properties. these properties enable the film to act as an antiseptic, to neutralize acid and alkali substances, and to interfere with the absorption of toxic agents. Because some soaps are highly alkaline, their excessive use should be avoided to prevent the removal of this protective surface film.

The epidermis, which partly consists of a layer of dead cells, serves as another defence mechanism. As the cells of the epidermis die, their protein material undergoes a change. The new protein form is called *keratin*, a tough, fibrous protein that causes the epidermis to become highly resistant to environmental elements, including bacteria, fungi, parasites, and most injurious chemicals. If this layer of skin (also called the horny layer) is broken, physical and chemical agents can enter the body. So protect yourself and the patient from scratches, cuts, and any breaks in the continuity of the skin.

Mucous membranes line cavities or passageways of the body that communicate to the exterior. These membranes secrete a fluid, *mucus*, which consists of several mucopolysaccharides, inorganic salts, water and epithelial cells. The membranes and mucus serve to decrease bacterial invasion and lessen the severity of chemical or mechanical trauma.

The surface of the stomach is lined with cells that secrete an alkaline fluid containing mucus. A layer of mucus 1.0 to 1.5 mm thick covers the gastric wall and serves as a protective barrier against various forms of chemical and mechanical irritants, such as digestive enzymes, hydrochloric acid and abrasive foods. The parietal cells of the gastric glands secrete a solution that contains hydrochloric acid. This acid environment acts as a barrier to destroy most pathogens that enter the digestive tract. The acid environment of the stomach can be diminished temporarily, however, by such foods as milk and eggs; thus the protective action of the acidity is decreased. Remember this when planning or instructing patients in diets that must contain large quantities of milk products and eggs.

Some mucous membranes in the digestive tract secrete substances that have bacteriostatic properties. Those in the intestines, for instance, secrete certain enzymes capable of destroying pathogens.

The genitourinary tract is also lined with mucous membranes. Pathogens entering the vagina are usually destroyed by the acid secretions produced by the cells lining this area. Frequent vaginal irrigations, or douches, will lower the acidity in the vagina and therefore lessen the protective function of the mucous membranes there.

A ciliated mucous membrane lines the respiratory tract. The external nares are surrounded by fine hairs that block pathogens from entering the nose; pathogens that do enter are trapped by mucus secreted by the cells lining the nasal passageways. Inhaled bacteria escaping these two defence mechanisms are usually blocked by *cilia* (hairlike projections), whose wavelike motions move the pathogens toward the pharynx, where they are swallowed or expectorated.

The eye is protected by several defence mechanisms. The skull provides a *bony orbit* that protects the eyeball (as well as the brain and vital centres) from mechanical injury. The *eyelids,* which are lined with a conjunctival membrane, serve as protective coverings for the eyeball. *Eyelashes,* lining the free edges of the lids, act to prevent foreign bodies from entering the eye. Tears or *lacrimal fluid,* secreted by the lacrimal glands, have a lavage action that serves to wash foreign bodies out of the eyes and to dilute irritant materials. Excessive tear formation occurs any time a foreign particle or other irritant gets in or near the eye. The lacrimal fluid also contains an enzyme, *lysozyme,* which functions to destroy bacteria.

Some *reflex* or *voluntary acts* assist the body to rid itself of pathogens. Sneezing and coughing eliminate pathogens from the respiratory tract whereas vomiting and diarrhoea help to eliminate them from the gastrointestinal tract. The reflex of blinking renews the tear film over the cornea and prevents the entrance of foreign material. Reflex muscular movement, such as removing the hands from a hot stove or foot from a sharp object, prevents injury.

One of the most important nonspecific mechanisms in the prevention of disease involves leukocytes (wandering cells) and certain pagocytic tissue cells.

*Phagocytosis* is performed by **phagocytes,** *special cells capable of ingesting and digesting bacteria and dead tissues.* In **phagocytosis** *projections of cytoplasm engulf solid particles external to the cells.* In order to promote phagocytosis, *opsonins* (globin molecules) combine with the bacteria and dead tissues and increase their cohesiveness with the phagocytes. Some pathogens may survive and multiply in the phagocytes, instead of being destroyed, and are transported in the bloodstream from one part of the body to another. Some phagocytes – for example, the stationary macrophages – are capable of forming immune bodies against foreign agents.

Phagocytic cells are classified according to size as macrophages and microphages. *Macrophages* are either stationary or mobile. The stationary cells, *tissue histocytes,* are permanently located in the interstitial tissues of the **reticuloendothelial system,** *which is composed of connective-tissue cells widely scattered throughout many vascular and lymph channels,* including the bone marrow, spleen, liver and lymph nodes. The reticuloendothelial system serves as the primary line of defence after bacteria have invaded the body. The mobile macrophagic cells are *lymphocytes* and *monocytes,* which are formed in the lymph nodes.[12]

*Microphages* are smaller and more numerous than the macrophages, and the phagocytic power per cell is greatly reduced. The microphagic cells are *granulocytes,* which are formed in the bone marrow. After their information, the granulocytes are transported throughout the body via the blood. Jointly, *the granulocytes, lymphocytes* and *monocytes are referred to as* **leukocytes,** mobile units of the body's defence system.[13]

*Any microorganisms that survive the action of the phagocytes trigger a second defence mechanism near the area of the invasion. This response is called the* **inflammatory response.** Because inflammation is one of the most common body responses to injury, knowledge of the inflammatory mechanism provides a basis for understanding many infectious and noninfectious diseases.

First, there is an accelerated blood flow to the site because of a dilatation of the adjacent capillaries. This process increases the amount of oxygen and nutrients in the area and produces *redness* and *heat* at the site. An accompanying increase in the permeability of the capillaries causes white blood cells and serum to escape into the surrounding tissues. The accumulated fluid (blood cells and serum) causes area *swelling,* and pressure on the nerve endings produces *pain.* Together the pain and swelling produce *limitation of movement.* Thus the cardinal signs of inflammation are redness, heat, swelling and limitation of movement. Pain as a subjective symptom results.[14]

Phagocytosis occurs with the increased number of localized white blood cells during the inflammatory reaction. The phagocytes engulf and destroy the pathogens. Dead phagocytes, pathogens, tissue cells and tissue fluid accumulate. This accumulation is known as *pus.* The dead pathogens and tissue cells are eventually carried away by the leukocytes via the blood and lymph. Those in the bloodstream are carried to the spleen, liver and bone marrow, where the phagocytic cells (macrophages) engulf and digest them. Those in the lymph stream are filtered out by the lymph nodes and ingested by phagocytic cells.[15]

An additional *nonspecific resistance to disease that inhibits multiplication of viruses may be found in the form of* **interferon.** Several types of cells in the body secrete the protein interferon. When a cell is infected by a virus, its secretion of interferon increases. Interferon does not benefit the cell that is already infected but causes other cells to enhance their defence posture and increase their resistance to the viral invasion. Interferon is not specific in its action against any particular virus but acts against viruses in general.[16] Human-derived interferon has been shown active against some human cancers as well as against human viral diseases. Drug companies, plus several independent research teams, are currently experimenting with methods to produce human interferon from bacteria, a feat that promises to make ample quantities of the substance available for testing against viral infections and cancer.[17]

**Specific resistance – specific immunity.** Specific immune responses are characteristic of vertebrate animals. Immune responses can be viewed in the same way as other adaptive processes in the body – as a stimulus-response sequence. The immune system, often referred to as the third line of defence (the first and second lines of defence being mechanical barriers and the various types of phagocytes), is an important companion to the nonspecific defence previously described.

The immunological response is initiated by the invasion of the body by foreign molecules. These foreign molecules are known as *antigens*. Antigens stimulate the body to produce either specific proteins, called *antibodies*, or defensive cells that interact with the antigens and make them harmless.[18]

The immunological response has two separate components. The cell-mediated component or *cellular immunity* is involved in the body's response to fungi, viruses, tumours and transplants of foreign tissue. *T lymphocytes* are responsible for mediating cellular immunity. Once stimulated by an antigen, these lymphocytes increase in size and then multiply. Eventually the lymphocytes leave the lymph nodes and make their way to the site of the invasion, where they destroy the invading cells. The sensitized lymphocytes are also capable of stimulating other lymphocytes at the invasion site and enhancing the local inflammatory response. It is hypothesized that the T lymphocytes do not actually produce antibodies.[19] The antibody-mediated component or *humoral immunity* is primarily involved in the response to bacterial infections. In humoral immunity *B lymphocytes* become activated by antigens. The B lymphocytes increase in size and differentiate into *plasma cells*; these cells produce large amounts of antibodies that circulate freely in the blood and the lymph. Once formed, the antibodies are contained in serum globulins, especially gamma globulins.[20]

Interaction and cooperation between antibody-mediated immune response and cellular-mediated immune response are important in eradicating infections and preventing their recurrence. The immune state, which results in humoral or cellular immunity, may be permanent or transient.

**Active immunization** *occurs when the body is sensitized by an antigen.* The antibody-mediated and/or cellular-mediated immune responses occur. An active immunity may last from 10 years to a lifetime.[21] The first encounter that an individual has with an antigen is characterized by the primary response. Initially there is a lag phase that may last from 20 hours to a few days. During the lag phase little or no response to the antigen occurs. A slow increase in antibody concentration in the body fluids follows and then a gradual decline as the antigen is overcome. With the second encounter with a particular antigen, the antibody concentrations or titers rise rapidly and often reach levels 200 times greater than the concentrations observed during the primary response.

**Natural acquired active immunity** *occurs when the host's body produces antibodies following the invasion of pathogens.* Natural active immunity can be acquired from subclinical forms of disease and from repeated contacts with pathogens not virulent enough to produce disease.[22] Chickenpox, mumps and smallpox usually confer permanent immunity after recovery from a single attack.

**Artificial active immunity** *occurs after an individual is inoculated with a specific antigen that stimulates the production of antibodies.* The two main agents used for these inoculations are vaccines and toxoids. *Vaccines* are prepared from microorganisms that are living, attenuated, dead or inactivated. Living vaccines are usually prepared with organisms of lower virulence; attenuated or weakened strains are used in the Bacillus-Calmette-Guerin (BCG) vaccine for tuberculosis. The vaccines for whooping cough and typhoid fever are prepared from dead bacteria and the vaccines for measles and influenza from inactivated viruses. A vaccine can be prepared from a strain that does not produce disease in humans but that compares with the antigenicity of human strains – for example, the use of cowpox vaccines for smallpox vaccinations.[23]

*Toxoids* are prepared from attenuated forms of toxins (poisonous chemical substances produced by certain bacteria). When introduced into the body, attenuated toxins stimulate the production of antitoxins. Toxoids are used to immunize the host to such diseases as diphtheria, scarlet fever and tetanus.

**Passive immunization** *occurs when the person acquires resistance to a disease by receiving antibodies or lymphocytes from an external source.* Passive immunization is immediate, but the duration of its effectiveness is no more than a few weeks. In **natural passive immunity** *antibodies pass from mother to the foetus by way of placental transmission.* This immunization is critical for the survival of the newborn, for significant antibody formation does not appear until a month or two after birth. Cellular-mediated immunity functions are also slow to develop in the newborn. The placental membranes are permeable to maternal immunoglobulins. Thus the newborn has partial immunity to those diseases to which its mother is immune.

The transmission of antibodies from mother to baby by colostrum and milk secreted by the mammary glands is still being investigated and sources vary in their interpretation of present data.[24]

**Artificial passive immunity** *occurs when immune bodies or antibodies for specific diseases are obtained from other human beings or animals and injected into a person who has been exposed to the same disease and who needs antibodies to prevent the establishment of the disease.* These antibodies provide temporary immunity, allowing the person time to produce his/her own antibodies. Tetanus antitoxin and gamma globulins for hepatitis and German measles provide this form of protection.[25]

Transfer of pathogenic microbes can be prevented and controlled through proper personal hygiene habits. Covering the mouth and nose when coughing or sneezing, disposal of contaminated tissues, and control of dust and particulate matter minimize the spread of airborne droplet infection. Thorough handwashing, use of individual equipment, and disinfection and sterilization of equipment prevent direct spread of microorganisms by touching of contaminated areas or articles. Foods and liquids require careful handling by few people so that they do not become sources of infection.

Immunization and various *medications* (such as antibiotics) also aid the human's natural defences by producing a desired effect on a particular body system. *Biological rhythms* are also increasingly understood as essential to adaptation.

Motion is synonymous with life and adaptation. When either the internal or the overall mobility of the person is interfered with, adaptation is inadequate.

*Biofeedback: new dimensions for the mind*

Bridging the gap between physiological and psychological controls has fascinated people for decades. Despite the wealth of biological and psychological scientific effort devoted to the control of physiological, behavioural, and emotional responses, little has been done to explore the capacity of the individual to hold the reins of control over his own body functions.

Biofeedback, a new and far-reaching discovery, has emerged from biological research. It is a mind-body technique that allows the person to communicate with his/her inner being. It is the feeding back of personal biological information to oneself in order to control voluntarily the automatic nervous system.[26]

Biofeedback permits a person to become familiar with internal functions, such as moving index of body temperature or a reading of brain waves. As with externally directed behaviour, the person is able with practice to learn how to control internal behaviour. Most people have experienced the doctor's interpreting for them, in an illness-health context, the results of physiological tests. If able to read the same information as it is occurring within you, you are using biofeedback.

Biofeedback has two aspects: the actual use of biomedical devices capable of taking a reading of one's physiological activity, such as temperature or heart rate, and the training in which one learns what to do with the devices. The client is linked to the instruments, which are modified to display the body information as visual or auditory signals, by delicate wires or tubes connected to special sensing materials taped to the skin. The body information is carried back to the devices, which continually read the signals reflecting the constantly changing activity within. As the client continues to work with biofeedback instrumentation, an association develops between changes in body signals and various subjective feelings that are either consciously or subconsciously recognized. The monitor gives information about the degree of success. Dependence on the instrumentation is temporary. Eventually the person should be able to monitor the fluctuations and thereby exercise some conscious control over physiological adaptation. Once learned, control over a physiological function is retained in the person's memory for a long time.[27]

Much success has been demonstrated in the use of biofeedback for the prevention and relief of such medical problems as tension headaches and Raynaud's disease. Work is being done to explore learned control over blood pressure, heart rate, and peripheral vasodilation and vasoconstriction. Control over some aspects of respiratory function could ease the discomforts of persons with obstructive pulmonary disease.

There are intimate interactions between the mind, emotion and body function. The process of biofeedback is essentially a mental function and it has relevance in most medical, psychological, psychosomatic and emotional problems.

For centuries Indian fakirs have performed such feats as lying on beds of nails or walking on live coals. In recent studies of such persons EEG readings have shown a preponderance of alpha waves, waves associated with deeply relaxed meditative states in which one is able to turn off distractions and free the mind of all invading thoughts or images. The practice of total relaxation is used in biofeedback training and is an example of a person's adaptive capacity. Proponents of a 'relaxation response' method suggest that periods of meditation, in a quiet environment with the mind shifted from external thought to a passive attitude and the body in a comfortable position, will produce a physiological adaptation. This state, tested at a Harvard laboratory, produces significant decreases in oxygen consumption, carbon dioxide elimination and rate of breathing.[28]

Helping patients relax when coping with stress has always been a nursing goal. Research in biofeedback may provide new techniques with which to assist patients in a variety of situations: the preoperative patient in a state of tense anticipation of the unknown; the mother in labour with whom we have already begun to recognize the value of relaxation; and the postsurgical patient whose pain is increased because of tension. The basic principles of biofeedback have become a necessary component in the education of today's nurse.


PSYCHOLOGICAL ADAPTATION

Whether life offers psychological threat involving loss and suffering or the challenge of goal attainment, adaptational tasks are necessary for psychological growth. The term **coping** is sometimes used to refer to *the psychological way in which a person deals with life's demands and goals.*


*Key concepts*

**Psychological adaptation** *refers to intrapsychic organization and behavioural adequacy in attaining appropriate human relationships.* Adaptation is achieved through the personality structure called the **ego,** *that part of the person concerned with the processes of judgment, thinking, memory, perception, discrimination, motor activity in response to perception, understanding, association, communication, control over behaviour, and use of adaptive of defensive behaviours.* The ego refers to what we commonly think of as the conscious self.

*Failure to satisfy basic innate or acquired needs or to reconcile conflicting value systems constitutes* **psychological stress.** Stressors may exist in the real world or only be perceived as real by the person. But three basic causes of psychological stress exist: (a) loss of something valuable; (b) injury or threat of injury, physical or emotional, and (c) frustration of drives. Each person's individual perception of events determines the reaction; this fact explains the wide variety of possible responses to a given situation.[29]

**Adaptive behaviour** *helps us to adjust to or cope with certain circumstances* whereas **defensive behaviour** *causes us to alienate ourselves from certain circumstances or to avoid life's demands and goals.* Patterns for both behaviours originate in the early formative years of childhood when anxiety and discomfort with people are first experienced and are learned without much awareness on our part. By adulthood these patterns are usually fixed, unconscious, and automatic. Current experiences sometimes reactivate feelings and behaviour associated with long-forgotten experiences and elicit responses similar to ones that were originally adaptive but may now be inappropriate, useless, or incapacitating. Thus what was once adaptive behaviour becomes defensive.

Generally **defensive behaviour** *is an exaggerated response to experience used too frequently or for too long when a situation is perceived or anticipated as a threat to self* or to a situation inconsistent with the existing self-image. The experience is temporarily rendered harmless by being distorted or denied to awareness. A normally active person who sprains an ankle, for instance, may insist on continuing routine activities, denying the implications of the sprained ankle. Such behaviour is defensive. To admit the necessity of staying off the sprained ankle is adaptive, for healing is fostered through resting the part.

Adaptive behaviour is maximum when the person is feeling a sense of discovery, a purposeful changing of self, or creativity. The adapting person is not necessarily happy, content, or a conformist. But he/she is living constructively and in as much harmony with the culture and others as possible to allow for a balanced satisfaction of needs.

The processes or functions of the ego help the person to delay gratification, presume a sense of reality, and feel a sense of mastery or achievement in the world. The ego also mediates among inner demands, needs, impulses and drives (the *id*), and the internalized prohibitions and rules of society, parents, and outer reality (the *superego*). As the ego becomes stronger in its role as mediator between inner demands and outer reality, more efficient and complex mechanisms are developed for adaptive behaviour. Thus the person can adapt emotionally to the physical or social surroundings.

The well-organized, adapting ego can recognize anxiety (feelings) as a signal in a situation and can cope with this situation and feelings. Mechanisms of adjustment are not used too frequently, too intensely, for too long a duration, or too rigidly. The underdeveloped, maladaptive ego has either no organized behavioural mechanisms for response to anxiety or uses the same defensive mechanisms rigidly in every situation, to an excessive degree, for too long a duration. Such a person is vulnerable to small amounts of anxiety and cannot adapt to his/her feelings. Mental illness occurs in such persons.

People generally use only certain mechanisms that work best for them, thus establishing styles of adjustment by which others can predict their behaviour. Nevertheless, a common core of needs, drives, patterns of responses, and other psychological phenomena can be identified. Understanding the similarities and general patterns of behaviour promotes an understanding of a person's psychological adaptive potential.

**Behavioural patterning,** *using a cluster of behaviours that have a common goal and are used with predictability and regularity when a person is faced with a similar stimulus or need,* is an adaptive process that minimizes the amount of energy needed to cope with changing surroundings and promotes stability or a steady state. Behaviours previously successful are repeated, usually without thinking, so that the myriad of daily routine activities are done automatically. The person does not substitute new behaviours unless they are advantageous; and the substitution depends on the source and intensity of stimuli and on a comparison of the satisfaction provided by the established pattern with the predicted satisfaction to be gained by changing behaviours. People vary in the ease with which they can change or adapt.

The interruption of these patterns during illness, whether related to eating, bedtime, work, socialization, or hygiene, constitutes a crisis. You will assess behavioural patterns and help the person cope or adapt to the changed internal environment (illness) and the changed external environment (health-care system).

The body usually maintains or regains internal constancy through automatic regulatory mechanisms without conscious effort. The person's relationships with others, however, depend on his/her behaviour, whether consciously or unconsciously motivated. Therefore the person is usually more concerned about others and the external environment than his/her body unless the malfunctioning body part interferes with daily activity. An illness is of secondary concern to someone who is about to experience a business loss or who feels great occupational obligations, for instance.

Although *stress* and *anxiety* are used interchangeably, the terms are not the same. **Anxiety** *is the psychological response to excessive unchannelled energy resulting from the stress reaction; it is a vague, diffuse feeling of dread, uneasiness, or general discomfort resulting from perception of a threat to the self, real or imagined.*[30]

Anxiety is the response to feeling helpless, isolated, alienated from others, insecure, an object rather than a unique, worthwhile person. Anxiety, like stress, is subjective and indirectly observable. Severe anxiety immobilizes the person. But using the energy generated from the stress state (as explained in the discussion of the Adaptation Syndrome) to create a plan of action or goal mobilizes or motivates the person under stress.

The energy aroused by the stress state, manifested in feelings of anxiety, can be dissipated or reduced in intensity by walking, talking, crying, or other physical and social activity. Yet frequently the ill person has limited ways of working off tension.

Certain variables alter the stress state and resultant anxiety: the physical and mental status, age, temperament, health status; the kind, nature, or number of stressors; the duration of exposure; and past experiences and reaction to similar stress.

*Manifestations of anxiety*

People use various behaviours to cope with anxiety or to attempt to change a stressful situation. Redistribution of energy is often not consciously recognized; thus a person may be unaware of any behavioural shifts, although others notice them. Certain behavioural changes may be the best the person can do at the time, although they seem inadequate to an objective observer. You must be observant of the responses that may indicate psychological stress.

**The General Adaptation Syndrome** described earlier can be modified to assess psychological adaptation. In the *Alarm Stage* the person has an increased ability to perceive data, comprehend relationships, and do problem solving. He/she feels mildly anxious but can cope with the situation. Should the feelings of alarm persist, the degree of anxiety heightens and other types of psychic behaviour that are less adaptive may be evoked: irritability, anger, demanding, denial, withdrawal, crying, hypersensitivity to noise and confusion, hallucinations, loquaciousness, silence, and eventual panic if the stimuli are overwhelming. Exposure to intense psychological stimuli can cause death.

During the *Resistance Stage* psychological adaptive mechanisms include the behaviours typical of moderate anxiety. The person has a narrowed perceptual field but the ability to focus on a delineated subject or situation while shutting out irrelevant distractions. He/she can comprehend relationships; has a strong feeling of persistence; shows stereotyped, rigid behaviour; but does problem solving to attack a problem directly. Various ego-adaptive mechanisms may be used, though not excessively – for example, sublimation, reaction formation, rationalization, selective inattention, displacement or overcompensation. The Resistance Stage involves some deliberative change of behaviour as the person gains control of self, others, or the inanimate environment.

Should the person's attempts at coping with the feelings involved in a situation be unsuccessful, the *Stage of Exhaustion* would be manifested by physical or mental illness (neurosis, psychosis). Now the person gives up coping attempts or uses inappropriate or ineffective behaviour. Without help, the person might indeed become chronically ill or even die.

Intervention for the person passing through these stages is crisis intervention, discussed in Chapter 6; relevant techniques or therapeutic communication are discussed in Chapter 2; and Table 5.1 shows some strategies which may be employed to reduce or handle stress and the rationale for their use.

ANTHROPOLOGICAL ADAPTATION

A culture makes adaptation possible through its ideas, inventions and customs. Together with physiological adaptive processes, culture is a powerful force. The human, for example, is able to live in a wide variety of climates because the body has adjusted gradually to permit survival. People also

*Table 5.1*   Various thought strategies to handle stress and their rationale

| Mental response | Definition and rationale |
| --- | --- |
| 1. Use of knowledge | Learn causes of stress and ways to prevent or manage situation. |
| 2. Objectivity (reality orientation) | Sort out, compare, and validate events, ideas, and emotions to get a total perspective and better understanding on basis of facts, not just feelings; maintain realistic perception. |
| 3. Analysis | Study logically and systematically the component parts of a situation to arrive at realistic explanations and answers; manage part if not all of situation. |
| 4. Concentration (mental self-control) | Deliberately set aside thoughts and feelings unrelated to the situation to master tension, save energy, find answers, and make necessary decisions for the task at hand. |
| 5. Planning | Think through situation prior to action to release tension, promote problem solving, and avoid unnecessary use of energy, error, and consequent frustration. |
| 6. Fantasize (daydream) | Visualize release of tension and successful achievement rather than dwelling on fear of failure, in order to plan strategy, ensure goal-directed action, cope with stressors, and relieve tension. |
| 7. Rehearsal | Fantasize or anticipate event or another's response prior to stressful event in order to practise coping mentally or behaviourally and to gain confidence in ability to manage. |
| 8. Substitution of thoughts and emotions | State ideas and feelings that are different than real ones in order to avoid adding to stressful situation or to meet demands of the situation. |
| 9. Suppression | Hold thoughts and emotions in abeyance or momentarily forget, in order to wait until it is more timely to change behaviour, attack a problem, or implement a solution. |
| 10. Valuing | Establish or reaffirm religious or sociocultural values to foster sense of balance and relaxation in face of stressors. |
| 11. Empathy | Imagine how others in the situation are feeling so that behaviour can take these feelings into account. |
| 12. Humour | Point out inconsistencies in situation, laugh at self, and use past feelings, ideas, and behaviour in order to be playful, keep objective distance from a problem, reduce anxiety, maintain self-identity, enrich solution and add enjoyment to life. |
| 13. Tolerance of ambiguity | Function in a way that lays the basis for eventual effective solutions when the situation is so complex that it cannot be fully understood or clear choices cannot be made now. |

(From Murray, Ruth and M. Marilyn Huelskoetter, *Psychiatric/Mental Health Nursing; Giving Emotional Care,* © 1983, pp. 410–411. Reprinted with permission of Prentice Hall, Inc., Englewood Cliffs, NJ.

heat and cool the environment for comfort, control predators and parasites, and domesticate animals and plants for personal needs. We have constructed a variety of livestyles and patterns of social relationships to guarantee our survival and to free ourselves from the limits of physical environments. Prescribed cultural norms are the most effective adaptive mechanisms that humans use: they affect physical, social and mental wellbeing; aid adaptation to diverse situations, environments and recurring problems; and teach about other environments to which we may have to adapt. In addition, some adaptive modifications are achieved through genetic, physiological, and constitutional capacities that have been transmitted for generations through natural selection or cultural conditioning. Physical mutation may also promote permanent changes in a group if it enables the person to compete successfully and live, promoting adaptation.

Different forms of physical or cultural selection are as follows:

1. Survival of the fittest, in which persons who cannot cope or who have dysfunctional mutant genes are most subject to an inability to reproduce or to early death. This condition is most intense when resources are scarce or competition is intense.
2. Modification of the environment to help the person with a condition that interferes with optimum health. An example is treatment of diabetes, inherited by a recessive gene, which permits a normal life span and adaptation in other spheres.
3. Cultural changes that strive to make the person diversified. Mass uniformity prevents adaptation to changing and diverse environments. Persons living in different regions of the same culture, for example, often live differently in some respects while adhering to the overall value system.
4. Cultural conditioning or teaching the person how best to survive in the environment and life situation.

Culture allows diversity within a framework of uniformity (customs, traditions). Today cultural differences are being recognized as factors to be dealt with in nursing practice, within a pluralistic society. Nursing care plans however, often fail to recognize the special care requirements of patients from diverse sociocultural backgrounds and have instead a strong reference to Anglo-American values. Lack of diversity in thoughts and actions prevents adaptation to the patient as a person as well as our aiding that individual's adaptation to the illness state.

## SOCIAL ADAPTATION

People need other people to become and remain socialized; consequently, **social adaptation,** *adjusting the self to a group,* is essential. Sensory-deprivation experiments indicate that a continual flow of changing sensory stimuli is necessary for a person's mental health. The infant needs stimulation through touch from another human being. Withholding caresses and normal human contact or similar emotional deprivation ultimately results directly or indirectly in physical as well as mental deterioration.

In developing, a person learns to accept symbolic rather than actual touch until the mere act of verbal recognition serves the purpose. The fact that people recognize one another's presence, and thereby offer the social contact necessary for the preservation of health, is more important than what is said.

Sensory stimulation that keeps certain parts of the brain active appears necessary in order to maintain a normal waking state. This need to be recharged by stimulation, especially by social contact, may be regarded as one of the biological origins of group formation. The fear of loneliness (or of lack of social stimulation) is one reason why people are willing to resign part of their individual desires in favour of group consensus while at the same time developing a high proficiency in getting as many satisfactions as possible from the socialization.

Through social adaptation the human being receives spiritual and emotional nourishment, obtains responses to love and creativity, and attains power and prestige. Threats to the ability to perform in these areas produce the everyday stresses that can cause disability and disease.


RESPONSES TO SOCIAL CHANGE

It is impossible to generalize about social adaptation or to define it as social striving or obtaining cultural goals. The individual's response must be considered objectively. Persons who are comfortable in a social climate of brotherly love and unworldliness, for example, would find it hard to survive or be happy in a competitive world.

The human being adheres to societal expectations, and social behaviour evolves from assuming particular social roles. Behaviour towards others is prescribed by **social norms,** *rules that define and prescribe performance and attitudes for persons in particular social positions.* There is a certain assumed degree of stability about norms so that each person knows what to expect from others. How norms are lived depends on the person's concept of his/ her role and the adaptive reactions of others as well as personal adaptive abilities. If mutual expectations are not met, adaptation to a situation is difficult.[31]

Social change is rampant in today's world. Unsuccessful social adaptation to rapid change can contribute to illness, such as ulcers, heart disease or arthritis. Illness, in turn, may force more social adaptations on the person.

Modern individuals are increasingly exposed to stresses of a symbolic nature. For this reason, goals and values determine the response of the whole being toward health or disease. As time evolved, values and goals became a way of life, and the person's performance has reflected the worth of chosen values. In both social and bodily health we have often been more maladapted than not, more sick than well.

Modern Western civilization requires the use of traditional adaptations, as well as new ones, to cope in a changing society. Conflict between the pressures of one's past and pressures newly encountered cause problems for those who change environments, whether the new one be another country, a different work climate, or a new social position. The social and cultural pressures that a person feels, the psychological drive, and innate abilities all influence his/her interpretation of and response to illness.[32]

The only stable thing in life is change. The human mind has created social change, ongoing and relentless. Reason has aided us in adaptation, but it has also created challenges. Power beyond the dreams of the past has built a scientific technology that protects us from the elements and from other destructive forces in the environment, but with this life has come new hazards of injury, death, and changes in the air breathed and the food eaten.

Illnesses related to modern technology and to social relationships are gaining attention. Society requires that people live together without destroying each other; differences in people and ideologies must be tolerated for survival. Adaptations fraught with stress accompany these developments. You will need to view the person in the context of biological tendencies, learned patterns of response, and the pressures, both tangible and intangible, to which he/she is exposed.

Toffler has confronted us with the concept of 'future shock', a force he predicts will ensure adaptational breakdown unless people can come to grips with rapid social change. Toffler describes the frequent shifting of families from one place to another, alterations in bureaucratic structures that may speedily engulf the worker in change, and diversity of options and continuing novelty in many life situations. The disposable, transient culture makes it difficult for people to establish roots or pass on culture as a guideline to future generations.[33]

Because of the 'futures hock syndrome', the risk of illness can be predicted from the amount of change present. If a person is in the equivalent of the Alarm Stage continually, body defences weaken. Extreme examples of persons caught in rapidly changing environments are the combat soldier, the flood victim, the culturally dislocated traveller. Other examples include the aged who are uprooted and the person who moves from a rural to an urban environment.

Constant adjustment to new surroundings, or creation of new ones is required in order to remain adaptive. In nursing you adjust in the work environment to changing client groups and the patient adjusts to the sick role, health-care system and workers. You can develop for yourself and teach others about adaptive behaviours to overcome the stress of constant change, because to deny change is occurring is to distort reality. Change seems easier if you are the one initiating the change or at least part of the changes. To begin with one can focus on a single aspect of the changing situation; eventually, however, awareness should expand to encompass the total situation.

## FAMILY ADAPTATION

**Adaptive responses in the family,** *a social system, represent the means by which it maintains an internal equilibrium so that it can fulfil purposes and tasks, deal with stress and crisis, and allow for growth of individual members.* Some capacity for functioning may be sacrificed in order to control conflict and aid work as a unit. But the best functioning family keeps anxiety and conflict within tolerable limits and maintains a balance between effects of the past and new experiences. Just as other social systems adapt, so must the family system.

Ideally, the family achieves equilibrium by talking over problems and finding solutions together. Humour, nonsense, shared work and leisure all help relieve tension. The family members know that certain freedoms exist within their confines that are not available elsewhere. Yet even the most stable family will briefly use the following behaviours to cope with stress, which, in turn, promotes more stress. However, these mechanisms are not overused in healthy families.[34]

*Adaptive mechanisms in family life*

Family conflict can be avoided or minimized through scapegoating, coalitions, withdrawal of emotional ties, fighting, use of family myths, reaction formation, compromise, or designation of a family healer. Two or more of these mechanisms may be used within the same family. If these mechanisms are used exclusively, however, they become defensive and are unlikely to promote resolution of the conflict so that the same issue will arise repeatedly.

**Scapegoating or blaming** involves labelling one member as the cause of the family trouble and is expressed in the attitude, 'If it weren't for you . . .' Or one member may offer himself as a scapegoat to end an argument by saying, 'It's all my fault.' Such labelling controls the conflict and reduces anxiety, but it prevents communication that can get at the root of the problem. Growth toward resolution of the problem is prohibited.

**Coalitions or alliances** may form when some family members side together against other members. Antagonisms and anger result. Eventually the losing party tries to get control.

**Withdrawal of emotional ties**, loosening the family unit, and reducing communication may be used to handle conflict, but then the family becomes rigid and mechanized. Family members are also likely to seek affection outside the family so that the home becomes a hotel with everyone superficially nice. In some families there is no show of emotion, for such emotion signifies loss of control or giving in to unacceptable impulses.

**Repetitive fighting** through verbal abuse, physical battles, loud complaints, curses, or accusations may be used to relieve tension and allow some harmony until the next round. The fight may have the same theme each time stress hits the family. The healthy family allows some 'blowing up' as release from everyday frustrations, but it does not make a major case out of every minor incident or temporary disagreement.

**Family myths or traditional beliefs** can be used to overcome anxieties and maintain control over others. Such statements are as follows: 'Children are seen, not heard.' 'We can't survive if you leave home.' 'Talking about feelings will cause loss of love.' In contrast the healthy family members encourage growth and creativity rather than rigid control.

**Reaction formation** is seen in a family in which there is superficial harmony or togetherness. Traumatic ideas are repressed and transformed into the opposite behaviour. Everybody smiles but nobody loves. No one admits to having any difficulties. Great tension is felt because true feelings are not expressed.

**Resignation or compromise** may provide temporary harmony when someone gives up or suppresses the need for assertion, affection, or emotional expression in order to keep peace. The surface calm eventually explodes when unmet needs can no longer be successfully suppressed.

**Designation of one person as family healer or umpire** involves using a 'wise one' (most often in the extended family), or a minister, bartender, or family friend, to arrange a reconciliation between dissenting parties. Part of the dynamics sometimes underlying the helper role is that the referee gets great satisfaction from finding someone worse off than self. The healer feels a sense of heightened self-esteem or omnipotence. A varient of the healer role is that of family 'protector'. Here one person takes on all the stresses in order to save other members stress or conflict. One person ends up fighting the battles for everyone else in the family.

You may find yourself in the role of the family healer. Help the family to develop harmonious ways of coping and avoid the protector or omnipotent role.

INADEQUATE ADAPTATION

Disturbances in adaptation (nonconstructive behaviour) result in illness or various disorders – physically, emotionally, socially. Some behaviours that are adaptive for a time become defensive or inadequate if used for prolonged periods. Illness or sensory distortions may, in turn, cause or further enhance disturbed adaptation. Inadequate adaptation may occur when there is:

1. Failure to sense change, present or coming; selective focusing on the here-and-now.
2. Adherence to values or beliefs no longer considered valid by the social environment.
3. Undue commitment to unrealistic, immoral, unethical, or inhumane goals.
4. Use of adaptive mechanisms no longer appropriate.
5. Resistance to rational change.
6. Presence of physical disease or disability.
7. Sensory distortion or deprivation.
8. Failure to discriminate because of thought disturbances or organic problems.
9. Severe anxiety feelings.
10. Overspecialization, limiting one's ability to adapt to new and changing circumstances.
11. Focusing on the involved body part or only one aspect of a situation rather than the entire body or situation.

Yet *apparently maladaptive behaviour should be considered as the best that the person is capable of at that time.* So-called deviant behaviour may actually be adaptive and may eventually promote constructive change in or for the person group. Adaptive deviance is seen in the client who demands control over herself and his/her treatment, for example, or in the nonconformist nurse who views a situation from a different perspective, acts accordingly, and improves nursing care as a result. Also, inadequate behaviour in one person may permit others in a group to function appropriately as a result. When a person is sick, the symptoms and problems may inadvertently preserve family equilibrium by drawing attention away from family conflicts.

The sick member may be designated the scapegoat or patient even though other family members are more socially or emotionally ill.


IMPLICATIONS FOR NURSING

Adaptation is a concept that can provide a unifying structure for nursing practice. It can link together the mass of information considered necessary to professional nursing practice. It helps you see how various factors affecting the person do not exist in isolation but in a multi-dimensional whole. It helps you more accurately predict and more effectively help each person adapt to a crisis, illness or disability.

If you are in a leadership position, teach your co-workers to report signs and symptoms of adaptational failure, such as restlessness, withdrawal, rigidity in behaviour, or inability to make a decision, just as they would note a disease symptom. Your knowledge of the patient's *accustomed* adaptive pattern, obtained through a nursing history, will help you formulate a plan of care to meet special needs. Assess needs, ways of coping, and the predominant stimuli affecting that person. If inadequate adaptation is occurring, attempt to modify or manipulate the stimuli to make a positive response possible. Adjusting the physical environment or using methods of purposeful communication is a way to enhance adaptation.

You can use adaptation theory as an independent nurse practitioner. You might be available in a community to promote adaptation where circumstances are making harmful demands – where a disease has broken out or a natural disaster occurred. Or you might do health teaching, diet counselling, support before surgery, discharge planning, and health maintenance among those persons in the community who have health problems in varying degrees.

Whatever the setting in which you practise, your assessments must be based on scientific knowledge, combined with an appreciation of the individual's behavioural responses. There are three basic forms of nursing intervention: (a) support and maintain adaptive behaviours; (b) teach and counsel in order to provide the person with additional or alternative behaviours that would enhance adaptation, and (c) modify physiological, emotional and behavioural patterns to reduce dysfunction. When your intervention influences adaptation favourably and promotes social well-being, it is *therapeutic*. If you cannot alter the course of adaptation and your best efforts only maintain the status quo or a slow downhill course, you are acting in a *supportive* role.

Adaptation as a concept is applicable to the nurse as well as the patient/ client for you will have to adapt to a new and different perspective and lifestyle as you involve yourself actively in the profession. You may feel threatened at times by the challenges. An understanding of yourself and your adaptive capacities will help you to keep faith in yourself and your ability to cope, adapt, learn, grow. You will become more comfortable with change and challenge, recognizing that they are part of normal adult living.

## REFERENCES

1. Murray, Ruth, and Judith Zentner, *Nursing Assessment and Health Promotion Through the Life Span*, 3rd edition (Prentice Hall Inc., Englewood Cliffs, NJ, 1985).
2. Langley, L.L., *Homeostasis* (Reinhold Book Corporation, New York, 1965).
3. McLeod, Dorothy L., 'Physiological Model', in *Theoretical Issues in Professional Nursing*, ed. Juanita F. Murphy, (Appleton-Century-Crofts, New York, 1971).
4. McKay, Rose, 'Theories, Models, and Systems for Nursing', *Nursing Research*, vol. 18 no. 5 (1969) pp. 393–9.
5. Byrne, M., and L. Thompson, *Key Concepts for the Study and Practice of Nursing* (The C.V. Mosby Company, St Louis, 1972).
6. Horowitz, Mardi, *Stress Response Syndromes* (Jason Aronson, Inc., New York, 1976).
7. See note 5, above.
8. See note 6, above.
9. Murray, Ruth and M. Marilyn Huelskoetter, *Psychiatric/Mental Health Nursing: Giving Emotional Care* (Prentice Hall Inc., Englewood Cliffs, NJ, 1983).
10. Luckman, Joan, and Karen Sorensen, eds., *Medical-Surgical Nursing: A Psychophysiologic Approach*, 2nd edition (W.B. Saunders Company, Philadelphia, 1980).
11. Norton, Cynthia Friend, *Microbiology*, Addison-Wesley Publishing Co. Inc., Reading, MA, 1981).
12. Ibid.
13. Ibid.
14. See note 10, above.
15. See note 11, above.
16. Marshall, Eliot, 'Gambling on Interferon', *Science*, vol. 216 no. 4550, (1982), pp. 1078–9.
17. See note 16, above; also Clark, Matt, and Sharon Behley, 'The Making of a Miracle Drug', *Newsweek*, January 28 1980, pp. 82–3.
18. See note 11, above.
19. Ibid.
20. Ibid.
21. Ibid.
22. Ibid.; also see note 10, above.
23. See note 11, above.
24. Ibid.
25. Beneson, Abram, *Control of Communicable Diseases in Man*, 12th edition (American Public Health Association Inc., Washington DC, 1975).

26. Brown, Barbara B., *New Mind New Body* (Bantam Books, New York, 1975).
27. Ibid.
28. Benson, Herbert and Mirian Z. Klipper, *The Relaxation Response* (Avon Books, New York, 1976).
29. See note 5, above; also, Engel, G., *Psychological Development in Health and Disease* (W.B. Saunders Company, Philadelphia, 1962).
30. Ibid.
31. Parsons, T., *Structure and Process in Modern Societies* (The Free Press, Glencoe, IL, 1960).
32. See note 29, above.
33. Toffler, Alvin, *Future Shock* (Random House, Inc., New York, 1970).
34. Messer, Alfred, *The Individual in His Family, An Adaptational Study* (Charles C. Thomas, Publisher, Springfield, IL, 1970).

# 6

# Crisis intervention: a therapy technique

Study of this chapter will help you to:

1. Differentiate between crisis and stress.

2. Identify the types of crisis and give examples of each.

3. Describe factors that influence coping with and the outcome of a crisis.

4. List the phases of crisis and discuss normal behavioural responses in each phase.

5. Compare and contrast reactions of a family, group, or community to a crisis or disaster.

6. Discuss examples of behaviour that indicate a crisis was not adequately resolved, including psychophysiological illness.

7. Discuss the necessity of integrating crisis theory into your philosophy of care.

8. Relate the steps of the nursing process to crisis therapy.

9. Discuss suicidal behaviour in relation to crises.

10. Assess and counsel the person in a suicidal crisis.

11. Work with survivors after intentional death of a loved one.

12. Define *loss, grief* and *mourning* and discuss the crisis of separation and loss as a part of life.

13. Describe the sequence of reactions and behaviours typical of the grief syndrome and mourning process.

14. List factors influencing the mourning process.

15. Explore your role in helping the person who has experienced loss.

16. Apply principles of crisis intervention with the client who has been a victim of physical assault.

17. Discuss factors contributing to the person's definition of and susceptibility to illness.

18. Identify the sick role and behaviours typical of the sick role.

19. Compare the reactions of the person who is ill at home to those of someone hospitalized for illness.

20. List and discuss the stages of illness and tasks of convalescence.

21. Define and discuss the characteristics of and reactions to impaired role behaviour.

22. Discuss reactions of the family to impaired role or to chronic illness or disability.

23. Explore how you can help a person and family resolve the crises of suicide, illness, disability, or loss, or assault.

24. Assess and care for a patient and family in a crisis.

## DEFINITIONS AND CHARACTERISTICS

Crisis theory provides nursing with a theoretical model of the processes of adaptation that follow certain kinds of stressful, disquieting, unmanageable events in the person's life. Its usefulness lies in its systematic organization of events that appear haphazard and unpredictable and in its potential to guide you when working with people in crisis.

**Crisis** *is any transient situation that requires the reorganization of one's psychological structure and behaviour, that causes a sudden alteration in the person's expectation of self, and that cannot be handled with the usual coping mechanisms.*
    The person's ordinary behaviour is no longer successful emotionally, intellectually or physically. Old habits are disturbed and the person feels motivated to try new responses in order to cope with the situation at hand. Even if the person's behaviour is inadequate or inappropriate to the present situation and may differ from normal, it should not be considered pathological. The crisis may also reactivate old unresolved crises or conflicts, which imposes an additional burden to be resolved. The crisis is a turning point, however, and with its resultant mobilization of energy is a second chance to correct earlier maladaptations or faulty problem solving. The time of crisis serves as a catalyst or opportunity for growth emotionally. There is a realignment of behaviour that, if all goes well, will lead to a

state of equilibrium or behaviour that is more mature than the previous status. On the other hand, because of the stress involved and the felt threat to equilibrium, the person is also more vulnerable to regression and mental or physical illness. The outcome – either increased maturity or illness – depends on how the person handles the situation and on the help that others give. Encountering and resolving a crisis are normal processes that each of us faces many times during life.

*Stress*, defined and discussed earlier, must be differentiated from *crisis*. **Stress** *is the everyday wear and tear on the body, the effects of the rate at which you live at any moment, positive and negative, physical, emotional, or mental.* All living organisms are constantly under stress, and anything, pleasant or unpleasant, that speeds up the intensity of life causes a temporary increase in stress or in the wear and tear on the body. A painful blow or a passionate kiss can be equally stressful, for example. Stress does not consist merely of damage but also of the adaptation to damage, and it can be positive and life promoting. During a stressful period the person can use normal coping mechanisms. The temporary upsets in equilibrium are solved by previously learned coping techniques and various mechanisms of tension discharge, such as talking. Stress, however, has a great potential for reducing the person's level of mental health, whereas crisis has a great potential for raising it. Yet both may have either a positive or negative outcome.

Not all persons facing the same hazardous event are in a state of crisis. But certain events or situations are viewed as a crisis by everyone in that some behavioural adjustment must be made by anyone facing that situation. Research by Holmes and Rahe has shown that the number and seriousness of certain types of life changes or crisis recently encountered increase the person's chance of facing other crises, including illness or accidental injury.[1] Crises also vary in degree; a situation may be perceived as major, moderate, or minimal in the degree of discomfort caused and the amount of behavioural change demanded.

Crisis in the person's life can be considered from the standpoint of adaptation theory discussed in Chapter 5. The total person responds to crisis in ways that affect adaptation or higher levels of integration of total body function. The response to crisis is also a way of adapting. Crisis, and one's reaction to it, affects physiological, intellectual, emotional, social and cultural aspects of the person's life as well as of the family unit.


## TYPES OF CRISIS

Two types of crisis affect the person and family systems: (a) developmental, maturational, or normative and (b) situational or accidental.

*Developmental crisis*

**Developmental crises** *are transition points, the periods that everyone experiences in the process of biopsychosocial growth and development and that are accompanied by changes in thoughts, feelings and abilities.* These are times in development when new relationships are formed and old relationships take on new aspects. Others have new expectations of the person and certain physical, emotional, intellectual and social tasks must be accomplished so that the person can move to the next phase of development. The onset of the developmental or maturational crisis is gradual because it occurs as the person moves from one stage of growth and development to another; the crisis does not last for the entire era, however.

Why does normal development leave the person vulnerable to crisis? Spiegel's description of role theory is helpful for understanding.

**Role** *is a goal-directed pattern of behaviour learned within one's cultural setting and carried out by the person in the social group or situation because both the person and the group expect this behaviour.* No role exists in isolation. It is always patterned to dovetail with or complement the role of another. When one person changes role, the role partners – other persons in the system – undergo reciprocal role or behavioural changes. The times of maturational or developmental crisis are mainly periods of many role changes, although they may be slow and gradual and vary from one culture or class to another. A maturational crisis occurs when the person is unable to make role changes appropriate to a new level of maturity. The stressful events are the social and biological pressures on the individual to see the self in a new and different role and act accordingly.[2]

There are three main reasons why someone may be unable to make the role changes necessary to prevent a maturational crisis:

1. The person's inability to picture the self in a new role. Roles are learned; adequate role models may not exist.
2. The person may be unable to make role changes because of lack of intrapersonal resources – for example, inadequate communication skills, realization that with life passing it is not possible to achieve certain goals, or inability to realize alternatives to the present lifestyle.
3. Refusal by others in the social system to see the person in a different role. When the adolescent tries to move from childhood to the adult role, for instance, the parent may persist in keeping him/her in the child role.

The primary developmental crisis are entry into school, puberty, leaving home, engagement, marriage, pregnancy, childbirth, middle age, menopause, retirement, and facing the death of others and of the self.

*Situational crisis*

The **situational crisis** *is an external event or situation – one not necessarily a part of normal living and often sudden, unexpected, and unfortunate – that is too threatening to the person's immediate resources or ability to cope and that requires a change in behaviour.* The self-concept is threatened. The person feels overwhelmed and helpless. There is a threat or danger to life goals; tension and anxiety are evoked; unresolved problems and crisis from the past are reawakened. The amount of time taken for healthy or unhealthy adaption to occur may take as little as 1 to 6 weeks, or as long as 6 months or a year, depending on the situation, its meaning to the person, and the inner resources and outer support system available. A situational crisis may occur at the same time as a developmental crisis.

Situational crisis include natural disasters, such as a hurricane, tornado or flood; loss through separation, divorce from, or death of a loved one; losing one's job, money, or valued possessions; and a change in job. Illness or hospitalization, a power struggle at work, a promotion or sudden change in role responsibilities, or a forced geographical relocation are other examples. Suicide attempts and violence, such as rape or being a victim of crime, can also be classified as this type of crisis.

Adaptation to loss of a loved one through death, divorce, stillbirth or neonatal death can be delayed for up to 5 years, in some cases. There are indications that the adaptive/coping mechanisms slow down with increasing age.

## FACTORS INFLUENCING THE OUTCOME OF CRISIS

Various factors influence how someone reacts to and copes with crisis situations:

1. *The person's perception of the event.* If the event or its consequences conflict with the value system or wishes for the future, the situation is defined as hazardous. The perception of the event is reality for the person regardless of how others might define reality, and determines behaviour. To illustrate, two persons live through the disaster of a flood. One loses a house and all possessions; the other loses a boat, but everything else is intact. Yet the latter may react with greater shock, denial, anger, or depression than the person who loses a home and possessions because of their different perceptions – the meaning to each of the loss.
2. *The physical and emotional status* of the person, degree of health, amount of energy present, age, genetic endownment, and biological rhythms.

3. *The coping techniques or mechanisms and the level of personal maturity.* If adaptive capacities are already strained, or if the stress is overwhelming, the person will cling to old habits and the behaviour will probably be inappropriate to the task at hand. The person who has met developmental tasks all along will adapt more easily in any crisis.

4. *Previous experiences with similar situations.* The person must learn to cope with stress and change. If someone resolved past crisis by distorting reality or withdrawing, then when similar crisis arise, the person must attempt to cope with a new situation while burdened with prior failure. Crisis of any kind are often cumulative in effect. The most recent crisis revives the denial, depression, anger, or maladaptation that was left unsettled or unresolved from past crises.

5. *The objectively realistic aspects of the current situation,* such as personal or material losses, and the number of life crisis changes encountered in the past year.

6. *Cultural influences.* How the person is trained and socialized in the home to solve problems and meet crisis situations, expectations of how the social group will be supportive during crisis, and the method established by the social system to provide help all influence present behaviour.

7. *The availability and response of family and close friends or other helping resources,* including professional persons. The less readily available the person's environmental or emotional support systems are to decrease stress or buttress coping responses, the more hazardous he/she will define the event. The family system, by its influence on development of self-concept and maturity, can increase or decrease vulnerability to crisis. When someone's involvement with others is concentrated on only a few family members – as, for example, in the nuclear versus the extended family support system – vulnerability is increased. The reaction to crisis is also increased in today's mobile, urbanized society because traditional support systems of long-term family and friends have been disrupted. Thus the professional person is more likely to be needed and sought. Even a small amount of influence exerted by a significant person can be enough to decide the outcome for mental health and against mental illness. Sustained mental health, however, is chiefly a result of a life history of successfully resolving crisis. The family, like the individual, may be **crisis prone,** *vulnerable to situational or developmental crisis that occur frequently and have a cumulative effect.*

The crisis-prone person or family often demonstrates the following characteristics:

1. Rapid encountering of one stressful situation after another, with inadequate time to adjust or to cope with any one situation.
2. A history of inadequate coping skills.
3. Lack of communication skills or inability to ask for help because of emotional isolation from others.

4. Feelings about solving problems alone because of loss of persons or things that were viewed as supportive or because of feelings of racial or ethnic prejudice, demoralization, or alienation.
5. Inadequate family, social, religious, economic or employment supportive resources.

Frequent illness or accidents, legal problems, or abuse of alcohol or other drugs may also increase the risk of other crises.
   Crisis effects are reduced by

1. Anticipating and preparing for the so-called unpredictable events, such as change of developmental stages, natural disasters or death.
2. Redefining or changing goals when something seems insurmountable.
3. Developing communication skills and a support system.
4. Seeking help to work through each crisis and unresolved past crises. [3]


PHASES OF CRISIS

All crises require a sudden and then later restructuring of biopsychosocial integration before normal function can be maintained. The phases involved are shock, followed closely by general realization of the crisis; then defensive retreat; acknowledgment; and, finally, adaptation or resolution.

**In the initial, impact, or shock phase** the person briefly realizes the seriousness and threat of the situation and then feels a high level of stress, helplessness, anxiety, chaos, and possibly panic. He/she feels overwhelmed and depersonalized. Self-esteem is threatened, and thinking and behaviour are disorganized. The person is unable to plan, to reason logically, or to understand the situation. Judgment is impaired. Habitual or automatic problem-solving behaviours are used without success, although the person cannot perceive any inadequacy. He/she may suffer physical illness or injury and either focus attention on them or completely ignore the physical status. Socially the person is unable to function appropriately, becoming withdrawn, docile, or perhaps hyperactive and chaotic. Basic needs cannot be met without help.
   The shock phase usually lasts a short time, perhaps a few hours or a day or two. The reactions of the alarm stage of the stress syndrome discussed in Chapter 5 cannot be tolerated for too long. On either perceiving or being told what has happened, the person copes with the realization of the sudden discontinuity in life through the second phase, defensive retreat.

**In defensive retreat** the person tries previously successful ways of solving problems and adjusting, but tension and discomfort are not reduced and the situation is not alleviated. He/she feels increasingly upset and ineffective. At the first try the problem is directly approached, but the behaviour does not work. Then he/she may try to redefine the problem (usually unrealistically), avoid the problem, or seek the support of others. Generally the person retreats into the self, avoiding reality, denying, fantasizing about what could be done or how well he/she once handled problems. The person may become disoriented, indifferent, apathetic or euphoric. Usually because of repression, the person will claim to feel all right and will not perceive the anxiety and ineffective behaviour. Changes suggested by others are resisted; a rigid manner of thinking and expressing the same ideas over and over are common. Behaviour is ineffective and disorganized; daily activities cannot be carried out. The person cannot devise alternate courses of action and cannot predict accurately the effects of behaviour. Physical symptoms are generally minimal; the person may feel better than usual. Socially the person may be withdrawn or superficial and hyperactive and unable to maintain social roles adequately. The phase of defensive retreat may last for a brief or prolonged period, depending on circumstances.

Denial is a mechanism used in defensive retreat and involves use of three other mental mechanisms:

1. Rationalization about discomfort or symptoms and the cause of the situation (for example, the person with chest pain says that it is indigestion).
2. Displacement of dangerous, disquieting, uncomfortable information onto the health team or family, often in the form of demands or complaints.
3. Projection of personal feelings of inadequacy onto others, saying how inept or neglectful others are.

The purposes of these mechanisms are to protect the self from painful information.

**The third phase, recoil or acknowledgment**, begins when the facts can no longer be denied. The person realizes the objective reality of the situation and slowly begins to redefine it, attempting to do problem solving. Tension and anxiety again rise. Reality may seem harsh; and depression, agitation, apathy, self-hate, low self-esteem, and the process of mourning occur. The person's coping abilities and self-concept may disintegrate before energy can be directed toward coping. Thinking may at first be disorganized, but gradually the person can make appropriate plans and find solutions for the situation by trial and error. Physically he/she may feel well or tension may be somaticized. The person will give up certain goals as unattainable. The person will recognize that he/she has been a social burden and make plans to resume former roles to the degree possible.

**The fourth phase, resolution or adaptation and change**, occurs when the person perceives the crisis situation in a positive way and integrates the painful event into the new self. Problem solving is successful and feelings about the event are expressed. A new sense of worth, a firm identity, a gradual increase in satisfaction in mastering the situation, and a gradual lowering of anxiety result. Thinking and planning are organized; appropriate resources and abilities are used. Physically the person is functioning at the optimum level. Socially he/she resumes status and roles and repatterns behaviour to cope and thus avoid future similar crises. In order to integrate the crisis into the personality, the person must develop a different concept of self and the lifestyle. The person does not feel bitter about the event encountered or changes made.

At this point the person should be at a higher level of maturity and adaptation than earlier. He/she has acquired new coping mechanisms.

Resolving the crisis is made more difficult by the negative influences discussed earlier and by additional hardships or complications caused by the crisis itself. Ineffective mastery or problem solving or lack of expression of feelings associated with the crisis may cause a restricted level of functioning in one or all spheres of the personality. The problem may be repressed and permanently denied and unresolved or major disorganization such as neurosis, psychosis, socially maladjusted behaviour, or chronic physical disability, may occur.

These are the predictable phases of crisis; however, each stage is not sharply demarcated. One stage may merge into another or certain behaviours may not appear at all, particularly in developmental crisis in which the person's functioning may be appropriate in one sphere but less so in another aspect of the personality. In addition, the person may be at the beginning of one phase and then return to the previous phase behaviourally. Thus the person may demonstrate some behaviours indicative of one phase – such as defensive retreat – and simultaneously demonstrate a few behaviours of shock or acknowledgment.

*Family reactions*

The family unit undergoes essentially the same phases of crisis and manifests similar reactions as the designated client, although the intensity and timing may differ.

If the source of trouble is from within the family, it is usually perceived as more distressing than an external source of trouble, for internal problems reflect lack of harmony and inadequacy in the members. Shock and defensive retreat reactions may be more pronounced during times of internal trouble. As acknowledgment of reality occurs, there is a strong tendency to scapegoat family members to restore family balance. Crisis events for the family include the developmental and situational crisis previously discussed.

*Group or community reactions*

A social group or entire neighbourhood may feel the impact of an individual or family in crisis.

The community is also affected by natural disasters, such as a flood, tornado, hurricane or blizzard; by disasters resulting from advances in our civilization, such as chemical or radiation spills and electrical blackouts; and by disasters for which humans are responsible, such as fire or war.

Community reactions to any of these disasters are influenced[4] by the following factors:

1. Element of surprise versus preparedness. If warnings are not given about an impending crisis – or if warnings are given without an action plan – panic, shock, denial, and defensive retreat are more likely to occur.
2. Separation of family members. Children are especially affected by separation; the family should be evacuated from a disaster area as a unit.
3. Availability of outside help.
4. Leadership. Someone must make decisions and give directions. Usually the police, Red Cross and Civil Defence workers, St John Ambulance, military, or professionals in a community are seen as authoritative persons. Coordination of the activities of all these groups is essential to deliver services and avoid chaos.
5. Communication. Public information centres must be established to avoid rumour, provide reassurance and direction, and ensure that all citizens get information about coping measures, evacuation, reconstruction, rehabilitation, and available financial aid. Otherwise citizens will later be bitter and suspicious when some learn that others benefitted more than they did.
6. Measures taken to help reorientation. Communication networks lay the foundation for re-identification of individuals into family and social groups and for registration of survivors.
7. Presence of plans for individuals and social institutions to cope with dis-

aster, including evacuation of a population from a stricken area if necessary. Emergency plans focus on the following concerns:

(a) Preservation of life and health through rescue, triage, inoculation and treatment of the injured.
(b) Conservation and distribution of resources, such as shelter, water, food and blankets.
(c) Conservation of public order by police surveillance to prevent looting and further accidents or injuries.
(d) Maintenance of morale through dispatching health and welfare workers to the disaster scene.
(e) Administration of health services.

Communities in crisis have characteristics in common with individuals in crisis. The most immediate social consequence of a disaster is disruption of normal social patterns and services; the community is socially paralyzed.

In a major disaster about 75 to 90 per cent of the victims will be in shock, followed by the phase of defensive retreat, in response to warnings of disaster, orders of evacuation, destruction of homes, and disruption of water, electricity, heat, food supplies, communication, traffic and transportation. Also, there is potential inability of the health agencies to care for the injured and ill because of manpower and supply shortages or damage. In addition to individual reactions, an atmosphere of tension, fear, confusion and suspicion exists; facts are distorted and rumours are rampant. Normal functioning is reduced as businesses, vital services, schools and recreational areas may be closed. Although some people are in shock or denial, there will be a few who take advantage of the chaos to loot and steal and a few businesses may profiteer.[5]

Response to external emergencies is often quicker than the response to internal stresses or crises. About 10 to 25 per cent of the victims remain reality orientated, calm, and able to develop and implement a plan of action; such people often are those with advanced training. But these crisis workers may react with at least brief periods of shock and defensive retreat after most of the immediate work is done.

When reality is acknowledged, people in the community at first become more cohesive as they help each other; then individual problems become the focus. People find shelter, look for someone to be with, want to be cared for, express a sense of loss through crying and talking, and share with others how they managed to survive. During this time, depending on the amount of damage, anger and frustration are keenly felt as the person evaluates the damage and feels robbed of possessions that have been worked for throughout life. The older, dependent, or incapacitated person may become seriously ill or die because he/she feels unable to start all over again. If loved ones were killed, grief and mourning for them, as well as for lost possessions, result. Guilt reactions as a result of being unable to save the loved one, of being spared death, and a relief at being alive are common. Reactive depression, anxiety reactions, regression, dreams, suicidal thoughts, physical illness, psychotic episodes, and neurotic reactions occur and may last for several months or a year after the disaster. The more severe the disaster, the longer these reactions last. Some people's psyches may be permanently damaged. Older people who suffer a disaster are statistically more likely to die within the year following the disaster. Also, psychological effects are more severe and slower to resolve when survivors perceive the disaster as a result of human callousness or error rather than as an act of God or nature.[6]

Resolution occurs in individuals as previously described and is related to the individual's psychological health before the crisis as well as to the kind of help given to the family unit during the disaster, the kind of crisis and extent of damage, and the ability of the community to repair damage and return to normal function. Perhaps the best sign of community resolution is a well-developed disaster plan of action, one that can be implemented in the event of another crisis, and community-wide education for individual and family preparedness for disaster.

If there is no adaptive resolution or change in behaviour to cope with the crisis, maladaptive or ineffective reactions occur as an attempt at resolution. There may be a delayed reaction in that the crisis event and its consequences are presently denied and repressed. A reaction is eventually precipitated when a future crisis occurs that recalls the buried feelings and that then renders the person ineffective in functioning. Various other reactions of distorted or inappropriate behaviour may occur, although neurosis, psychosis, or socially ineffective behaviour occur only in a small percentage of people. The person may be euphoric if denial is prolonged. In the crisis of death of a loved one the person may prolong identification with the deceased by developing symptoms like those in the last illness of the deceased. And eventually the organic pathological changes specific for the disease may occur. Sometimes such illness occurs on the anniversary of the loss. Or the aggrieved person may develop a different disease, caused by the **mind-body relationship** – *in which physiological changes result because of the effects of emotional states on body parts and which eventually cause organ damage. (Illness resulting from the effects of the emotional state is also called* **psychosomatic illness**.)

Statistics show that bereaved relatives are found to have a higher mortality rate during the first year of mourning, a rate that increased further for widowed persons. The risk of the close relative dying from the effects of anxiety, hostility and guilt during that first year was significantly increased when the loved one had died at some place other than home.

Personality significantly mitigates the illness-providing effects of stressful life events. Two groups of executives had comparably high degrees of stress over a 3-year interval as measured by the Holmes and Rahe schedule of recent life events. One group suffered high stress without becoming ill; the other reported becoming ill after an encounter with stressful life events. Illness was predictably related to personality. In comparison with high-stress, high-illness executives, high-stress, low-illness executives show more control, commitment to the job, and interest in change as a challenge rather than change as stress. Individuals with a high need for power who are inhibited in expressing feelings are more likely than others to report severe illnesses, apparently related to chronic overactivity of the sympathetic nervous system, with above-average epinephrine excretion and lower concentrations of immunoglobins.

Sudden death has occurred in persons who feel depressed, helpless, hopeless, acutely anxious or angry following a crisis situation, apparently from disequilibrium in the hormonal and autonomic nervous systems.

Maladaptation may include expressing hostility for an excessively prolonged time against authority figures – doctors, nurses, police officers, parents or teachers. Prolonged sadness, apathy, lack of initiative, irritability, suspicion, and withdrawing from others because of internalized anger or shock can be equally detrimental to relationships with others and to overall conduct. Feelings of isolation, worthlessness, hopelessness and guilt may become magnified to the point of inducing suicide attempts. Then again, the person may suppress his/her own personality, taking on traits of the lost person.

The person who stays compulsively busy or is ritualistic may become ineffective in attempts to cope. Alcohol, drugs, or excessive eating may become a crutch or escape when activity no longer provides adequate tension release.

The person may engage in action detrimental to the self economically or socially through excessive generosity or foolish financial dealings (which represent self-punishment) or through delinquency. The latter invites apprehension, punishment and, at times, someone else making the decisions.

After loss of a loved one, the person, through extreme denial, may continue to act as though the lost person is still alive and present. The survivor, for instance, may continue to set a place at the table for the deceased or keep all the possessions of the lost one. Or the person may acknowledge the death but deny the significance of the loss emotionally or intellectually. He/she may not take care of business matters because the deceased person was the person who previously did so.

You have an opportunity to help prevent maladaptive resolution through appropriate crisis intervention. When assessing the person in any illness situation, determine if the problems and needs could be the result of an earlier crisis that is now causing symptoms or inappropriate behaviour.

Working with someone who has maladaptive behaviour can be a slow process. You should not expect too much of yourself or the other, for in your disappointment and frustration you may withdraw from him/her, thus preventing crisis resolution. Recognize your strengths and limitations and decide whether the person can use help beyond what you can offer. Accept the fact that because this person is unique, available knowledge and techniques may not be of sufficient help. On the other hand, a possibility of failure should not preclude an attempt to help.

Provide an environment in which the person can experience the phases of recovery from any maladaptive behaviour or illness. Help him/her reminisce about what he/she used to do, express fear, look forward optimistically but realistically to the future, and use appropriate rehabilitative measures.

## THE NURSING PROCESS AND CRISIS INTERVENTION

You will encounter crises in a variety of settings: the emergency room, recovery room, coronary-care unit, surgical intensive-care unit, industrial or school clinics, and the obstetric, paediatric, and psychiatric units. In most of these settings you will collaborate with the physician and other health-team members. In the mental or neighbourhood health centre you may function as primary carer within the agency policy or with other health-team members.

Your philosophy of care must include the concept of crisis. The person in crisis is at a turning point and ready for great changes in a relatively short period of time because of the tension, pain and disequilibrium associated with crisis. These feelings motivate efforts to alter the situation. Distress creates an openness to assistance and change. The person expects expert help and perceives the nurse as an expert. A minimal amount of support and help can influence the outcome of a crisis significantly.

Crisis therapy is based on the theory that aid during crisis will help the person to adapt in a healthy manner. The minimal goal of therapy is psychological resolution of the immediate crisis and the restoration of coping mechanisms to at least the level of functioning that existed before the crisis event. The maximal goal is to bring about a change in behaviour that is more mature than that of the precrisis level. Crisis work involves reinstating earlier stress-reducing behaviour or developing new adaptive techniques. Underlying these goals is the assumption that the person seeking help has unused resources that, with minimum assistance, can be called on to function effectively in everyday living.

Factors influencing the course of crisis therapy are as follows:

1. Attitude of the therapist and the value placed on crisis work.
2. Use of time, in that assessment is done as quickly as possible to define

accurately the nature of the crisis, identify the person's response to the event, and devise a course of action for resolving the crisis.

3. Use of nontraditional treatment practices, for appointment time and place are determined by the degree of stress and impaired functioning that the person is experiencing, the skill of the therapist, and the number and kind of resources in the community available to assist the person.

4. Differences between the value systems of the therapist and the individual concerned. The therapist must be open to what constitutes a problem for another. The person's lifestyle and values may be foreign to or in conflict with those of the therapist, but the person needs acceptance in order to maintain a basic lifestyle and value system.

*Assessment*

Collecting information must be systematic and yet flexible, rapid enough to interrupt the crisis, but thorough enough to define the problem and phase of crisis and identify and achieve the desired outcomes.

The following factors should be assessed: the anxiety level and feelings of the person; ego functioning (perception, judgment, memory, problem solving); presence of symptoms; whether the person is suicidal or homicidal; and usual living patterns, work arrangements, and interpersonal and social situation. Nonverbal behaviour and the consistency between verbal and nonverbal behaviour must be noted. The person does not always mean what is said and will not always act in a way that directly expresses true feelings. If the person cannot identify the problem because of disorganized thinking, focus attention on what was occurring just prior to the situation and onset of symptoms. Constructing a sequence of events aids reorientation.

After determining the extent of the problem, focus the person's perception on the event – for example, the illness or loss. What does this situation mean to him/her? How does he/she see its effect on the future? Is the event seen realistically? What hardships have been created by the crisis? For example, job loss due to depression or mental illness, which, in turn, causes financial and family problems and loss of self-esteem.

Ascertain if the person is suicidal or plans to kill another person. If so, try to learn how and when. If the intention is carefully planned and details are specific, hospitalization and psychiatric evaluation must be arranged to protect the person and others.

Your next questions should be directed to the availability of help and supportive others or the extent of isolation from significant relationships. What is the person's relationship with supportive other? Crisis intervention is sharply limited in time. The more persons who are helping, the better. Then, too, when crisis therapy is terminated, if helpful others are involved, they can continue to give support to the person. Assess the adaptive capacities of the others involved in the situation who have not sought help but who might also be experiencing crises. If no helpful resources are available, you become a temporary support system while helping the person to establish a relationship with a person or group in the community or work setting.

Ascertain what the person usually does when confronted with an unsolvable problem. What are the coping skills? Has anything like this happened before? What was done to decrease tension? If the person is trying the same method now and it is not working, what *would* decrease stress symptoms? Any past activity that proved successful could be tried again. Determine strengths and not just problems and limitations.

Through assessment you can determine why this situation is a crisis to this person, why he/she is unable to alter lifestyle to cope with the situation, and what in the lifestyle can be altered so that the crisis can be resolved.

*Planning intervention*

As you study the data collected in the preceding manner, the person should also be actively involved in seeking a potential solution. You cannot solve the problem for the person; you can only help that individual to help the self.

The problem should be clarified and the immediate situation put in focus. The plan for intervention is determined by assessing the nature of the crisis (whether acute or chronically recurring), the reactions of others significant to the person, and the strengths and resources of all persons involved. The plan for intervention must extend beyond the person to others involved less directly in the crisis. To understand the person's adaptive capacity in comparison to precrisis adaptation, some attention must be paid both to past experience and to current personal and environmental resources.

Several alternate solutions should be explored. Positive guidelines for action should be given to the person before leaving each session, including the first one, so that alternate solutions can be tested. This step permits evaluation of coping behaviour at each successive session so that additional solutions can be sought if necessary.

*Intervention*

Some help can be provided during the first interview by clarifying the problem with the person and encouraging verbalization of feelings. Getting a hold on a problem by talking it through is the first step in problem solving. The person can begin to recognize what this situation means, how to cope with it, and what or who can help. The resultant increase in self-confidence motivates further coping behaviour.

Use primary, secondary, or tertiary preventive intervention, depending on the person and the crisis.

**Primary prevention,** *or preventing a crisis,* can be achieved by helping the person work through developmental periods or anticipated situations.

The anticipation of life crisis is an important concept in health promotion and so has broad implications in nursing. If able to prepare for what is potentially in store, the person will be less vulnerable to physical or mental illness. The more thorough the thinking, planning, or 'work of worry' before a crisis, the more adequate is the subsequent adjustment and the less severe is the impact felt. Persons with either excessively high or excessively low levels of fear or worry, however, are ineffective in preparing for crisis. The high-level worrier feels so much fear that something bad will happen that it is impossible to effectively plan ahead. The low-level worrier does not adequately contemplate impending stress and feels anger and resentment when it comes. The moderately worrisome person can express tension physically, emotionally and verbally, but maintains self-control and thus rationally plans and adjusts behaviour to the situation.

You can help the person do the 'work of worry' or anticipatory grieving in the following ways: through premarital counselling to increase the chance of healthy resolution of stressful marital events and the achievement of appropriate developmental tasks; teaching and counselling in prenatal classes to prepare for childbirth and child care; talking with a mother whose child will soon enter school or be married; preretirement counselling to help the person plan ahead to meet the problems and developmental tasks associated with retirement; counselling the family of a terminally ill patient; and talking preoperatively with the person who is undergoing major surgery and body-image changes. Can you think of other situations in which primary prevention can promote health?

Preventive intervention is not designed to cause major changes in the maturity of personality structure of the person but rather to maintain the usual level of functioning of equilibrium.

**Secondary prevention** *involves early identification of the crisis so the person can avoid maladaptive behaviour.* The person is helped to adapt to the crisis, thereby reducing the intensity and duration of reaction to it. He/she is quickly given support, encouraged to use energies and available resources constructively, and helped to understand that his/her feelings and behaviour are a normal response to the situation.

Examples of secondary prevention in crisis therapy are working with women who have not resolved the crisis of motherhood and extending help to the person who is mourning the loss of a significant person, object or role.

**Tertiary prevention** *is aimed at preventing further decompensation or impairment, after the person has partially resolved a crisis, so that he/she can continue to live a useful role in the community.* The person's behaviour may initially interfere with rehabilitation. When able to resolve the meaning or implications of the crisis and feelings about it, the person will be able to become involved in rehabilitation. Progress depends strongly on the counselling role of the nurse and on continuity in the nurse-client relationship. Through this kind of intervention, the person may eventually rework the crisis and become more effective behaviourally. Examples of tertiary prevention are group therapy with chronically ill or disabled persons to help them cope with their health problems, counselling to help a person work through delayed mourning, and remotivation techniques to prevent further disengagement in the aged.

Crisis therapy is basically brief and specific to the present situation and involves placing attainable goals directly before the person. Thus the principles of crisis intervention are relevant to all people, including those concerned primarily with the here and now, who prefer brief, concrete intervention, and who seek assistance for specific problems.

The person or family in crisis becomes more susceptible to the influence of significant others. A little help directed purposefully and with the right timing is more effective than greater help given at a period of less emotional accessibility. View yourself as intervening in a social system, into a network of relationships, and not as a single resource to the person. Use the skills of other health-team members – the doctor, social worker, chaplain, psychologist and occupational therapist – either directly or for consultation.

**Principles of intervention**, discussed next, can be accomplished by using your knowledge of crisis theory, therapeutic communication and establishment of a nurse-client relationship.

Show acceptance of the person and establish a positive, concerned relationship so that he/she feels a sense of hope, self-worth and lessened anxiety.

During crisis you are often confronted by an angry, bitter or accusatory person or family who berate you, other health-team members, or the agency for negligence. Keep two points in mind: their statements may be accurate and justified or that may be the only way they can cope with their own aggression, helplessness or guilt at the time. Provide the best care possible, show genuine concern, and do not become verbally involved in the dispute. Do not take the behaviour personally if it does not apply to you.

Help the person confront the crisis by talking about present feelings of denial, anger, guilt or grief. Catharsis lowers tension, clarifies the problem, promotes comprehension of the reality and consequences of the situation, and mobilizes energy for constructive action.

Help the person confront the crisis in amounts of 'doses' that can be managed, being cautious not to soften the impact of the event too much. The reality of the situation must be kept in the foreground, although periods of relief from facing the whole situation are needed. Help the person first gain an intellectual understanding of the crisis; then encourage an emotional understanding and adjustment. In this way, he/she can more objectively handle the real situation.

Recognize denial as a normal reaction. Cope with personal feelings about the person's behaviour and situation; observe such behaviour objectively; avoid reinforcing denial; and gently represent reality. Work with other resource persons for information, collaboration, maintenance of support, and representation of reality.

Explain to the person the relationship between the crisis situation and the present behaviour and feelings. People feel less overwhelmed and better able to manage when they understand that the feelings are normal in the context of crisis.

Help the person find facts, for facts are less awesome than speculations or fantasies about the situation or the unknown.

Explore past life occurrences only in relation to the existing crisis, particularly if feelings aroused in past crises have been unresolved and are influencing present behaviour. The present experience can produce defensive behaviours used in the past that are no longer useful.

Avoid giving false reassurance. Acknowledge the validity of fears and other feelings. Show faith in the person's ability to manage, but do not reduce motivation to cope and adapt by saying that everything will be fine.

Do not encourage the person to blame others for the crisis event, for this process avoids the truth, reduces motivation to take responsibility for personal behaviour, and discourages adaptation. Listen initially to rationalizations; then raise doubt about such statements through questioning.

Anticipate that people facing loss may behave in a grossly maladaptive way and need to be treated with tact, patience, warmth and empathy, as well as encouraged to express feelings without feeling guilty about doing so. Set limits on behaviour that would be destructive to the person or to others.

Explore coping mechanisms to assist the person in examining alternate ways of coping and in seeking and using new behaviours or alternate ways of satisfying needs. Help him/her to learn or relearn basic social skills as necessary and to fit the personality to the demands presented by the crisis.

Strengthen or reinforce previously learned behaviour patterns that can be effective but are not presently being used.

Clarify and reemphasize responsibility for personal behaviour, decisions and way of life. For example, the person in crisis from illness and hospitalization should be assisted in learning the patient role. Thus, any uncertainty about expectations for self and others is replaced by the feeling of being a participating member of the treatment team. Therefore orientation to the hospital division's policies and routines, the room, personnel, diagnostic procedures, and preoperative and postoperative care is necessary. When aware of the possible outcomes of the illness, the person can make decisions about present care goals and future health needs. When he/she knows what to expect from the health-team members, behaviour can be adaptive. Health-care workers can be resources to improve the health status.

Help the person establish necessary social relationships and change personal behaviour accordingly. If someone has lost or is otherwise removed from all significant persons, as might be true for the elderly or new immigrants, introduce the person to new people to help fill the void and obtain support and gratification.

Assist the person in seeking and accepting health. By acknowledging that trouble exists, he/she is more likely to use personal resources and the help offered by others. If necessary, encourage acceptance of help with the everyday tasks of living and mobilization of inner strengths as well as concerned others in the environment.

Although you work with a person or family in crisis therapy, some crises may upset an entire community, such as natural disasters. Use of support systems and role redistribution is then more complex.

Beware of creating dependency or be prepared to withdraw support very slowly.

**Crisis resolution and anticipatory planning** terminate crisis intervention. Crisis work is then reviewed and the accomplishments of the person in working through the predicament should be emphasized. Adaptive coping mechanisms and appropriate behaviour that the person has successfully used should be reinforced. Positive changes in behaviour should be summarized to allow reexperiencing and reconfirming the progress made. Give assistance as needed in making realistic plans for the future and discuss with the person ways in which the present experience may help in coping with future crises. The person should leave with self-confidence in managing his/her life and with the awareness that assistance will be available in the future if necessary.

**Evaluation.** In order to continue to do effective crisis intervention, the step of evaluation in the nursing process must be carried out as discussed in Chapter 3.

## CARE OF THE HOSPITALIZED SUICIDE ATTEMPTER

The client who regains consciousness after a suicide attempt may severely test your attitude and beliefs about suicidal behaviour. A wide range of behaviours may be seen: anger and dismay at still being alive, euphoria, denial, apathy, belligerence – in fact, almost any behaviour seen in the first three phases of active crisis. Because these clients are in active crisis as well as psychological pain, they are unable at this point to make an informed and rational choice about their 'right to die' – in the authors' opinion. Your role is to see alternatives and hope for the client when he/she cannot.

Here are some general guidelines to follow:

1. A current suicidal assessment should be recorded and communicated.
2. Detailed data on the actual attempt, steps of the attempter took to avoid discovery, *the attempter's notion of the toxicity of the drug, likelihood of rescue,* and so on need to be recorded. (Too often we base our conclusions about intent on *our* notions of toxicity, rescue, and so forth).
3. Be aware that the behaviour that you see immediately postattempt may be highly altered by the physiological effects of the attempt or the psychological effects of rescue and may tell you almost nothing about the psychological status of the client prior to the attempt.
4. Observe and interact! Don't leave a vulnerable client more isolated than he/she was prior to hospitalization. Simply offer your quiet presence at frequent intervals if that is all the client can tolerate.
5. Accept the attempter's perception of his/her life situation as valid for him/her at that point in time.
6. Attend to the family and significant others. Are they in a phase of crisis? Minimizing or denying the event? Seemingly suicidogenic or helpful?

### THE CRISIS OF SEPARATION AND LOSS

The crisis of separation and loss can be either developmental or situational in origin and both may occur simultaneously.

*Life – a series of losses*

Loss and the universal reaction to loss, grief and mourning are experienced by everyone at some time in their lives and frequently you are the one most involved with and available to the person who is experiencing loss.

As one's interdependence with others grows, the likelihood increases that separation, loss of something valuable, or death of a loved one will induce a crisis. The capacity to have warm and loving relationships also leaves one vulnerable to sadness, despair and grief. The more one has emotionally invested in what is lost, the greater the threat felt to the self.

Every person is also subjected to separations or losses that are subtle and may not be recognized. Any crisis, developmental or situational, involves some degree of loss. If nothing else, there is a loss through change in old behaviour patterns and the addition of different coping mechanisms. The process of achieving independence in psychosocial development in the course of normal upbringing involves a whole series of separations. The way these early separations are dealt with affects how later separations and loss, including death, will be resolved.

1. Period of weaning in infancy; learning to wait.
2. First haircut, even when it involves pride and anticipation.
3. Period of increasing locomotion, exploration, and bowel and bladder control and resultant loss of dependency.
4. Loss of baby teeth, baby possessions, toys, clothes or pets during development.
5. Change in the body, body image and self-attitude with ongoing growth and development.
6. Change in body size and shape and in feelings accompanying pregnancy and childbirth; loss of body part or function, external or internal, through accident, illness, or aging.
7. Departure of children from the home when they go to school or marry.
8. Menopause and loss of childbearing functions.
9. Loss of hearing, vision, memory, strength, and other changes and losses associated with old age.
10. Changes and losses in relationships with others as the person moves from childhood to adulthood – loss of friends and lovers; separation from or death of family members; changes in residence, occupation, or place of business; promotions and graduations.
11. Losses that have symbolic meanings, such as the loss of a symptom that attracted others' attention, a loss or change that necessitates a change in body image, or 'loss of face', honour or prestige.
12. Loss of home due to natural disaster or relocation projects; loss of possessions or money.
13. Loss experienced with divorce or incapacitation of a loved one.

Thus the person brings to any major crisis a backlog of experience that predisposes either successful integration of a personal tragedy or failure to absorb another loss or change. The significance of the present reaction may become clear only when you understand the person's earlier separations and losses.

*Definitions*

**Loss** can be defined as giving up external or internal supports required by the person to satisfy basic needs. In regard to loss, the term **object** may mean a person, thing, relationship or situation.

**Grief** is a sequence of subjective states, a special intense form of sorrow caused by loss, either through separation or death of a loved person or loss of an object that is felt to be a part of the self or that provides psychological gratification. Grief is the emotion involved in the work of mourning. Absence of what is lost is felt as a gap in one's sense of continuity and self-concept.

Grief reaction differs from depression in that cognitive disorders, such as gross distortion of events, are not normally present in grief; also, the reaction is more directly proportional to the amount of loss. In depression, the feeling of sadness and self-depreciation affects the person physically, intellectually, cognitively, emotionally, socially and spiritually; it is out of proportion to the apparent situation and it is more greatly influenced by developmental and symbolic changes.

**Mourning** is a broad range of reactions, a psychological process that follows either loss of a significant or valued object or person, or realization that such a loss could occur. It is the process whereby the person seeks to disengage self from an emotionally demanding relationship and reinvest emotionally in a new and productive relationship.

*Grief and the mourning process*

A review of the grief syndrome described by Lindemann and the stages of grief and mourning described by Engel help us understand the dynamics involved when any crisis results in a grief and mourning reaction.[7]

On becoming aware of the loss, the person is likely to feel somatic distress and an altered sensorium. The somatic symptoms last from 20 minutes to a few days and may include shortness of breath, choking, sighing, hyperventilation, chills, tremors, fatigue, anorexia, tightness in the throat, emptiness in the abdomen, and loss of strength. The altered sensorium exists during the stages of shock and disbelief or defensive retreat. Included may be feelings of unreality, emotional distance from people, intense preoccupation with the image or occasional hallucination of the lost object or person, helplessness, loneliness and disorganization. In spite of apparent intellectual and verbalized acceptance of the loss, the implications of the loss are not comprehended. The person may overtly behave as if nothing happened or may be unable to carry out ordinary activities of living, lacking energy, organization and initiative in doing daily tasks. The person may at times seem out of contact with reality and express feelings of despair and anguish as the reality of loss penetrates awareness.

Increased preoccupation with the lost object, a heightened desire to talk about the loss, a search for evidence of failure 'to do right', verbal self-accusation, and ambivalence towards the lost object become manifested with increasing awareness of loss.

The greater the ambivalence felt towards the lost object or person, the greater are the feelings of guilt and shame. With any love relationship, the person will also at times feel anger or dislike towards, or desire to be rid of, the person, along with love feelings towards him/her. In addition, the grieving person may feel angry at the lost (deceased, divorced or separated) person for having left him/her. Guilt and anger feelings, a normal part of grieving, are frequently displaced onto others: the doctor, nurse, employer, family member or God. If guilt is not resolved, self-blame for the loss and preoccupation with it, with future losses, or with his/her own death will occur. Unsuccessful attempts at expiating guilt and anger may be made by blindly identifying with the lost object, by quickly seeking a substitute relationship or object, by absorbing oneself in work, by overindulging in alcohol or drugs, or by literally fleeing from the situation. The person may fear going crazy because of felt despair, helplessness, hopelessness and guilt. Early crisis therapy can reduce the intensity of some of these reactions.

Crying (the intensity of which depends on the culture) helps to express some anguish and is a form of communication that engenders support from others. In Britain, loss through death is one situation in which adult tears, even in the male, are acceptable and cause no loss of respect.

**The importance of ceremonies**. Restitution for or adaptation to the loss, the actual work of mourning, is assisted by religious, cultural or legal ceremonies.

The funeral ceremony, for instance, with the gathering of people who share the loss of the dead person and who either need or can give support to the grieving survivors, serves several purposes. It helps to emphasize the reality of the death, to minimize the expression of anger, and to expiate guilt. In addition, support is sought from a more powerful figure (God, Allah). Emphasis is placed on the possibility of life and reunion after death in some religions, and the process of identification with the deceased is initiated. Through the ceremony, the person *symbolically* expresses triumph over death and denies fear of death. The shared fellowship of a meal before or after the funeral, common in some subcultures, symbolically expresses return to life through the oral incorporation of eating and talking. The ceremony is the public way of adapting to the loss. But the persons closest to the deceased will continue to suffer for some time after the ceremony.

Other ceremonies dealing with separation or loss and involving the work of mourning may not be as extensive, obvious, or sad as a funeral. Each culture, however, provides ways to help the person acknowledge separation or loss. In fact, some ceremonies are joyous occasions, for the loss or separation means leaving behind old ways of behaviour and being promoted or progressing to a new stage of life or adopting new behaviour. Consider the baptism or circumcision; the birthday or graduation party; the first communion, confirmation, or Bar Mitzvah; the engagement or baby shower; and the retirement party. Although varying in degree of over expression and intensity of feeling, each represents essentially what the funeral represents after the death of a loved one.

**Stages in the mourning process**. Resolving loss, whether the death of a loved one or the loss of a significant object, status or job, involves a number of steps.[8]

The loss is first felt as a defect in the psychic self as the mourner becomes aware of innumerable ways in which he/she was dependent on the lost object as a source of gratification, for a feeling of wellbeing, for effective functioning, and for a sense of self. The mourner is not ready to accept a new object in place of the old one, although passively and transiently he/she may accept a more dependent relationship with remaining objects, roles or persons.

The mourner becomes increasingly aware of his/her own body. In addition to developing symptoms that are a normal part of grieving, the person may develop symptoms similar to those suffered by a deceased loved person. This identification process maintains a tie with the deceased loved one and appeases some of the guilt felt for harbouring earlier aggressive or angry feelings toward the dead person. How such symptoms are expressed depends on the person's constitutional factors as well as on past learning about which symptoms are most likely to get attention or to be defined as illness by the self and others.

The person is preoccupied with the lost object; there is a strong wish to have a continuing experience with the lost object. The mourner frequently talks about that which is lost, the pleasant memories and events associated with it. Constantly talking about the loss and its meaning is one way of reinforcing reality as well as of expiating guilt through repeated self-assurance that all possible action was taken to prevent the loss. This repetitious talking continues until the person forms a mental image almost completely devoid of negative characteristics of the lost object to replace that which no longer exists in the real world. This process of idealization follows difficult and painful experience of alternating guilt, remorse, fear and regret for real or fantasized past acts of hostility, neglect and lack of appreciation, or even for personal responsibility for the loss or death.

Through identification following idealization, the mourner consciously adopts some of the behaviour and admired qualities of the dead person.

He/she changes interests in the direction of activities formerly enjoyed by the lost loved one, adopts that person's goals and ideals, or even takes on certain mannerisms of the deceased. As this final identification is accomplished, preoccupation with the deceased, ambivalence, guilt and sadness decrease and thoughts return to life. If strong guilt is present, the person is more likely to take on undesirable characteristics, including the last disease symptoms, of the deceased. This negative identity may lead later to seeking a substitute relationship or object, absorbing self in work, overindulging in alcohol or drugs, literally fleeing from the situation by moving to another location, or psychopathology, especially depression.

Feelings are gradually withdrawn from the lost object. A yearning to be with the person is replaced by a wish to renew life. The person gradually unlearns old ways of living and learns new life patterns. The lost object becomes detached from the person and is enshrined in the form of a memory, memorial or monument. At first the person's renewed concern for others may be directed towards other mourners or other persons in crisis. It is easier to feel closeness with someone who has experienced a similar loss.

Finally, the person becomes interested in new objects and relationships and allows self new pleasures and enjoyments. At first the replacements must be very much like the former object, but eventually new relationships are formed and objects acquired that are equally or even more satisfying.

**Acceptance – the successful work of mourning** – may take 12 months or longer. Complete resolution of or adaptation to the crisis of loss is indicated by the ability to remember comfortably and realistically both the pleasures and disappointments of the lost relationship. When the mourning process is adaptive or successful, the person is capable of carrying on life with new relationships without mental or physical illness.

This syndrome of feelings, thoughts and behaviour, although varying somewhat in sequence or intensity from person to person, is characteristic of grief and mourning. Resolution of mourning is delayed whenever the person confronts a chronic situation, such as birth of a defective child. Acute grief is manifested at birth of the child (or onset of the situation), but mourning is drawn out as long as the child lives (or the situation continues).

*Factors influencing outcome of mourning*

In addition to the factors that affect the resolution of any crisis mentioned earlier, the duration of reaction and manner in which the person adjusts to the changed social environment after loss also depend on the following factors:[9]

1. Degree of dependency, for support from the lost object. The greater the dependency, the more difficult is emancipation from the lost object and resolution of loss.
2. Degree of ambivalence toward the lost object. Because ambivalence in a relationship determines the amount of felt guilt, this emotion slows the process of idealization, identification and reinvestment of emotional energy in new objects.
3. Preparation for loss ('anticipatory grieving'), whether the loss was expected or had only been briefly thought of some time in the past.
4. Number and nature of other relationships. If prior to loss, the person derived satisfaction from a variety of other objects, persons or roles, he/she now has more bases of support and can more readily form new relationships.
5. Age of the mourner or the deceased person. The death of a young person generally has a more profound effect on mourners than the death of an aged person in our culture. There is the feeling of great social loss for the young person who has had inadequate time to fulfil him/herself. Among mourners, children generally have less capacity for resolving loss than adults because of their relative inexperience with crises and abstract thinking.
6. Changes in the pattern of living necessitated by loss of a person, money, job, pet, valuable possessions, role or status.
7. Social and cultural roles of the mourners as defined by society. Mourning dress, fasting and sacrifice are indefinitely prescribed in our culture. The role of mourner may also conflict with other roles – for example, with masculine or wage-earner role. Society makes little provision for replacement of the loss or for the discharge of hostility and guilt created by loss.

In general, obstacles to the normal progression of grieving arise when the person tries to avoid the intense distress connected with the grief experience and the expression of related emotions.

*Nursing process for the person experiencing loss*

The nurse's role with the person experiencing any kind of significant loss is essentially the same as with the person and family experiencing the greatest loss, death.

Reactions to loss are not always obvious. In assessing the patient who is admitted for a medical or surgical illness following a serious loss, direct your assessment and intervention to the mourning process as well as to the illness. Recognize the necessity of grief work for this person to achieve an optimum level of wellbeing.

The principles of crisis intervention described earlier and the concepts of primary, secondary and tertiary prevention are applicable to the person experiencing loss.

You can help the person finish the mourning process by giving support during disengagement from the significant object and the seeking of new and rewarding relationships and patterns of living. The person cannot be hurried through mourning to resolution of the crisis. Encouragement and a time and place to talk, weep and resolve grief are needed. The person will need help in developing a philosophy about life to the point where he/she can again tolerate stress, changing behaviour to meet the situation rather than using behavioural mechanisms excessively to protect self from reality. Encourage the person to do what he/she can for self. Help him/her experiment with new modes of living and behaving and with new relationships. At times you may be a source of anxiety to this person as you attempt to encourage change and growth, but your simultaneous support will aid resolution.

The person who has been in mourning for some time may exhibit inappropriate behaviour. Denial, feelings of emptiness, self-depreciation, anger at self and others, self-pity, somatic complaints, hopelessness and helplessness may be expressed. Although such behaviour may be disturbing, this person needs respect and acceptance from you and others before he/she can again respect self and accept the life situation.

## THE CRISIS OF PHYSICAL ASSAULT OR RAPE

To be helpful to the assaulted victim, you must understand that the significant event is that the victim *perceives self* as having been violated.[10] A sense of control of the body and destiny becomes part of our psyches once we successfully master the independence strivings of early childhood. Few events can so overwhelmingly and suddenly undermine that essential sense of body integrity as being the victim of bodily or sexual assault. For example, D.K. Ipema identifies loss of choice as a central issue facing rape and other assault victims.[11]

Reports of clinical studies of rape victims seemingly date back only a decade or so to that of Sutherland and Scherl in 1970. Later references add information and also describe the silent rape reaction.[12] There is an even greater lack of clinical information in considering male victims of sexual abuse, although male victims suffer reactions similar to female victims. Further, any of the following persons may feel like violated victims: the wife forced into sexual submission by her husband, the youngster intimidated into 'sexual play' by older children or into an incestuous act, or the adolescent (male or female) psychologically coerced by another into sexual activity not freely willed. Their needs may be similar if not identical to those of rape victims. The following intervention principles, along with crisis intervention principles previously described, will apply to the victim of assault:

1. Emotional cartharsis.
2. Exploring self-blame.
3. Active support and encouragement on a short-term basis.
4. Assistance in identifying the situational supports available.

In counselling the sexually assaulted victim, try to get your own biases out of the way and *hear* what that individual's experience *was for her/him*. Put aside your beliefs, such as the victim's role in inviting or encouraging the assault. Avoid vicariously fabricating in your own mind what the experience must have been like. The client will need you to provide opportunities for sorting through her/his own conflicting reactions, whether they are vengeful rage, guilt regarding some element of satisfaction, crippling anxiety in the face of such vulnerability, or some combination of all these and more. Emergency care of rape victims involves very specific kinds of assistance.

Notman and Nadelson help us consider some special factors that are relevant when the sexual assault victims are children or adolescents. Rape as the first sexual experience may leave a victim quite confused about the relationship between sexuality, violence and humiliation. To be sexually assaulted during the years of independence strivings can leave a victim anxious that desired independence is not a safe pursuit. Adolescents have to deal with peer group issues. School phobia and truancy may result.

Parents may feel guilt that they did not somehow protect the child or adolescent. They have a need to blame someone, whether attacker, child or themselves. Sexual assault may be the proverbial straw in a family where members are already crippled by a general inability to discuss sexuality. Acute family crisis may result. Parents who are anxious about sexuality may react defensively to a fear that their child provoked the assault.

*Rape prevention*

Frequently rape prevention is not possible. Victims may only have a choice between submission or survival. They may react with paralyzing fear, especially when weapons or physical brutality are involved. The victim is usually at a disadvantage in terms of physical strength. 'Fighting back' requires not only physical self-defence skills but also a psychological overcoming of cultural inhibitions.[13] Rapists typically are opportunists and generally preselect a victim, or type of victim, and an environment conducive to their success.

Some women increase their odds of avoiding rape by massive security arrangements for their apartments or homes. Some feel safer by remaining aloof, unfriendly, and doing nothing that may draw attention to themselves. Some refuse to give or accept help from strangers. Some potential victims avoid actual rape by not showing intimidation or submissive behaviour. By striving for a cool, problem-solving mentality, the person may sometimes realize possibilities for escape. It is important to be prudent, discrete and self-directed. When all that fails, most of us would endure physical abuse to preserve life.

## ILLNESS: A SITUATIONAL CRISIS

In order to further relate crisis theory to nursing practice, the most common type of family crisis, illness, is discussed. Chapter 1 furnished a basis for the discussion in this section.

**Illness** may be defined as *an experience, manifesting itself through observable or felt changes in the body, that interferes with the person's capacity to carry out minimum functions appropriate to the customary status.*

The sensory quality of the illness experience is the result of nerve receptors. Exteroceptors include the organs of reception for visual, gustatory, olfactory and auditory sensations. Interoceptors include organs of reception for sensations of pain, touch, pressure, warmth and cold. Proprioceptors respond to impulses for tension, position and movement. Illness can be experienced as a change in the intensity, extension, preciseness, or duration of sensation from any of these receptors, accompanying various pathological states.[14]

*Influences on illness susceptibility*

In addition to the influences on health and illness discussed in Chapter 1, the difference in illness and susceptibility from person to person may arise either from differences in perception and evaluation of the environment or from innate constitutional differences, or both. There is usually a relationship between the frequency of a person's illness episodes and the manner in which life situations are perceived. Those who see their life experiences as challenging, demanding, and conflict-laden suffer more disturbances of bodily processes, mood, thought and behaviour. Susceptibility to illness may also be influenced by actions taken to avoid illness and by age, for adaptive defences are not well developed in the very young and are less effective in the very old. Developmental level also influences perception and response to environmental demands.[15]

Every person is active in a number of social roles that place various demands on the person and call for shifts and flexibility in attitude and behaviour. At times, however, the kinds and nature of the roles in which the person is involved are demanding or stressful to the point of contributing to illness. The occupational role is important; for example, a farmer, nurse, steel-mill worker, or office clerk all are predisposed to different types of illness.

The family contributes not only to genetic predisposition but also to the actual etiology of specific diseases through the transmission of social values, the socialization process of the child, and the family pattern of daily living and behaviour.

Because health is a multidimensional concept involving varying degrees of feelings, performance and symptoms, the family places a certain value on health as well as a definition, often unspoken, of what they consider to be illness. For the person from a low socioeconomic background, symptoms are important only if they interfere with everyday functions and work. Therefore such a person goes to the doctor only when severely ill. Perhaps only after the symptoms are corrected does he/she admit the extent of illness, for previously the pressure to earn a living wage kept him/her going. Some people value health so highly that they are acutely aware of many body sensations and any unusual ones are considered symptoms of illness and reported promptly to the doctor. While the latter value system can signal hypochondria, it is also the system that permits early diagnosis and a greater degree of health promotion. The family attitude toward money and spending directly affects its value on health. For some, the new car or television set is more important than the elective surgery or treatment that can be postponed, thus preventing loss of earnings.

The definition of illness is learned by the child through family values. For example, if the father is a construction worker who uses his back muscles considerably on the job, he and his wife are likely to express concern verbally and nonverbally when he suffers backache. His back represents a job, status, money and masculinity to him. The child perceives the situation; later, if he/she feels uncomfortable, backache may be the complaint. He/she soon learns such a complaint will get the parents' attention because of their value on this part of the anatomy. Backache is defined as illness in this family whereas other symptoms or signs of equal or greater intensity or potential severity may go unattended. The child is likely to keep this orientation into adulthood. Similarly, the pianist, minister and editor will emphasize their hands, voice and eyes, respectively. Such attitudes should be recognized and worked with in health teaching and care. Just telling the person which symptoms are regarded as a threat to health is useless. The person's behaviour depends on a personal definition of illness.

The family pattern of living and the socialization of family members are influential in contributing to and defining illness – for example, through eating and rest habits, housing and sanitation standards, leisure-time pursuits and hobbies. The family that places a high value on food or that has learned to use food for tension release is more likely to contain obese members who develop illnesses related to obesity. The athletic family is more likely to suffer sprains, bruises, and fractures. A tension-filled family life may contribute to mental illness and indirectly to physical illness or socially malajusted behaviour.

Research increasingly shows that the mind-body relationship is a key factor in many illnesses. The emotional status and personality of the person affect physiological processes.

Organic changes and various diseases that occur as a result of stress and emotional factors include peptic ulcers, ulcerative colitis, hypertension, cardiovascular disease, migraine headache, diabetes, asthma and other allergic conditions, eczema and other skin rashes, arthritis, muscle and joint conditions, insomnia, premenstrual tension and menstrual disorders. Some of these diseases can predispose to more serious conditions; for example, hypertension can predispose to heart failure, cerebral vascular accident, or renal damage. It is also possible that most illnesses, including cancer, infections, the common cold, gingivitis and dental caries, have their basis in psychological factors. Various references at the end of the chapter describe these psychophysiological illnesses and their effects in adults. Children, as well as adults, may suffer psychosomatic illnesses.[16]

The site and types of symptoms do not necessarily remain the same in the person over time. A symptom may have different effects for the same person at different times in life and in different family, group, or cultural circumstances. The Theory of Somatic Weakness explains why emotional stress affects each person differently, or some not at all. Genetic inheritance, previous illness in a body organ, prior strain of a body system, and learned behaviour responses all influence which organ-body system will be vulnerable to symptoms or disease when the person experiences distress. A person is more likely to develop a psychosomatic disorder if there is a previous family history of such a disorder. Or a person may develop a psychosomatic disorder by observing and learning a pattern from another family member with the same disorder.[17]

*Factors determining the definition of illness*

People in our society perceive illness as an obstacle to goal achievement, an interruption in the rhythm of life, a personal crisis, a frustration of normal life patterns and enjoyments, a disruption in social relations, or a punishment for misdeeds. Thus illness is considered a deviant role because the culture enforces an unusually high level of activity, independence and responsibility on the person. Illness is closely related in people's minds to the role of childhood dependency. Moreover, resorting too frequently to illness as an escape poses a threat to the stability of social systems. Thus the institutionalized role of illness involves important mechanisms of social control: during illness certain behaviours are expected of the sick person and his/her caretakers.

Being ill involves more than being admitted to a hospital or visiting the doctor. When you first see the person during the diagnostic process, the disease may be at midpoint. The diagnosis or definition of illness does not usually occur until after the symptoms are felt and described by the person to someone, usually in the family; both the person and family agree that he/she is ill; and a course of action is planned.

The person recognizes self as ill from the cues given by the illness, such as uncomfortable sensations, or the statements, facial expressions, or actions of others. Recognition of illness is usually made when present cues are seen to agree with past experience. In the absence of familiar cues the person may fail to recognize illness or become so apprehensive that he/she denies it. Even familiar cues may cause sufficient anxiety so that the person denies them and the illness experience.

In one study of 563 patients psychosocial factors were found to influence the amount of time that elapsed between the first sign or symptom of cancer and the search for medical help. Detection of cancer through routine physical examination ensured the least delay. In self-discovered signs of cancer worry about the condition reduced delay time more than pain, incapacity or other factors. Patients of higher social class sought help significantly earlier than the less privileged. Persons who openly used the word *cancer* had less delay than those who used the word *tumor* or another euphemism. Delay in seeking help appears to be conscious and deliberate rather than caused by failure to perceive the neoplasm or comprehend its consequences.

Whether the family or others validate the person's definition of illness depends on their pattern of interaction with and expectations of him/her and their past experience with being ill. Does he/she 'cry wolf' too often? Malinger? Act 'like a baby'? Such interpretations are likely to cause the family to prod the person to persevere in his/her independent, healthy role. The person's role within the family is also crucial. The breadwinner of the family may feel that he/she cannot afford to recognize illness unless it is severe enough to interfere with ability to work.

So the family can either accept or reject the person as ill. In turn, the person will accept or reject the family definition of the situation, depending on how he/she feels. If he/she continues to define self as ill, help is sought. When he/she declares self to be ill, the sick role is entered.

The person's course of action is dependent on previous illness and health-care experience, the kinds of help traditionally sought by the family, the knowledgeability about illness and the health-care system, value

⌐igion, and a variety of other factors. Such factors include the na-
⌐ility, seriousness, and intensity of the illness; the body part in-
⌐he extent to which symptoms interfere with daily patterns of liv-
⌐ anticipated consequences of the illness; the person's tolerance for
abno⌐⌐nality; the tendency to be concerned about self; and the availability,
cost and convenience of treatment facilities. Social class, culture, age, sex,
and occupational status are additional determinants of this behaviour.[18]

The person may seek help for the illness from any one of a number of resources: a family member, neighbour, local pharmacist, chiropractic or
osteopathic physician, a medical 'quack', soothsayer, religious advisor,
herbalist, midwife, nurse or medical doctor.

Perhaps the best way to ensure that a patient/client will seek a qualified
health-care worker in any *future* crisis of illness is to treat and care for him/
her in a way that is perceived as helpful in the *present* crisis.

*The sick role*

Illness forces the person to assume an unaccustomed social posture called
the *sick role*. In the sick role one comes in contact with the caretakers – doctors, nurses, or other health workers – whose jobs are defined by society. In
addition, society defines who is sick and who is well. What is considered illness in one culture is not so considered in another.

In the sick role the person has declared self to be in a position in which
he/she must be taken care of. Society and the health-care system reinforce
that he/she is not competent to care for self. He/she cannot do – and supposedly does not know – what needs to be done. Thus a person must follow
the orders of others and let others make decisions for and about the self.
The sick role frees the person from responsibility for the illness, but it carries the obligation to cooperate with caretakers and to get well. Medical
workers get frustrated, angry, or judgmental when it appears that the person will not or cannot get well. While 'working' to return to an independent, healthy status, society frees the person from ordinary duties, obligations and responsibilities. Thus the sick person's two rights are (a) exemp-
tion from usual responsibilities and (b) absolution of blame for illness.
Three obligations are to (a) view illness as undesirable; (b) want to get well,
and (c) seek competent help from and cooperate with caretakers.

Although some health-care professionals approach the ill person as a
client rather than as a patient – seeking the person's point of view about
care rather than being authoritarian – the health-care system as a whole
treats the ill person (patient) as a child or an object rather than as someone
capable of self-care and decision making.

**Certain adaptive behaviours** normally unacceptable to society are common during illness and are considered helpful in promoting rest and recov-

ery. By accepting illness, the structure of the person's world becomes simpler and more constricted. The person becomes somewhat dependent and regressed because of the unpleasant sensations, physical weakness and helplessness caused by the illness; because of society's expectations; or from egocentricity, feelings of helplessness and concerns about body functions and routines administered for his/her welfare. Withdrawal into self rather than interest in others, a focus on the present rather than on the past or the future, and a reduced ability to concentrate and to think abstractly are all typical behaviours of the sick person. Routines may seem too burdensome so that daily activities, such as taking a bath and personal grooming, may be avoided, if possible, by the sick person. Through social, emotional and physical regression, and in compliance with the medical plan, the sick person redistributes energies to encourage the healing process.

The patient is simultaneously in a position of great power and of extreme weakness. This combination of domination and dependence provokes a difficult inner conflict, a certain ambivalence similar to what young children feel at times. The patient in essence loves the authority figure (the nurse or doctor) for taking care of him/her while simultaneously feeling angry toward the medical worker for being powerful while he/she is essentially helpless.

**Certain deviant or maladaptive behaviours** in the sick role may occur and be so labelled by the medical team because the behaviours do not assist the person in getting physically well or regaining independence. Someone who uses illness for secondary gain, attention, escape from responsibility, control, or manipulation of others in the environment will not move through the sick role to return to health at the expected pace or in the expected way.

The health team also considers the ill person as deviant if he/she is unable to accept the dependent sick role. Often this pattern occurs when the person has unresolved dependency-independency conflicts. The patient may fear becoming dependent or may actually long to be dependent and feel guilty about this urge. Strongly independent behaviour, such as protracted denial of illness, unwarranted physical activity, or refusal to cooperate with health-care workers, may be a signal of such inner conflicts. Recognize, however, that in some cultures the ill person may refuse a dependent role because of expectations of self and others. On the other hand, excessive dependency, using illness as a refuge, and refusing to engage in self-care activities within one's strength limitations are as detrimental to getting well as is excessively independent behaviour.

The patient may hinder progress by becoming apathetic or uninterested in recovering. Overly compliant, submissive, docile behaviour should not be mistaken for cooperation with the treatment plan. Rather, the person's feelings of powerlessness and hopelessness, the lack of initiative and enthusiasm, signs of physical and emotional depression, or an apparent retreat as if waiting for death appear to diminish natural body responses for recovery.

In addition, any maladaptive response noted in this chapter's discussion of crisis may occur and can hinder progress to recovery, at least from the point of view of the medical team.[19]

## The culture of illness

Although the prescribed medical care may be identical, a person acts and is treated differently whether sick at home or sick in the hospital. In the home the person is in a familiar environment; it is possible to retain a sense of dignity, rights and privileges and to insist on being treated on one's own terms. The sick one is reinforced by family and friends, who accord special concessions. These prerogatives are generally disregarded when the sick person enters a hospital.

**Hospitalization** *may be defined as confinement of a person to an institution, away from the family, for a varying amount of time. Its purposes may be diagnosis; care or treatment that is palliative, rehabilitative, or curative in nature; or restoration of the person to a previous state, such as return to a nonpregnant state after delivery.*

Upon hospitalization, the individual is stripped of personal possessions. Gone are familiar surroundings that afford a sense of security. Instead there are various strange, disquieting, and bothersome odours, noises and sights. At home the health-care worker rings the bell and waits for the door to open. In the hospital the patient rings the bell and waits for a nurse to come. At home the doctor is on call, the nurse is a visitor, and relatives belong. In the hospital the patient is admitted and discharged, the health-care workers perform their duties, and relatives are the visitors. At home everyone present acknowledges the patient's wishes. In the hospital all health-care workers are in a distinct position to grant or withhold small and very precious favours from the patient, often depending on their personal judgment of the latter and his/her behaviour.[20]

## Reactions to hospitalization

In the best of settings the person is overwhelmed by many strange, foreboding, conflicting, or frightening feelings. In spite of the many people around, he/she feels isolated and lonely. In fact, lack of privacy, with the intrusion of these many workers into the room, often unannounced, is a frequent complaint. Compartmentalization of care, bureaucracy, and other characteristics of the hospital within the health-care system, combine to strip the person of individuality and identity. He/she is robbed unnecessarily of decision-making power, a sense of responsibility, and significant communication by a rigid schedule, ritualistic routines, and staff who appear to hurry, won't answer questions, talk too fast, or use words not understood. Moreover, the body rhythms are disrupted.

The hospital often means separation from valued persons, objects and activities. It may seem to be a place where one is sent in retaliation for inappropriate behaviour or at least a place that inflicts undesirable controls and forced conformity. There is endless waiting and the feeling of boredom, aimlessness and sameness every day. On the other hand, some people may consider the hospital more as a source of relief. It may seem a secure place, with its emergency equipment and trained concerned personnel, where basic needs can be met without effort of the self. For still others, the hospital is a place to go to die.

Health-team members should consider some of the possible undesirable side effects of hospitalization on the patient:

1. Enforced dependency on strange authority figures.
2. Dramatic changes in the physical environment.
3. Disruption of daily routines and preferences.
4. Separation from family.
5. Different behavioural expectations imposed by the sick role.
6. Forced adjustment to an interaction with a variety of strangers at a highly vulnerable time.
7. Depersonalization, loss of privacy and freedom, and fostered regression.
8. Increased anxiety from all of these effects, which may cause further physical and mental changes and further impede progression towards health.

Thus illness, especially if it necessitates hospitalization, is a crisis. The person is moving from familiar into strange territory and the usual patterns of behaviour are not adequate to cope in the strange situation. The crisis becomes greater in its impact when, as a result of the illness, the person must thereafter live with a chronic debilitating or disabling condition or when a structure or function of the body has been altered.

*Stages of illness*

The crisis of illness does not occur as an isolated event in the life of the person. The psychological states that occur during illness do not represent a change of difference in the person as much as temporary adaptive behaviours that maintain or promote restoration of the pre-illness self. The reactions to illness must be understood in terms of the person's prior personality organization. Thus adopting the sick role and going through the phases of crisis during the stages of illness are maladaptive only when the person is *not* ill by commonly accepted standards.

The stages of illness described by Janis, and listed next, fit into the phases of crisis described earlier.

**Transition from health to illness, the first stage**, lasts from the time the person first considers that he/she might be ill until he/she and others acknowledge that the person is ill. During this period the person may show signs of emotional shock if the illness is acute or severe and the disruption to normal life is considerable. Then denial is used, at least briefly, to minimize or ignore the symptoms. If denial is strong, the person has a feeling that nothing can happen to him/her, that he/she never felt better, and he/she may engage in more than the usual amount of activity. Denial is usually impossible to maintain for a prolonged time because of pressure from others, feelings of extreme discomfort, or manifestation of more symptoms when the person tries to maintain normal behaviour.

**Acceptance of illness, the second stage**, occurs when the person feels the reality and impact of the illness, acknowledges the illness, seeks validation from significant others, seeks help from a caretaker, and enters into the sick role with all the related behaviours previously described. During illness the person may go through a mourning process for loss of body function or structure, even if such loss is temporary. During this time the person has many worries – job, finances, ability of the family to manage without him or her, fidelity of the spouse, child care and loss of status. The patient may become aggressive or haughty, displacing anger on others, even though feeling weak or inadequate. Or the person may be passive in order to control fears and anger.

The stigma, embarrassment, or shame felt because of illness begins to be worked through, along with the emasculating or defeminizing effects felt as part of the illness. Feelings of rejection, of being abandoned, and self-pity gradually diminish.

Different body parts and certain body functions may have great significance to the person. If altered by illness of the treatment plan, the distortion in body image that occurs must be resolved before the patient can enter the last stage of illness, convalescence. Gradually the coping mechanisms are reorganized and perception becomes more realistic.

**Convalescence, the last stage**, is analogous to the adaptation or resolution phase of crisis. Now the person returns to health. Or, in the case in which there is a permanent disability and no further physical improvement is possible, convalescence marks a gradual increase in satisfying experiences. The person's new sense of worth and reduced anxiety enable him/

her again to use those abilities typical of health. This period is like moving from adolescence to adulthood. The person is reassessing the meaning of life and is becoming increasingly independent, stable, outward looking, and involved in decision making.

There are many variations in convalescence. Physical convalescence frequently occurs before emotional convalescence or resolution of the illness. The person's level of maturity, the kind of crisis intervention given, and the environment in which the person must function combine to determine progress. If others encourage constructive activity instead of passive, less adaptive behaviour, the person can more easily resolve feelings about having been ill. Then again, health may represent more of a threat than illness due to the pressures of life. If illness justifies irresponsible behaviour, provides an escape from obligations, or satisfies emotional or financial needs, then the person may actively (although perhaps unconsciously) resist convalescence.

*Tasks of convalescence*

Certain tasks must be accomplished, in addition to solving the practical problems of returning home from the hospital, in order to go from illness to full emotional and physical health. The minor adaptations in the physical environment of the home and in the daily routine can usually be easily made. Then the family and friends expect the newly discharged patient to be grateful for recovery and for what they have done for him/her, to be cheerful about rejoining loved ones, and to be eager to return to the usual way of life. However, they may soon find the person is unable to live up to these expectations.

Before resuming the usual activities and making the transition back to health, the person must first accomplish the task of convalescence. Only then will crisis be resolved.

**Reassessment in life's meaning** is one of the primary tasks for the convalescing patient. He/she thinks about life goals, purposes, and perhaps even the meaning of death and redirects energies toward developing a full potential for living.

**Reintergration of body image** becomes a second major task after the acute phase of illness, when the patient is less concerned about any threat to life. Scarring, deformity, impaired functioning, or removal of valued organs must be dealt with and integrated into the self. The person must work through feeling dependent, 'dirty', repulsive, unattractive, or possibly totally unacceptable to certain others. Moreover, he/she may not feel the same even if there has been no actual change in body structure or function.

Moving from the dependent patient role to independent adult status takes time and help. The person must feel self-interest, assertiveness and persistence. Independence cannot be demanded; it is the result of work, usually between the nurse who views the person as a unique individual and a client and the person who trusts the nurse as a caregiver.

**Resolution of role changes or reversals** that have occurred during the illness is a third major task and must be worked out within the patient and in relation to family members. After illness, there are no prescribed behaviours for convalescence, but the person usually does not fully assume normal responsibilities for some time. Seeing the family members carry out some of his/her responsibilities may be difficult and family members themselves usually look forward to a return to the normal pattern of living with less burden.

Added to the problems of continued role changes are the mood swings and other unpredictable responses of the convalescing person – behaviour that may be very unlike the pre-illness personality. Some distance still exists between the convalescing person and the rest of the activities going on around him/her.

Today the sick person normally returns home early in the illness for convalescence or rehabilitation. Before the person's discharge, you must learn if there is a family to help with care or at least a place to go, whether transportation to get home is available, and how the person will manage within specific limits, such as restrictions on mobility or diet. Every ill person comes from a culture and a community and returns to the same. Do not make assumptions; instead ask about the situation so that realistic plans can be made. If you listen and use nondirective interviewing techniques, you can help the person and family reexamine their lives, marshall their strengths, and focus their energies on convalescence.

The person who has a fatal illness will not truly convalesce and yet may enjoy periods of essentially good physical health. The reaction of the person who is terminally ill must be understood in terms of numerous and sometimes conflicting factors, taking into account previous relationships and previous experiences with crisis, particularly illness and loss. There must be an understanding of the significance of family, social group, occupation, and religion as well as of the other sources of love, comfort and support. The person's self-concept and body image, ability to recognize and cope with reality, and responses to dependency, pain and uncertainty will influence the overall reaction. Other crucial factors are the nature of the specific illness; the organ or body system affected, along with its symbolic as well as real significance to the person; the type of treatment required; and the degree of functional loss and disfigurement.

*Impaired role behaviour related to illness*

Following illness or surgery, the person may not regain complete health; he/she may remain chronically ill. The person then reaches a state where he/she gets neither better nor worse but is no longer viewed by self or by society as being ill. He/she may even be disabled by a condition that imposes a restriction on activity and provokes social prejudice and stigma.[21] Examples of such conditions include blindness, deafness, and cases in which some body part or function is congenitally or surgically absent or malfunctioning. The disability may or may not be obvious, but the person considers self well most of the time. He/she has emotionally resolved the crisis that surrounded the disability; limited ability to carry on usual roles and responsibilities remains. For the disabled person who is not experiencing illness, social pressures serve to aid in maintaining normal behaviour within the limits of his/her potential. This situation is called *impaired role behaviour.*

The behaviour of the person depends on his/her perception of the disability as well as on the perceptions of others. Some persons who are chronically ill or congenitally or surgically disabled will remain in the sick role indefinitely. Such persons have not resolved the crisis of illness; the person with impaired role behaviour has.

**Characteristics of impaired role behaviour** differ from those of the sick role. Thomas suggests that **impaired role behaviour** *is an extension of the sick role. The disabled person, however, is not considered by society to be exempt from normal behaviour or responsibilities within the limits of the condition.* He/she is expected, as far as possible, to improve or modify the life situation in the light of his/her disability, to make the most of remaining capabilities to overcome the disability, and to accept limits realistically. The person is then considered rehabilitated and no longer in the sick role.

The behavioural responses of the disabled person also depend on his/her feelings of being accepted or rejected. Schutz describes the basic human need to be included rather than excluded from others, to feel lovable, worthwhile, significant, competent and responsible. The disabled person desires and needs to have close relationships with nondisabled persons and needs to be accepted by others for what he or she is, in spite of the disability.

Disability often forces the person to modify the self-concept and self-image. New and different body sensations, changed appearance or body functions, and changed or reduced abilities challenge the person's self-confidence. He/she may feel shame, worthlessness, and inferiority, often to a degree not justified by the condition. Negative responses from others intensify low self-esteem and a negative self-image results, for everyone learns to incorporate the image that others have of him/her into the self-concept.

The disabled person is expected to learn to adjust and respond to being dependent on the aid of others to complete tasks or meet his/her needs, in spite of our cultural emphasis on self-reliance and independence. The person is expected to share in the management of the medical condition and be involved in decisions regarding treatment and care. He/she will be asked to explain the disability to others, often revealing considerable personal information, and accept that he/she is an object of curiosity medically and socially. The person recognizes that through these explanations he/she is helping to reduce social stigma, pity and prejudice, and this will eventually permit greater opportunities to realize his/her potentialities.

The primary reason for considering impaired role behaviour is that some people are neither ill – and therefore governed by sick-role norms – nor healthy in the usual sense. The well-adjusted disabled person views the self as physically or psychosocially restricted rather than ill.

In contrast, not accepting one's disability and its attendant limitations results in behaviour that interferes with maintenance of health, prevention of further illness, and performance of social roles. Such a person is considered deviant in his/her behaviour in that he/she remains in the sick role.

Although acute illness causes worry about outcome of the disease, financial status, and staying abreast of the demands of daily living, family reactions to disability or chronic illness is even more complex.

Family reactions may include a sense of shame, lowered self-esteem, and a sense of family instability as roles and responsibilities are shifted. Members may blame each other for the condition. A sense of depression or grief may be constantly present because the ill or disabled person cannot achieve certain developmental tasks. Family members may fear that they will not be able to meet care demands or financial obligations. Anger may be verbalized or indirectly expressed to the ill person or among family members because of the burdens and stresses encountered. The uncertain future may cause a feeling of hopelessness. Further, family members may feel guilty about their feelings toward the ill person, and yet resent the life changes caused by the chronic illness in the family.[22]

*Nursing responsibility*

**The nursing process and principles described earlier** in this chapter are applicable to the care of the sick person and the family. The principles of crisis intervention, combined with the necessary physical care, will help the person reach maximum potential.

**Reactions of the nurse to loss, disability and intentional death**. Just as patients and families experience various emotional reactions, the stress of being a health-care provider can also provoke anxiety. You may identify with the client because of age, sex, disease type, or professional or cultural background. Perhaps you are in a health-care field as a counterphobic reaction, as a way to deal with your fears and anxieties related to illness. You may also become very attached to the client and feel a sense of loss on discharge or death. Concerns about failure in doing the job correctly, causing damage to the client and receiving criticism from colleagues, are common sources of anxiety. Anticipating stressors and their effects, and realizing that you are not the only nurse who feels anxious, is an important step in coping with your anxiety and other unpleasant emotions.[23]

You are a model of health to your clients. If you cannot cope effectively with stressors, you will not be effective.

**The meaning of the illness and related care determine behaviour.** Diagnostic and treatment activities that the ill person encounters can be classified into four categories, according to the amount of threat perceived in each activity:

1. Intrusion or forceful entry into a body orifice, such as in an enema, catheterization, irrigation, gastric intubation or injection.
2. Invasion of privacy, as in a probing interview, a vaginal, or rectal examination, or undue exposure of the body during care.
3. Threat of pain, suffering, or annihilation, such as represented by surgery or any other care procedure that threatens to distort, alter, or destroy the person's body image.
4. Little or no threat, as in taking routine vital signs or bedmaking.

Because these activities carry certain meanings, you can predict with some degree of certainty the person's behaviour. For example, surgery may have any or all of the following meanings to a patient: pain, the unknown; fear of not being told the truth; mutilation and changes in the body image caused by incisions and removals; fear of death; disruption of life plans including occupational and recreational; and fear of loss of control under anaesthesia.

**Establishing a frame of reference** is helpful in preparing the person for diagnostic, treatment or care measures. If he/she can compare a familiar event or sensation to the event about to be experienced, the event will seem less strange. He/she will feel less threatened and more in control of the situation and illness can be better tolerated and perceived more realistically. Of course, the frame of reference must have meaning for the individual. For example, a breast biopsy could be compared to the removal of a mole. If a procedure is going to hurt, the sensation should be described to the person – for example, as feeling like the pain of a burn from a hot stove, a needle prick, a toothache, or abdominal pressure from having overeaten. A patient/client usually will not engage in a comparison of the sensation or experience of illness without prompting; his/her main concern is to get relief from it.

If the person has been prepared intellectually to expect certain consequences, such as the possible outcome of a diagnostic procedure or the complexity of a tentative treatment plan, the emotional reaction will be less disorganized when he/she learns that the possibilities have become reality. He/she needs help in thinking about the possibilities of what might happen so that he/she can use certain behavioural mechanisms that aid coping with potential and actual danger. Behaviour will become more cooperative with the health-care team, whereas when the person's perception of the diagnostic or treatment plan is anxiety-laden and negative, behaviour is likely to be negative and uncooperative.

You will be the health-team member best qualified to do this preparation.

**Consider the less obvious but equally important needs of patients,** such as aesthetic needs. Eliminate or at least control unpleasant sights, sounds and odours whenever possible. Consider the likes and dislikes of the person and the family. Let the family or individual make decisions about 'the little things that count' as long as they do not interfere with the treatment plan. Help the person maintain identity by using the proper title and name. Encourage bringing some personal possessions from home and instruct the person and family about hospital routines and policies in order to reduce feelings of strangeness, isolation and powerlessness. Flexible visiting hours can reduce loneliness and anxiety related to separation from loved ones.

As a nurse, you will coordinate various activities of other health-care workers as well as perform the unique functions of care called *nursing*. Often you are the only caregiver prepared to understand the total person and his/her many unique needs while engaging in a therapeutic process with the patient.

**The tasks of convalescence** can best be accomplished when patient, family and nurse collaborate, with the patient doing most of the work. Promote realistic adaptation by explaining the meaning of the crisis of illness and the tasks of convalescence. With shorter hospitalization the rule today, some resolution of feelings traditionally accomplished in the hospital must now be done at home. Be supportive and accepting and help both family and individual prepare for the tasks of convalescence to be managed at home after discharge. This preparation is as important as the discharge planning that helps the person make necessary physical adaptations or learn self-care. The person may never be able to do the latter satisfactorily if he/she is given no help with the former or has unrealistic expectations about treatment outcomes.

Therapeutic communication is essential in helping the person resolve convalescence. Pick up verbal cues. Reflect pertinent statements. Do not feel you must give answers. Encourage him/her to talk about thoughts and feelings so that he/she will arrive at personal answers and decisions.

Much of the physical care given in the hospital, such as bathing, changing dressings, guiding range-of-motion exercises, and positioning, could be done with greater thought directed towards helping the person acquaint self with and accept the changed body. Preserve and emphasize his/her strengths, but do not ignore or minimize problems. Realistic, pertinent teaching is essential for the person to adapt to a changed body. Recognize the signs of independence and promote it – without forcing the person to be independent before he/she is ready.

*Final discharge planning and preparing for termination* of the nurse–client relationship should be started long before the day of discharge. When you and the person jointly work through feelings about termination, both of you feel less cheated or rejected when he/she leaves the hospital.

You can evaluate the effectiveness of care and preparation for convalescence best through follow-up home visits or interviews with the person and family on their return to the clinic or doctor's surgery. Convalescence and the crisis of illness have been resolved when the person can talk about illness or surgery with equanimity and acceptance. Convalescence is not resolved when the person needs to talk continuously about the illness experience or states that he/she 'never did get over it!' You can help to prevent or minimize such responses.

By intervening as a crisis therapist, you are involved in promoting the health of the person and family in the present situation as well as in future crises. In turn, the health and functioning of the community are indirectly enhanced. Thus a number of systems are positively affected.

## REFERENCES

1. Holmes, T., and R. Rahe, 'The Social Readjustment Rating Scale', *Journal of Psychosomatic Medicine*, vol. 2 no. 8 (1967) pp. 213–17.
2. Spiegel, John, 'The Resolution of Role Conflict With the Family', *A Modern Introduction to the Family*, eds., Norman Bell and Ezra Vogel (The Free Press, Glencoe, IL, 1963).
3. See note 4, below; also Hoff, Lee Ann, *People in Crisis: Understanding and Helping* (Addison-Wesley Publishing Co. Inc., Reading, MA, 1978).
4. Murray, Ruth and M. Marilyn Huelskoetter, *Psychiatric/Mental Health Nursing: Giving Emotional Care* (Prentice Hall Inc., Englewood Cliffs, NJ, 1983); Skeet, *Home From Hospital* (The Macmillan Company, New York, 1974).
5. See notes 6 and 9, below; also, Hargreaves, Anne, 'Coping with Disaster', *American Journal of Nursing*, vol. 80 no. 4 (1980) p. 683.

6. See notes 4 and 5, above; also, Ferguson, Tom, 'Coping with Disaster', *Medical Self-Care*, vol. 19 (Winter 1982) pp. 32–7; Maxwell, Christopher, 'Hospital Organizational Response to the Nuclear Accident at Three Mile Island: Implications for Future-Oriented Disaster Planning', *American Journal of Public Health*, vol. 72 no. 3 (1982) pp. 275–6.

7. Engel, George, *Psychological Development in Health and Disease* (W.B. Saunders Company, Philadelphia, 1962).

8. Ibid.

9. Jackson, Edgar, *Understanding Grief* (Abington Press, New York, 1967).

10. Hilberman, Elaine, *The Rape Victim* (Basic Books, Inc., New York, 1976).

11. See note 4, above.

12. See note 4, above; also, Brownmiller, Susan, *Against Our Will: Men, Women and Rape* (Simon & Schuster Inc., New York, 1975).

13. Wu, Ruth, *Behaviour and Illness* (Prentice Hall Inc., Englewood Hills, NJ, 1973).

14. See note 7, above.

15. See notes 2 and 7 above; also Bonami, M., 'Overt and Covert Personality Traits Associated with Coronary Health Disease', *British Journal of Medical Psychology*, vol. 52 no. 1 (1979) pp. 77–84.

16. See notes 2 and 13, above.

17. See note 13, above.

18. Stockwell, E. *The Unpopular Patient*, Royal College of Nursing, 1972.

19. See note 2, above.

20. Ibid.

21. See notes 9 and 18, above.

22. See note 4, above.

# UNIT II

Factors influencing health in a pluralistic society

# 7

## The person's relationship to the environment

Study of this chapter will help you to:

1. Explore the scope of environmental pollution, both outdoor and indoor, and the interrelationship of the different kinds of pollution with one another and with people.

2. Observe sources of air pollution in your community and identify resulting hazards to human health.

3. List types of water pollution and describe resultant health problems.

4. Describe substances that cause soil pollution and the effect of these substances on the food web as well as on other facets of health.

5. Discuss the types of food pollution and ways to prevent food contamination.

6. Listen to noise pollution in various settings and discuss its long-term effects on health.

7. Discuss health hazards that are encountered by workers and the major effects of these contaminants.

8. Discuss and practise ways that, as a citizen, you can reduce environmental pollution.

9. Discuss your professional responsibility in assessing for illness caused by environmental pollutants and in taking general intervention measures.

10. Demonstrate an ability to help establish a therapeutic milieu for a patient/client.

Often the physical environment in which we live is taken for granted, overlooked as a direct influence on people and their health, although ecology is a well-publicized subject. You may wonder why a unit discussing major influences on the developing person and that person's health begins with a chapter about humans and their environment. Yet where we live and the condition of that area – its air, water and soil – determine to a great extent how we live, what we eat, the agents of disease to which we are exposed, our state of health and our ability to adapt.

Some environmental factors, both external and internal, that affect health status are discussed in Chapter 1. This chapter focuses primarily on noxious agents in the external environment to which many people are exposed, agents that are detrimental to health. Because of the interdependence of people, only those living in isolated rural areas escape the unpleasant effects of our urban, technologically advanced society. Yet even the isolated few may encounter some kind of environmental pollution, whether through groundwater contaminated from afar, food shipped into the area, or smog blown from a nearby city.

Nursing in the past was concerned primarily with the patient's immediate environment in the hospital or home. Today the nursing process is increasingly extended to include assessment of and intervention measures directed toward promoting a healthy environment for the person and family, well or ill. Understanding some specific environmental health problems, their sources and effects, will enable you to work both as a citizen and as a professional nurse to help prevent or correct those problems.

## HISTORICAL PERSPECTIVE

The natural components of the environment were once considered dangerous. In most instances, people dealt successfully with any environmental problems encountered. In their quest to conquer nature early people discovered fire and the wheel. Fire was essential to survival; but with its advent, natural or manmade sparks and pollutants were sent into the atmosphere – the beginning of environmental pollution.

The fire and the wheel played major roles in the early civilization and industrialization of the world. With the Industrial Revolution came many technological advances that gave people increased power and comforts. These advances also introduced artificial, chemical and physical hazards into the environmental. Soon after the start of the Industrial Revolution, the population of cities grew; disease spread with the crowding of people, and food distribution became more complex. It became apparent that the natural components of the environment were not as dangerous as the manmade components.

Antipollution and environmental health legislation can be traced back to the last century in Britain. Legislation in force currently is enacted under the aegis of the Department of the Environment. Concern about atmospheric pollution has a long history in the UK – a proclamation by Edward I in 1306 prohibited the use of sea coal in furnaces on pain of execution. In the eighteenth and nineteenth centuries the industrial revolution brought increasing problems of atmospheric pollution with the smoke from factory chimneys, but over the years the public showed little interest in this form of pollution and 'smog-type' fogs were accepted as the norm. A dramatic attitude change came about in 1952, when a London smog coincided with a dramatic rise in the number of deaths. A committee was set up which examined comprehensively the pollution arising from the burning of solid fuels. The link between pollution and respiratory disease and the economic cost of pollution on property was emphasised. The recommendations formed the basis of the 1956 Clean Air Act. Most other forms of pollutants and environmental health hazards are dealt with under the 1974 Control of Pollution Act. The Clean Air Act 1956 was updated by a further Act in 1968.

The entire environment has been and is a vital part of our existence. Human skill in manipulating the environment has produced tremendous benefits; but none has been without a price, the high price of pollution.

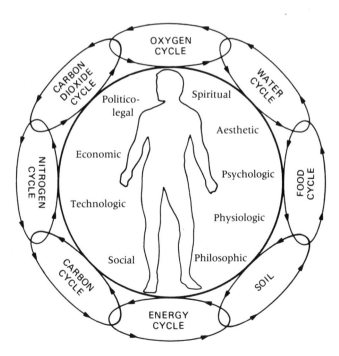

*Fig. 7.1*　The person's interrelationship with the environment

Pollution of our environment is not only a health threat but also offends aesthetic, spiritual, social and philosophic values. Environmental pollution is a complex, significant problem requiring multiple solutions.

The following discussion is divided into categories of air, water, soil, food, noise and surface pollution. Keep in mind, however, that these categories overlap. To illustrate, when a person inhales harmful particles from the soil that have become airborne, soil pollution becomes air pollution. And soil or surface pollution becomes water or food pollution if these harmful particles are swept into the water, consumed first by fish and then by people.

*Problems of air pollution*

Air pollution, 'aerial garbage', is not a new problem. Natural processes, such as forest fires and volcanic eruptions, or burning cities set afire during war, have long contaminated the air. Smog and the byproducts of coal burning have long been recognized as irritating disturbances plaguing many areas and clouding the skies.

Air and water pollution act interchangeably; together they present a world problem. All people on the earth share the oceans and the air. Significant local pollution of either can greatly affect distant areas, especially if the oceans cannot, by the processes of precipitation, oxidation, and absorption, cleanse the atmosphere before harmful effects occur. Given enough time, the ocean can cleanse the atmosphere. But if the amount of pollution exceeds the ocean's capacity to neutralize the waste, then the harmful effects are dispersed into the atmosphere and we realize the effects by breathing contaminated air.[1]

*Sources of air pollution*

The five most common pollutants found in the air are suspended particles, sulphur oxides, nitrogen oxides, hydrocarbons and carbon monoxide.

A major cause of air contamination is imperfect combustion. **Perfect combustion** exists only in the chemistry books and is *the result of hydrogen and carbon uniting completely with oxygen, thereby relinquishing heat, water vapour, light, and carbon dioxide to the air.* **Imperfect combustion** refers to *the additional liberation of carbon monoxide, sulphur oxides, and nitrogen oxides into the air.* Car exhausts in heavy traffic produce a significant amount of **carbon monoxide,** *a colourless and odourless poisonous gas produced during the incomplete combustion of carbon.* This gas combines with the hemoglobin of red blood cells in place of oxygen and can produce a **hypoxic state,** *a decreased amount of oxygen* in the body. The severity of this state depends on the ratio of carbon monoxide to oxygen in the air inhaled. The deficiency of oxygen in the blood caused by carbon monoxide primarily affects respiration and the function of the brain and heart. Carbon monoxide in high concentrations can cause death: in small amounts it can cause dizziness, headache, fatigue, and impaired perception and thinking. Carbon-monoxide pollution can be especially dangerous for persons who suffer from heart disease, respiratory disease, or anaemia, for they already have a physiologically impaired oxygen-carrying capacity,[2], and for the foetus because it can cause retardation of growth and brain development.

**Sulphur oxides** *are poisonous gases that come from factories and power plants that burn coal or oil-containing sulphur,* eventually producing dangerous sulphur dioxide. *Sulphur dioxide combines with water to form* **sulphuric acid (H$_2$SO$_4$),** *a heavy, corrosive, oily, colourless liquid* that irritates the sensitive mucous membranes of the eyes, nose and throat and injures the mucous membrane that lines the lungs and the delicate structures accessory to the lung tissue. Besides directly affecting our health, sulphur and its byproduct, sulphuric acid, indirectly jeopardize health by damaging plant life and contributing to rust on metals. In the process of trying to control these harmful effects through technological means, a new industrial pollution is sometimes created. Rust-proof cans may contain some elements that contaminate the environment, for instance, and they also add to waste-disposal problems.

Other gaseous end products from burning fuels are the nitrogen oxides, especially nitrogen dioxide. While this gas hovers in the air, producing an unpleasant, characteristic odour, it causes irritation to the mucous membranes and creates a haze that destroys the view and blocks out necessary and helpful rays from the sun.

Another air contaminant is **particulate matter,** *minute particles, such as dust, dirt, air, smoke and fly ash.* Particulate matter, suspended in vapours and fumes, may hover for annoying and dangerous periods of time, depending on atmospheric conditions. These pollutants may soil surfaces, scatter or distribute light rays unevenly and, most dangerously, enter the lungs of people breathing the air. The severity of the lungs' response depends on the percentage of particulate matter or fumes and vapours in the air mixture and on preexisting lung disease.

Breathing in asbestos particles released into the atmosphere from certain construction industries and from the wearing of brake lining and clutch facings in cars can cause cancer. Asbestos was also widely used for fire-proofing and insulating homes and public and private buildings. When the asbestos material becomes damaged or starts to deteriorate, asbestos fibres are released into the air. Inhaled beryllium, used in making metal alloys, also is known to cause a debilitating form of lung infection. Cigarette smoke has been identified as an air pollutant, causing increased carbon-monoxide content in the blood. In addition, numerous other chemicals make up the particulate matter in tobacco smoke. Tobacco smoke can produce cardiovascular, respiratory, and other symptoms in nonsmokers as well as smokers. Second-hand smoke can produce cancer in the nonsmoker as well as smokers. Sufficient exposure to any type of particulate pollution may lead to pulmonary emphysema.

Unlike the other forms of pollutants mentioned, ozone is not emitted directly by specific sources. **Ozone** *(triatomic oxygen $O_3$) is a pungent, colourless, toxic gas.* In the upper atmosphere ozone forms a protective barrier that prevents excessive ultraviolent light from reaching the earth. In the lower atmosphere ozone is *formed in the air by chemical reactions between nitrogen oxides and hydrocarbons (volatile organic compounds),* such as the vapours of petrol and chemical solvents. These reactions are stimulated by sunlight and produce a type of *photochemical smog.*

Ozone severely irritates the mucous membranes of the nose and throat. Normal functioning of the lungs is impaired and the ability to perform physical exercise is reduced. Individuals with chronic lung disease are more severely affected. Ozone also irritates the eyes.

Four additional air pollution problems should be mentioned: depletion of the upper atmosphere ozone layer, increasing levels of atmospheric carbon dioxide, acid rain and radioactive substances. As noted, a small layer of ozone surrounds the earth and blocks much of the ultraviolet radiation from reaching the earth's surface. The ozone layer is in danger of being depleted by the continued use of fluorocarbons (freon) and chlorofluoromethanes that release chlorine into the stratosphere to combine with ozone. The continued use of fluorocarbon-propelled aerosol products and supersonic transport planes would add to that danger. In Caucasians short-wavelength ultraviolet sunlight is thought to cause melanoma and nonmelanoma skin cancer that would increase in incidence if there were a reduction of the ozone layer.[3]

The *atmospheric content of carbon dioxide* has increased by 15 per cent in the past century. $CO_2$ is added to the atmosphere by burning fossil fuels and clearing forests. The increased level of atmospheric $CO_2$ alters the heat balance of the earth. Areas of the world are becoming warmer and wetter. Such changes might eventually result in polar ice caps melting, flooding of large coastal plains areas, and disrupting agriculture with altered food production.

**Acid rain** *is the end product of chemical reactions that begin when sulphur dioxide and nitrogen oxides enter the atmosphere from coal-, oil-, and gas-burning power plants, iron and copper smelters, and car exhausts.* These gases undergo changes and eventually react with moisture to form sulphuric acid and nitric acid. One-half to two-thirds of the pollution falls as acid rain or snow; some of the remainder is deposited as sulphate or nitrate particles that combine with dew and mist to form dilute acids.

The full effect on the environment is not understood as yet. Certain freshwater ecosystems are particularly sensitive to acid; fish, frogs, and certain aquatic plants die. Acid rain may actually increase the yield of several crops, such as corn and tomatoes. It will be years before the full effect of acid precipitation is known. At present, the only solution is to decrease the emissions of sulphur and nitrogen oxide to the atmosphere.

*Radioactive substances are produced by mining and processing radioactive ore and by nuclear-fission and radiation procedures* used in industry, medicine and research. Pollution from radioactive materials poses a serious threat to our ability to reproduce and to our gene structure. It is also related to an increase in leukaemia, as demonstrated in persons working with radioactive materials over long periods without adequate safeguards and in survivors of Hiroshima and Nagasaki. A small fraction, 1 to 3 per cent, of all cancers in the general population is attributable to natural radiation. Occupational irradiation produces an increase of less than 1 per cent over the natural incidence.[4]

All forms of air pollution are physically irritating and present a potential hazard to our long-range health either by direct harm to the mucous membranes of the respiratory tract or by the indirect effects of continuously breathing contaminated air. Only in becoming aware of these factors as personal health threats will we seriously consider alternatives to using two or three cars, seek to know the serious hazards in our jobs, and become concerned about houses downwind from an industrial site or the amount of ultraviolet light we receive.

*Indoor air pollution*

Recent air samplings in new energy-efficient homes have shown that many pollutants are more concentrated indoors than out. Nitrogen dioxide and carbon monoxide accumulate when gas stoves and heaters are burning. **Radon,** a *natural radioactive gas produced by the decay of radium,* seeps into basements through cracked floors and diffuses out of brick and concrete building materials. Formaldehyde escapes into the air from foam insulation, particle board, and furniture made of plywood. Formaldehyde gas in newly insulated homes has reached concentrations high enough to cause dizziness, rashes, nosebleeds and vomiting. Indoor radon may be contributing to thousands of lung cancer cases each year.[5] Particles, such as dust, soot, ash or cigarette smoke, may be inhaled into the lungs.

Indoor air pollution can be controlled by several measures: proper venting of gas stoves and heaters, painting over materials that emit radon and formaldehyde, and daily airing of the house.

## WATER POLLUTION

Pollution of the water from the natural processes of aquatic animal and plant life, combined with man-made waste, constitutes another hazard to the delicate state of human health. Man-made water pollution has two major origins, *point sources* and *nonpoint sources*. Point sources are those that discharge pollutants from a well-defined place, such as outlet pipes of sewage treatment plants and factories. Nonpoint sources consist of runoff from city streets, construction sites, farms, and mines. The water pollutant list is long: phosphates in laundry detergents; acid contamination from mine drainage; and industrial effluent of toxins, acids, radioactive substances, and mineral particles, such as mercury. Increasingly obvious causes are salinization of water from evaporation in the arid American West, land erosion, heat from industrial processes and oil spills.

*Types of water pollution*

Water pollutants causing much of the problem can be categorized as common sewage, infection-causing organisms, nutrients, synthetic chemicals, inorganic chemicals, sediment or heat. The common denominator of major water pollutants is called biologic oxygen demand (BOD), which is the amount of free oxygen that extraneous substances absorb from water.

**Common sewage,** traditional waste from domestic and industrial sources, is a significant problem because oxygen is required to render this waste harmless. This waste thus uses up oxygen needed by aquatic plant and animal life. With increasing amounts of sewage, the problem is even more serious because of the inability of the water to deal successfully with the waste. When bacteria in the water can no longer decompose the waste, widespread aquatic death results. Waste will then accumulate, and the water will become useless as a personal or industrial resource.

**Infection-causing organisms** pollute water when sewage carrying these bacteria enter a river or stream. A human or animal drinking this water can become ill. Microbiology and pharmacology have done a great deal in helping prevent and treat such diseases by identifying the responsible microorganisms and developing appropriate vaccines and antibiotics. Occasionally a whole community or area may be negatively affected, however, because of a gross error that contaminates a large body of water with diseased microbes. These microbes may spread infectious hepatitis or typhoid fever, especially in rural and urban fringe areas where population density is high and public utilities are limited.

**Nutrients** that nourish plant life, especially phosphates and nitrates, are produced by sewage, industrial wastes and soil erosion. These nutrients are not easily removed by treatment centres because they do not respond to the usual biological processes. Moreover, treatment centres may inadvertently change these substances into a more usable mineral form that stimulates excessive plant growth. This growth, in turn, becomes a problem by interfering with treatment processes, marring the landscape, producing an unpleasant odour and taste in the water, and disturbing the normal food web in a body of water. Because humans depend on many lower forms of life for food, this process could eventually affect their wellbeing if it occurred on a large scale.

**Synthetic chemicals** that are used in everyday household chores, especially chemicals found in detergents, pesticides, and other cleaning agents, affect the water. They may be poisonous to aquatic life even in small proportions. When resistant to local treatment measures, they can produce an unpleasant taste and odour in the water. The extent of the long-term problem is not known, but the possibility of human poisoning over a long period by the consumption of small doses of these chemicals taken in drinking water cannot be ignored. This problem is discussed later in the chapter.

**Inorganic chemicals** or mineral substances from mining or manufacturing processes can destroy land animals (including people) and aquatic life when ingested. Industries sometimes improperly and illegally empty large quantities of toxic materials into sources of local water supply. This group of pollutants corrodes water-treatment equipment and makes waste treatment an even more expensive problem.

**Sediment** – particles of earth, such as dirt and sand – consists of pollutants that are becoming a problem because of the magnitude of its debris. Sediment causes a nuisance and a hazard by covering food sources for aquatic life (and thereby eventually reducing sources for other life), by filling streams, and by preventing natural reservoirs from filling during rainy seasons. Resultant floods destroy animal and plant life and property and can cause epidemics of such water-borne diseases as typhoid and salmonellosis. Because of its sheer volume, sediment also increases the cost of water treatment.

**Heat** becomes a problem because it reduces the ability of the water to absorb oxygen. If significant amounts of water are heated through industrial use, the water becomes less efficient in providing oxygen for aquatic life and in assimilating waste. Even more dangerous, the ecological balance of lakes and rivers can be permanently upset through prolonged alteration

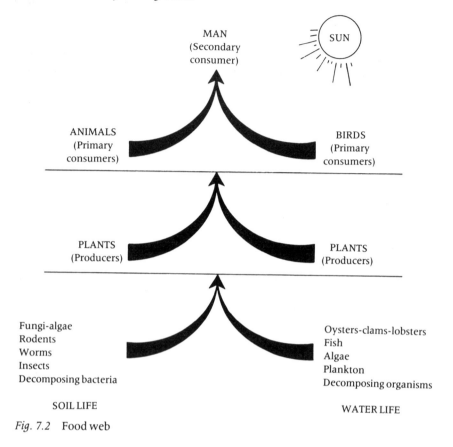

*Fig. 7.2*    Food web

of water temperature. The food that people eat either comes directly from water or has fed on aquatic life somewhere in the food web. Faced with an expanding world population, we must increasingly be aware of the significance of every organism in the food web (Fig. 7.2) and its relationship to us.

One of the most frightening results of water pollution is the threat to the oceans. The collective discharges of the world's nations and the practice of ocean dumping of sewage sludge may permanently pollute the oceans. Research on the effects of deep ocean dumping and the development of a waste management plan for coastal areas and pretreatment techniques that reduce the danger of sewage sludge should be continued before major investments in other forms of disposal are made.

*Problems in water purification*

The natural water purification process involves the action of bacteria using oxygen to decompose organic matter. If too much waste is dumped into a given body of water, this natural cleansing process cannot take place, or at least does not take place fast enough. Further, once the water in the underground aquifer is contaminated, it is nearly impossible to guarantee a safe water supply.

The ultimate problem of water pollution stems from our using natural resources in greater and greater amounts because of additional industrialization, population growth, a greater dependence on appliances, and a subsequent increase in the need for sewage disposal. The problem of dissolving waste has put a real strain on waste-disposal systems. Even excessive amounts of treated waste now obstruct the waterways. Current engineering research is attempting to solve some of the problems of water pollution by developing different types of waste-disposal systems.

Water is essential to life. When it contains such a variety of pollutants in ever-increasing amounts, it becomes a threat to human health. It poses a threat, first, because of its increasing unavailability for consumption, and second, because of the harmful proportion of dangerous pollutants contained in what does remain.

Pollution of marshes and shorelines has severely impaired breeding habitats for many types of shellfish and deep-water species, thereby subsequently affecting the nation's food supply. Polluted water cannot be used for recreational purposes. The odour of decay and the unsightliness of polluted water destroy the beauty of any natural setting.

Misuse of our water has far-reaching consequences, threatening people all over the world from every age group and culture. Therefore we must take definite personal responsibility for stopping needless pollution of the water by exercising careful personal use of agents that can ultimately destroy it and by using legal procedures to prevent undue dumping of wastes into streams.

## SOIL POLLUTION

*Substances used to kill weeds, rats, mice, worms, fungi and insects are called* **pesticides**. Soil pollution can occur as a result of excessive or improper use of pesticides (insecticides, herbicides, fungicides) or crop fertilizers. Many chemicals used in these preparations are highly toxic and can remain in the soil for long periods of time without being degraded, thus setting the stage for pollution of food, water and, ultimately, people.

Farmers are the largest users of pesticides, but they are also used by industry; central and local governmental agencies; and individual people in their homes and gardens. Actual toxic effects of the different compounds vary and some effects occur before the chemicals reach the soil. Vertebrates usually will not suffer acute poisoning from these substances except through accidental ingestion, direct skin contact, or inhalation of the dust or spray of the more toxic pesticides. Workers in pesticide manufacturing plants, agricultural workers, and commercial pest-control operators applying the chemicals to crops or soil can all inhale pesticide dust or spray. Inhalation exposure can occur in a subtle manner at times – for example, by inhaling the dust from storage bags during the filling and emptying process or from cultivated soil previously treated with pesticides. Symptoms occurring as a result of such exposure may not be attributed to the pesticides. Therefore many episodes of acute poisoning go undiagnosed. Direct skin contact can occur when solutions are spilled accidentally or when the moist spray touches exposed skin. An occupational history aids early diagnosis of such problems.

*Effects of soil pollution*

Reports from epidemiological studies indicate that various acute illnesses and physiological changes were observed in farmers after handling agricultural chemicals. Such effects on the central nervous system as forgetfulness, decreased attention and interest span, hyperirritability, anxiety, depression, nervousness and insomnia have been reported. Skin diseases, eye and respiratory conditions, and digestive disorders have also been identified. In some instances, these problems occurred after a single exposure to a toxic chemical.[6]

Pesticides have an immediate toxic effect on birds, bees and rodents, thus curtailing the necessary natural agents of cross-pollination and insect destruction which, in turn, can affect the food supply. Surface water may be contaminated during spraying or dusting; or rain may wash pesticides or fertilizers into streams and lakes, again affecting food supply.

Edwards shows that earthworms are capable of concentrating toxic chemicals from the soil and storing these chemicals in their fatty tissues. Because earthworms provide food for other animals that are also capable of concentrating these chemicals, they may prove to be an important source of undesirable chemical residues in higher animals and humans.[7]

The effects on people of long-term exposure to pesticides by inhalation or by ingestion of food and water containing residual chemicals are unknown. However, lower activity values of serum lactic dehydrogenase (an enzyme present in large amounts in liver tissue); inhibited cholinesterase activity; and altered hemoglobin, hematocrit, and amino acid levels have been shown to exist in people occupationally exposed to pesticides.[8] Experimentally, small doses of pesticides have caused such metabolic changes as lowered estrogen levels, altered glucose metabolism, and inhibition of adenosine triphosphatase (ATP) in a wide variety of vertebrates, including humans. In addition, potent **herbicides,** *substances used to kill weeds or plants,* such as 2,4,5-T, have produced spontaneous abortions, birth defects, and skeletal and tissue changes *after birth* in animals and humans.

The widespread contamination by dioxin in Missouri in 1983 following massive flooding illustrates the complexity and extent of the problem. Chemicals were used without awareness of harmful effect. Unregulated use of chemicals for dumping various chemicals by industries has occurred for some time and has only become apparent later. Furthermore, chemicals may not remain where originally used or dumped. Flood waters, underground water and wind transport chemicals or their residues from one soil site to another. People are now learning that their past and present symptoms or diseases are related to or caused by hazardous pollutants in the environment to which they did not know they were being exposed.

Dioxin, for example, is considered the most toxic synthetic compound known to science. A complex organic chemical compound, it is insoluble in water but dissolves in organic solvents mixed with water. It is strongly attracted to lipids: fatty tissue in the body, oils, or related lipid substances. It becomes strongly attached to soil particles. The chemical remains in lipids or soil for many years and can move through water with solvents, soil particles, or colloids to which it is attached, such as during a flood or with soil erosion. Dioxin is also part of many other chemical compounds – for example, chlorophenols, herbicides, and the antiseptic hexachlorophene. It can be generated by incineration of industrial, commercial and municipal wastes that contain chlorinated aromatics, chlorophenols, or PCBs. It produces a wide range of harmful effects in humans and animals, including:

1. Fatal liver damage.
2. Birth defects.
3. Spontaneous abortions and sterility.
4. Many types of cancer.
5. Nerve and brain damage.
6. Disturbed enzyme production.
7. Reduced immunity to infections.
8. Chloracne, a disfiguring and painful affliction of the skin.
9. Damage to the urinary, genital, and gastrointestinal tracts, the thymus and spleen.

Many effects are chronic and long term.

Dioxin is not only a problem for residents along Missouri rivers outside of St Louis, however, although that was the scene of much publicity in 1983.

Dioxin was a contaminant in Agent Orange, the herbicide sprayed in Vietnam, to which many US service personnel were exposed. These servicemen are also suffering a variety of health problems. Where else dioxin contamination may be found is not yet known.


FOOD POLLUTION

Some of the same chemicals found in pesticide preparation are used as **food additives**. These purposely used additives are not designed to be toxic but rather *to preserve, improve and protect nutritional value.*

Artificial flavours and colours make up 80 per cent of all chemicals used in our food; preservatives, sweeteners and thickeners, a total of 11 categories of substances, make up the rest of the additives. However, determining their potential health hazard over a life span is difficult. Certain food additives interfere with intestinal mucosa absorptive ability and therefore affect availability of nutrients and drugs. Also, some nontoxic substances or chemicals used as food additives are metabolized into toxic substances in the body. Adverse reactions to synthetic flavours and colours include gastrointestinal, respiratory, neurological, skeletal and skin disorders. Removal of artificial flavours and colours from the diet has been found to reduce hyperkinesis and certain learning disabilities in 50 per cent of the children with these disorders.[9] Under certain physiological conditions nitrites used to inhibit bacterial growth in processed foods can combine with certain amines to form chemicals that are potentially mutagenic and carcinogenic.

Unexpected side effects due to antibiotic and hormone residues from drugs given to animals for growth promotion and disease prevention have resulted. In people these residues have resulted in (1) allergy and increased drug toxicity or resistance to pathogens when the *same* family of antibiotics is later administered therapeutically, and (2) change of normal bacterial flora in a body area so that invasion by pathogens is more likely, causing infection or disease. Synthetic estrogen diethylstilbestrol (DES) was used to cattle feed to promote rapid weight gain. Studies have linked DES to increases in a rare genital tract tumour in young women whose mothers were given DES when pregnant. As a result of these studies, use of DES has been restricted. An attempt to ban its use and the use of other sex hormones as feed supplements for cattle is underway.

Other food pollution hazards are radioactive materials, such as strontium 90, which has been traced in milk; mercury found in swordfish; worms; and mould, which may be present without noticeable change in the food's appearance, taste or smell. Food handlers may introduce their infectious diseases into food by touching it or the equipment with soiled hands or by coughing onto it. Prolonged storage of highly acidic foods in aluminium cookware or aluminium foil may cause more aluminium than usual to enter the body. Using unlined copper utensils for cooking or storing food may also be harmful. Food sources may become contaminated by the chemicals and metals used in fertilizers and pesticides. In the future, diseases from food additives may assume as much significance in humans as do the **zoonoses,** *diseases transmitted between animals and humans,* such as trichinosis, brucellosis, tuberculosis, psittacosis, salmonellosis, typhus, roundworms and rabies.


NOISE POLLUTION


Sensory stimulation plays a major role in psychological and physiological development and is therefore directly related to physical and mental health. Sound is but one form of sensory stimulation. **Sound overload,** *unwanted sound that produces unwanted effects,* as well as sound deprivation, can be hazards to health.

Sound overload can produce temporary or permanent hearing loss by affecting the tympanic membrane and by slowly deteriorating the microscopic cells that send sound waves from the ear to the brain. The effects produced on each person's hearing vary, depending on the sound intensity and pitch, the location of the source in relation to the person, the length of exposure, and the person's age and history of previous ear problems.

One means of determining the potential hazard of any sound is to measure its loudness. *The measurement of sound loudness is stated in* **decibels.** The faintest audible sound is designated 1 decibel; ordinary conversation, measured at 40 to 60 decibels, is considered adequately quiet. 55 decibels is considered to be the level above which harmful effects occur. Studies have shown that moderately loud sounds of 75 to 80 decibels, such as those produced by a washing machine, tabulating machine, or home waste-disposal unit, can be discomforting to human ears and can, over a period of time, produce temporary or permanent hearing loss. Here are examples of common sound pollutants and their decibel readings:

|  | Decibels |
|---|---|
| Vacuum cleaner | 72 |
| Dishwasher | 76–96 |
| Minibike | 76 |
| Heavy city traffic | 90–95 |
| Food blender in home | 93 |
| Pneumatic hammer | 95 |
| Air compressor | 95 |
| Power lawnmower | 95 |
| Farm tractor | 98 |

| | |
|---|---|
| Outboard motor | 102 |
| Jet flying over at 1000 feet | 103 |
| Riveting gun | 110 |
| Motorcycle | 115 |
| Live rock music | 120 |
| Jet plane at takeoff | 150 |
| Rocket engine | 180 |

Sound louder than 130 decibels, such as that produced by a nearby jet plane, gunshot blast, or a rocket at the launching pad, may cause actual pain. Persons who work regularly with any of the machines listed should realize the potential long-range effects of such noise levels, and understand why protective measures are important.

*Effects of noise pollution*

Sound overload affects everyone at some time by intruding on privacy and shattering serenity. It can produce impaired communication and social relationships, irritability, chronic headache, depression, fatigue and tension, in addition to hearing loss. Research indicates that less obvious physiological changes can also occur. These changes include involuntary responses in the digestive, cardiovascular, endocrine and nervous system. They can produce blood vessel constriction, pallor, dilated pupils and visual disturbance, increased and irregular heart rate, hypertension, headache, gastrointestinal spasm with nausea and diarrhoea and eventual peptic ulcer, hyperactive reflexes and muscle tenseness. These responses do not subside immediately but continue up to five times longer than the actual noise. Noise has also been associated with elevated blood cholesterol levels, atherosclerosis and accident proneness.

We do not adapt to excessive sound, as was once thought; we learn to tolerate it. Even when a person is asleep, noise cannot be shut out completely. We are exhausted by our efforts to remain asleep in the midst of this external stimuli. Perhaps being aware of these environmental stress factors can aid in reducing or coping with them.

Although not every harmful form of sound can be avoided, certain measures, such as wearing protective ear coverings, shortening exposure time, having regular hearing examinations, and seeking immediate medical attention for any ear injury or infection, will decrease the possibility of permanent damage or hearing loss. Noise can be brought under control without excessive cost. You can educate the public about the hazards of excess noise and ways to reduce noise in the home environment. Some suggestions to reduce noise are: hang heavy curtains over windows closest to outside noise sources, use foam pads under blenders and mixers, use carpeting in areas of heavy foot traffic, use upholstered instead of hard-surfaced furniture, and install sound-absorbing ceiling tiles in the kitchen.

The hospital, considered a place to recuperate and rest, may actually contribute to symptoms because of the noise levels in certain areas. One study showed that noise levels in infant incubators, the recovery room, and acute care units were high enough to act as a stressor and stimulate the hypophyseal-adrenocortical axis. Peripheral vasoconstriction affecting blood pressure and pulse, threats to hearing loss in patients receiving aminoglycosidic antibiotics, and sleep deprivation were noted. Noise pollution in the operating rooms, causing vasoconstriction, pupil dilation, fatigue, and impaired speech communication, has also been found.

*Nuclear waste*

One type of hazardous waste product that has attracted considerable attention is radioactive waste. Some fission products that must be stored are cesium-137, strontium-90, iodine-131, and plutonium-239. Some decay rapidly in hours or days while others require thousands and millions of years to lose their radioactive potency (136). No satisfactory method of permanent disposal has been developed; the cost and fear of leakage from the storage area have been stumbling blocks.

The use of nuclear energy or power produced by fission reactors has caused much concern and debate among the people of the United States. The concerns centre around two major issues: the long-term disposal of radioactive wastes and the safety of the actual reactors.

When a utility shuts down a reactor at the end of its period of usefulness, the utility is faced with the problem of what to do with intensely radioactive materials. At present, only three means of disposal exist: dismantlement of the reactor with the debris shipped to a burial site, entombment of the reactor in a concrete structure, and protective storage that would prevent public access for 30 to 100 years. Even though nuclear power is a quarter of a century old, the problem of safe disposal of radioactive waste is not yet critical.

The seriousness of problems associated with the safety of nuclear reactors for generating electricity is well illustrated by the following highly publicized event. In Pennsylvania, in March 1979, an accident occurred at the nuclear reactor site known as Three Mile Island. In retrospect, the accident was preventable and was less severe than originally reported. Residents near the site, however, were exposed to the radioactive isotope xenon-133, which has a half-life of approximately 5 days. The radiation release has the potential for causing the death, by cancer, of less than one person in the next 30 or 40 years. The major health effect of the accident appears to have been on the mental health of the people in the region. The fear, anger and confusion felt by the Three Mile Island community are shared nationally and internationally. The majority of citizens now have serious second thoughts about the safety and reliability of nuclear power.

The full effects of the nuclear accident at Chernobyl in the USSR in 1986 are still being evaluated. Movement and sale of cattle, sheep and other forms of produce in parts of the UK, for example, Wales and Cumbria, is still restricted because of excessively high levels of radioactivity in animals and soil as a result of contamination from Chernobyl.

Diminishing resources lead to the need for alternative energy sources. The problems in this area must be explored.[10]

*Lead poisoning*

*Lead* is another surface pollutant. We inhale lead as an air pollutant and ingest traces of lead daily through a normal diet. Because lead wastes have increased during the past century, particularly from industry and motor vehicle use, exposure and intake into the body have multiplied. Consequently, the rate of absorption by soft tissue exceeds the rate of excretion or storage by bone.[11] An urgent problem is controlling the lead exposure that occurs from drinking or eating from improperly lead-glazed earthenware, using leaded petrol, consuming lead-contaminated 'moonshine', or working in or living near industries where lead exposure is not controlled. Two-thirds of the lead found in canned foods comes from solder. This source of lead constitutes one-third of the lead that the average person ingests from food.

Individuals who work in areas with high lead levels show evidence of chronic lead poisoning. Persistent abdominal pain is the cardinal symptom in adults. They also exhibit fatigue, nervousness, and sleep disturbances as well as cognitive deficits and peripheral neuropathy. Kidney damage occurs slowly and may not be detected until two-thirds of the kidney function is destroyed. The male workers have a decrease in the quantity and quality of sperm, and the female workers have an increased risk of foetal damage and/or abortion.

Another urgent problem arises when young children, mainly in urban slums, form the *habit of eating nonfood substances, including peeling paint, plaster, or putty containing lead. This behaviour is called* **pica**. The precise cause of pica is not completely understood, but it may be related to nutritional, cultural and emotional factors. Acute or chronic lead poisoning, an insidious disease, results from this eating pattern and is a major source of brain damage, mental deficiency and behaviour problems. The pathological changes that occur affect the nervous, renal and hematopoietic systems. Kidney damage is usually reversible, but chronic lead poisoning in childhood may lead to gout or kidney disease later in life. Damage to the hematopoietic system is evident by the reduction in the number and quality of red blood cells produced, thus leading to severe anaemia. The most serious effects are on the nervous system. The mortality rate from lead encephalopathy (disease of the brain) is 5 per cent. Of the children who survive acute lead poisoning, 40 per cent have convulsive disorders and another 20 per cent have significant neurological deficits.

The sale of lead paint and lead in children's toys or furniture was banned in the UK over a decade ago.

## OCCUPATIONAL HAZARDS

Increasingly we learn of the health hazards that many workers face daily at their jobs. Monotony, paced work, and performance pressures are major sources of stress in many jobs and can contribute to disease pathology. The muscle strains, backaches, fractures, burns, eye injuries and other accidental emergencies are taken for granted by the public. But workers may not suffer the consequences of the hidden environmental hazards – the chemicals or radiation they work with directly or indirectly – until years later. Often in the past the etiology of the physical illness remained unsolved. Not only do miners and factory workers become ill because of their work environment, hospital workers also may suffer. Those who work regularly with certain anaesthetics, for example, may develop cancer, leukaemia or lymphoma. Those who work with high levels of radiation risk sterility or defective offspring if adequate protection is not maintained. Nurses may suffer infections, back and muscle injuries, varicose veins, and any of the other physical or emotional effects of stress.

The Health and Safety At Work Act, which updates the Factories Act and adds to previous legislation seeks to ensure that proper safety measures are taken in industry and public places. Regulations are issued which must be adhered to and inspections are carried out by officers of the Health and Safety Executive. All major unions have a Health and Safety representative at the shop-floor level to ensure that agreed safety measures are being kept by the workers and the management.

Hazards of the factory or mine can extend beyond the workplace and endanger workers' families and other residents of the community. Workers carry out dust particles on skin and clothing; wind currents also deposit particles. Even if workers shower before leaving work, the total removal of all dust particles of some chemicals or elements is difficult. As a result, some communities become well known for a high incidence of certain types of cancer or skin or respiratory disease.

Another group of health hazards related to a large industry is cosmetics, including aerosol preparations, hair dyes and feminine sprays, which increasingly are related to skin and other diseases, including cancer. As with other occupational chemicals, effects of the use of these products are usually not known until years after their regular usage.[12] The World Health

Organization estimates that 75 to 85 per cent of all cancers are environmentally caused. No one knows how much occupational factors contribute to the causes.[13]

Laryngeal cancer has been found among workers exposed to asbestos, cutting oil, wood dust, grease and oil; among workers in the paper, metal, construction, leather, food and textile industries; and among barbers, sheet metal workers, electricians and naphthalene cleaners.

Often occupational health hazards are taken for granted. They are seen as part of the job. Employees in laundries and dry cleaning establishments, for example, suffer hazards of excess heat, humidity, and noise; falls and accidents from slipping on wet floors; back injury and muscle strains from lifting; and circulatory problems from standing. Caretakers may have contact with dangerous chemicals in cleaning agents. Asthma is an occupational hazard for animal workers, vets, farmers, bakers, carpenters, welders and many other workers.

Industrial nurses and safety engineers emphasize wearing protective clothing and using protective equipment. Yet there are problems. The employee may not want to be bothered with cumbersome protective clothing. Or the protective clothing and equipment given to the female employee may be too large or too heavy, thus ill-fitting and not protective, for it is designed for the male employee. (However, a few companies do specialize in protective clothing designed for females.) Hard hats, safety shoes and gloves, and ear muffs that fit improperly may actually contribute toward an accidental injury.

To compound the problem of prevention, length of exposure to an industrial substance often determines if it will cause disease. The amount of exposure to the worker often depends on the production phase involved. Additionally, each substance appears likely to produce disease, such as cancer, in a specific body part; such information becomes available after workers become ill. Sex is also a factor, for some substances affect the reproductive organs of the female (or foetus) but do not affect the male. Some substances do not affect the male reproductive organs, but the father's genes may contribute to foetal damage.

Table 7.1 summarizes common industrial agents (various substances, elements or chemicals) and their major known effects.

Knowing that the worker may come in contact with a variety of harmful substances and that presenting symptoms may often seem unrelated to the occupation should help you be more careful and thorough in assessment. Also, as a citizen you can work for enforcement of preventive measures for known hazards and for continued research.

*Table 7.1*     Effects of some common industrial agents upon the worker

| Agent | Type of industry or occupation | Body area affected |
|---|---|---|
| Acetaldehyde | Chemical, paint | All body cells, especially brain and respiratory tract. |
| Acetic Anhydride | Textile | Exposed tissue damage, especially eye and respiratory tract. |
| Acetylene | Welding, plastic, dry cleaning | Respiratory tract asphyxiant. Explosive, especially when combined with certain substances. |
| Acrolein | Chemical | Skin, eye, respiratory tract. |
| Allyl Chloride | Plastic | Skin, respiratory tract, kidney. |
| Ammonia | Chemical, leather, wool, farmers, refrigeration workers | Eyes, skin, respiratory tract. |
| Anaesthetic Gases | Medical, dental, and veterinary workers | Reproductive (increased rate of spontaneous abortions and congenital anomalies whether male or female exposed). |
| Aniline | Paint, rubber | Skin, hematopoietic system. |
| Arsenic | Mine, smelter, leather, chemical, oil refinery, insecticide makers and sprayers | Skin, lung, liver (cancer). Nervous system damage. |
| Asbestos | Mine, textile, insulation, shipyard workers, construction | Respiratory and gastrointestinal tract (cancer) as well as asbestosis (lung scarring). More harmful to people who smoke. |
| Benzene | Rubber, chemical, explosives, paint, shoemakers, dye users, office workers | Skin, liver, brain, hematopoietic system (cancer, leukaemia). |
| Beryllium | Foundry, metallurgical, aerospace, nuclear, household appliance production | Skin and eye (inflammation, ulcers), respiratory tract (acute inflammation and berylliosis – chronic lung infection), systemic effects on heart, liver, spleen, kidneys. |
| Butyl Alcohol | Lacquer, paint | Eye, skin, respiratory tract. |
| Carbon Disulfide | Rubber, viscose rayon | Gastrointestinal, heart, liver, kidney, brain. |
| Carbon Tetrachloride | Solvent, dry cleaning | Skin, gastrointestinal, liver, kidney, brain. |
| Chlorine | Industrial bleaching, laundry workers | Eye, respiratory tract, skin. |
| Chloroform | Chemical, plastic | Heart degeneration, liver, kidney. |

*Table 7.1*    (cont.)

| Agent | Type of industry or occupation | Body area affected |
|---|---|---|
| Chromium | Chrome plating, chemical, industrial bleaching, glass and pottery, linoleum makers, battery makers | Irritating to all body cells. Skin, eye, respiratory tract, (cancer) liver, kidney. |
| Coal combustion products (soot, tar) | Gashouse workers, asphalt, coal tar, or pitch workers, mine, coke oven workers | Skin, respiratory tract, scrotum, urinary bladder (carcinogenic to all areas). |
| Cotton, flax, hemp, lint | Textile | Respiratory tract (byssinosis-chest tightness, dyspnea, cough, wheezing; chronic bronchitis). Cigarette smokers especially affected. |
| Creosal | Chemical, oil refining | Denatures and precipitates all cellular protein. Skin, eye, respiratory tract, liver, kidney, brain. |
| Dichloroethyl ether | Insecticide, oil refining | Respiratory tract. |
| Dimethyl sulphate | Chemical, pharmaceutical | Eye, respiratory tract, liver, kidney, brain. |
| Ethylene oxide | Hospital sterilization | Possible foetal damage. |
| Formaldehyde | Textile | Liver, lung, skin (infection and cancer). |
| Fungus, parasites, microorganisms | Food, animal, outdoor workers, clinical laboratory workers | Skin, respiratory tract (infection, including hepatitis B). |
| Germicidal agents | Health-care workers, maintenance/cleaning workers | Skin (contact allergy, dermatosis). |
| Hydrogen chloride | Meat wrappers | Respiratory tract (irritation and asthma). |
| Iron Oxide | Mine, iron foundry, metal polishers and finishers | Respiratory tract (cancer). |
| Lead | Auto, smelter, plumbing, paint, metallurgical, battery making. Exposure in 120 different industries | Hematopoietic, liver, kidney, brain, muscles, bone, gastrointestinal tract. Causes foetal damage during first trimester of pregnancy. |
| Leather | Leather, shoe | Nasal cavity and sinuses, urinary bladder (carcinogenic for each). |
| Manganese | Mine, metallurgical, welders | Respiratory tract, liver, brain. |
| Mercury | Electrical, laboratory workers. Exposure in 80 different types of industries | Toxic to all cells. Dermatosis. Respiratory tract, liver, brain damage. Exposure of pregnant woman causes congenital defects and retardation. |

*Table 7.1* (cont.)

| Agent | Type of industry or occupation | Body area affected |
|---|---|---|
| Mica | Rubber, insulation | Respiratory tract. |
| Nickel | Metallurgical, smelter, electrolysis workers | Skin, respiratory tract (infection and cancer). |
| Nitrobenzene | Synthetic dyes | Skin, hematopoietic system, brain. |
| Nitrogen dioxide | Chemical, metal | Eye, respiratory tract, hematopoietic system. |
| Organophosphates | Agriculture | Brain dysfunction, memory loss, disorientation, ataxia, liver and kidney damage. |
| Petroleum products | Rubber, textile, aerospace, workers in contact with fuel oil, coke, paraffin, lubricants | Skin, respiratory tract, scrotum (carcinogenic to each); dermatosis. |
| Phenol | Plastics | Corrosive to all tissue. Liver, kidney, brain. |
| Polyurethane | Plastics and most other industries | Respiratory tract (asthma, cancer). Dermatosis. |
| Rubber dust | Rubber | Respiratory tract (chronic disease). Dermatosis. |
| Silica | Mine, foundry, ceramic or glass production | Respiratory tract (silicosis). |
| Talc dust | Mine | Respiratory tract (cancer), calcification of pericardium. |
| Tetraethyl lead | Chemical | Hematopoietic system, brain. |
| Thallium | Pesticide, fireworks or explosives | Skin, respiratory and gastrointestinal tract, kidney, brain. |
| Toluene | Rubber, paint, clerical workers, printers | Skin, respiratory tract, liver, hematopoietic system, brain (may cause drunken state and accidents). |
| Trichloroethylene | Chemical, metal degreasing | Skin, liver, kidney, brain. |
| Vinyl chloride | Plastic, rubber, insulation, organic-chemical synthesizers, polyvinyl resin makers | Skin, respiratory tract, (asthma), cancer in the liver, kidney, spleen and brain. Exposure of pregnant woman to polyvinyl chloride causes defective foetus. |
| Wood products | Furniture | Respiratory tract (asthma). |

NURSING RESPONSIBILITY

*Personal responsibility*

Consider the environment, the various social institutions, and the population as a complex of interacting, interdependent systems. Environmental problems are a concern to everyone and are of equal consequence to every part of the world. Each of us shares the earth and so we are all responsible for its wellbeing. Environmental pollution is our collective fault and requires our collective solutions. In the United States alone discarded materials amount to 4 billion tons yearly and the quantity is growing by 8 per cent annually.

Linton describes a fourfold environmental protection system for continuously identifying, analysing and controlling environmental hazards:

1. Surveillance – maintaining an awareness of what people are doing to the air, water and land, and of the effect of these actions on health.
2. Development of criteria for the detection of pollution.
3. Research
4. Compliance – getting local government and industry to accept and implement new standards.

An informed public can help establish such a system, but the financial support and legislative and administrative guidance of central and local governments seem to be the most feasible solution.

As citizens we should conserve natural resources to the best of our abilities and learn about the environmental pollution in our own areas. Remember that metallurgical and chemical companies are the greatest source of hazardous waste. Campaign for minimized waste and for safe disposal of unavoidable waste. Encourage the development of additional burial sites for long-term safety as well as the monitoring of present sites for escape of wastes.

Avoid unnecessary use of water, electricity and fuel. Don't litter. Buy beverages in returnable bottles and save cans and papers for recycling. Most towns have community tips for domestic waste materials, bottle collection points, etc.

Avoid high-phosphate detergents and aerosols. Don't carelessly dispose of used batteries, used engine oil, or empty pesticide containers. Walk or bicycle instead of driving a car when feasible. Avoid cigarette smoking in closed, crowded areas. Avoid contact with pesticides by thoroughly scrubbing or peeling food stuffs and, if possible, maintain your own garden without use of pesticides. Quiet surroundings are a natural resource, too. Make your own quieter through personal habits. Help plan for local recreation sites that offer natural surroundings. Campaign for adequate acoustical standards in homes, apartments, hospitals and industrial buildings, and for noiseless kitchen equipment. Participate in local governmental planning to decrease town and city noise in relation to transportation routes, zoning, and industrial sites. Don't burn leaves; contribute to a natural resource – soil – by composting plants or organic content in garbage. Plant a rooftop or patio garden to contribute to the oxygen cycle. Limit the number of pet animals. Join citizens' crusades for a clean environment or a conversation organization to learn more about problems, preventive measures, and means of strengthening legislation. Support antipollution and noise-control laws. Be an involved citizen!

The momentum that surrounded much of the environmental effort in its earliest stages has lead to some degree of apathy. It is a never-ending task to make the environment safe for the public and attitudes must be positive to maintain this serious concern.

*Professional responsibility*

Although nursing responsibilities have been interwoven throughout this chapter, consider that your primary responsibilities are detection through thorough assessment, making suggestions for intervention, and health teaching. You can play a significant role in the early detection of lead poisoning, for example. Assessment of a child's health should include observation for physical signs, such as tremors, abdominal discomfort, decreased appetite and vomiting, as well as questions related to a pica behaviour. Ask the mother about her child's interest in play, ability to get along with playmates, coordination, and level of developmental skill attainment. Phrase your questions and comments carefully, in a nonjudgmental manner, so that the mother will not feel that her fitness as a parent is being judged. If the persons for whom you are caring live in unsatisfactory, low-income housing, work for improvement through local legislation. Emphasis must be placed on repair and deleading of dwelling places, not just on moving the present dweller to a new house or apartment. You can encourage the formation of screening and case-finding programmes, already started in many cities, and you can assist with their activities. Be as thorough in assessment as possible.

Natural or manmade chemical pollution in soil, water and food products can produce various adverse effects, ranging from slight health impairments to death.

Another dangerous problem associated with chemical pollution is its possible carcinogenic effect (as seen on Table 7.1). Incidence of specific forms of cancer can be higher or lower, depending on exposure to specific compounds, a common example being the high incidence of lung cancer in the USA and the UK because of heavy tobacco use. Be aware and knowledgeable of the incidence of chemically produced cancer in your particular locale. Health teaching can then be directed at trying to eliminate or control the responsible carcinogenic chemical. Radiation is also carcinogenic. Encourage the use of protective clothing and sunscreen lotions to prevent overexposure to the sun. Prevent overexposure to ionizing radiation by making certain that unnecessary X-rays are not taken, by keeping a record of the frequency of X-rays, and by using a lead shield when X-rays are given.

The biochemical response to chemical pollution or radiation can influence the cell in various ways. *Teratogenic* (producing malformations) and *mutagenic* (producing hereditary changes) are two such changes in cells. Be aware that these changes can occur in both the client and the health-care worker who are exposed to radiation. Genetic counselling might be indicated for couples who have been exposed to radiation. Citizens should know of the possibility for dealing effectively and therapeutically with biochemical changes, whether prenatally or in any stage of growth and development.[14]

In the past 100 years disease and death have been reduced because of preventive public health measures in the form of environmental control, such as water and waste management, rodent and insect control, development of housing codes. Now we are again faced with problems and diseases that have an environmental impact. Prevention can begin with informed consumer groups who have educational and work projects as their goals. It can begin with your responsibility for the patient's environment.

*The patient's immediate environment*

Besides a feeling of responsibility for the community and physical environment in which the patient lives, you also have a responsibility for that individual's immediate environment while receiving health care. The patient's *surroundings should constitute a* **therapeutic milieu** *free of hazards and conducive to recovery, physically and emotionally.*

The patient's surroundings should be clean and adequately lighted, ventilated and heated. Precautions should always be taken during care to prevent injury, such as burns from a hot-water bottle. Falls should be prevented by removing obstacles from walking areas and having the person wear well-fitted shoes and use adequate support while walking. Lock the bed or wheelchair while the patient is moving to and from them. Be sure that electrical cords and scatter rugs are not so placed that the patient could fall. Wipe up spilled liquids immediately. Use sterile technique and proper handwashing methods to ensure that you bring no pathogenic organisms to the patient. Avoid excessive noise from personnel and equipment to the degree possible.

The aesthetic environment is also important for rest. Arrange articles on the bedside table in a pleasing manner if the patient is unable to do so. Keep unattractive equipment or supplies out of sight as much as possible. Electrical equipment should be in proper repair and function. Minimize offensive odours and noise. Place the person's bed or chair by a window or door so that the person can watch normal activity rather than stare at the ceiling and walls. As a nurse, involve yourself in making the entire ward as well as the patients' rooms look pleasing. Consider colour combinations and the use of curtains, furniture, clocks, calendars, pictures and various artifacts to create a more homelike atmosphere. The committee in charge of decorating and building should include at least one nurse. You may need to volunteer to ensure that nursing and, indirectly, patients are represented in such programmes.

The patient's surroundings should not only be safe and attractive, but the emotional climate of the unit and entire institution affects patients and staff as well. The patient and family are quick to respond and react to the attitudes and manner of the staff. Here are some questions you might ask yourself. How do I treat delivery workers who bring gifts and flowers to patients? Do I participate in the joy such remembrances bring to the patient? Do I help arrange the flowers into a pleasant pattern or just stick them quickly into whatever can be found? Do I treat visitors as welcome guests or as foreign intruders? The emotional climate should radiate security and acceptance. A sense of warmth should prevail that promotes a feeling of trust, confidence, and motivation within the patient as he/she and the staff work together to cope with problems. The emotional relationship between the patient and the health-care staff should help the patient reach the goal of maximum health.

In a truly therapeutic milieu the staff also feel a sense of harmony among themselves. There is mutual trust and acceptance between staff and supervisors, and supervisors recognize work well done by the staff. As a result, staff feel motivated to continue to learn and to improve the quality of patient care. Staff members are not likely to give individualized, comprehensive, compassionate care in an agency where they are not treated like individuals or where their basic needs are not met.

Be aware of environmental pollution in the health-care environment. 'No Smoking' should be the rule not only when oxygen is in use but also in any health-care setting. Often the conference of dining rooms or lounges for health-care workers are polluted with cigarette or cigar smoke and ashtrays are full. It is difficult to teach a client the adverse effects of smoking and nicotine when an odour of cigarette smoke hangs on the uniform. Moreover, health-care workers will benefit from practising what they teach others. Health-care workers and clients may also come in contact with agents listed in Table 7.1. Constant vigilance is necessary to detect harmful agents and prevent or reduce their usage. Early assessment of harmful effects to reduce the symptoms and proper intervention for dermatoses, allergens, or other symptoms is essential.

There are times when the treatment for the client may also affect the health-care worker – for example, radiotherapy. Proper precautions should be taken to protect the worker from excess exposure and to protect any body areas of the client that should not be exposed. Constant monitoring of the dosage and duration of exposure to radiation, whether from a portable X-ray machine or a radium implant, is essential.

Patients who are receiving radiotherapy[15] should be assessed for the following side effects:

1. Redness, edema, itching, denuding, and atrophy of skin.
2. Inflammation, dryness, pain, and impaired physiological function of mucous-lined areas of the body, including the oral cavity, esophagus and vagina.
3. Sloughing of epithelial cells in various body areas, such as the esophagus, stomach, intestine and genitourinary tract, resulting in ulceration, chronic inflammation, pain, necrosis and impaired physiological functions of the organ system affected (vomiting, diarrhoea, cystitis).
4. Depression of bone marrow, resulting in reduced white and red blood cells and platelets which, in turn, causes infections, anaemia, and haemorrhagic tendencies.
5. Inflammatory and fibrotic damage to the lungs and heart, causing pneumonitis, pericarditis and occasionally myocarditis.
6. Temporary or permanent loss of hair, depending on dosage and duration of exposure.

Intervention for these side effects includes skin and mouth care; dietary modifications; use of mild analgesics, antiemetics, and antidiarrheal drugs; and reverse isolation techniques.

If you are caring for a person in the home, you are limited in the amount of change you can make. You can point out such hazards as electrical cords in the walking area, however. You can make suggestions for furniture rearrangement if you think that the person could function more easily with the change. You can put a clock in sight, pull the curtains or put needed materials within the patient's reach if feasible.

Specific ways of meeting the patient's environmental needs also differ for various developmental stages. The components of a therapeutic milieu are different for the baby than for the middle-aged man. However, a safe, secure environment, physically and psychologically, must be present for both. Accurately determining the factors that make up the environment and making appropriate changes may be the first step in promoting health.

## REFERENCES

1. Waldbott, George, *Health Effects of Environmental Pollutants,* 2nd edition (The C.V. Mosby Company, St Louis, 1978).
2. Ibid.
3. 'Cancer, The Environmental Connection', *Science Challenge,* vol. 5, no. 3 (1982).
4. Ibid; also see note 1, above.
5. Gold, Michael, *The New Genetics and the Future of Man,* (William B. Eerdmans Publishing Company, Grand Rapids, MI, 1972).
6. World Health Organization, 'Most Cancers are in the Developing World', *The Nation's Health,* vol. 11, no. 12 (1981) p. 18.
7. Edwards, Clive, 'Soil Pollutants and Soil Animals', *Scientific American,* vol. 220, no. 4 (1969) pp. 88–99.
8. Ibid.
9. Duffus, John H., *Environmental Toxicology* (John Wiley & Sons Inc., New York, 1980).
10. Purcell, Arthur, 'Three Mile Island's Three Fateful Dates and the Fate of Nuclear Energy', *Science Digest,* vol. 87, no. 4 (1982), pp. 41–9.
11. See note 9, above.
12. See note 1, above.
13. See note 6, above.
14. Yasko, J., *Care of the Client Receiving Radiation Therapy. A Self-Learning Module for the Nurse Caring for the Client with Cancer* (Reston Publishing Co., Reston, VA, 1982).

# 8

# Sociocultural influences on the person

Study of this chapter will help you to:

1. Define *culture* and *subculture* and describe various types of subcultures.
2. Discuss the general features of any culture and how they affect the persons under your care.
3. Discuss influences of culture and social class on the health status of the person and group.
4. Describe how knowledge of cultural and social class values and attitudes toward daily living practices, health and illness can influence the effectiveness of your health care.
5. Discuss ways to meet the needs of another with cultural and social class values different from your own.
6. Apply knowledge about the teaching-learning process to a health education programme for a person or family from another culture or social class.
7. Assess and care for a person or family from another culture and social class and identify your own ethnocentric tendencies.

The great divide between humans and animals is culture. Culture includes using language, art forms, and games to communicate with others; cooperating in problem solving; deliberately training children; developing unique interpretations; forming organizations; and making, saving, using and changing tools. Humans are heir to the accumulation of wisdom and folly of preceding generations and, in turn, they teach others their beliefs, feelings and practices. The patient, family and you are deeply affected by the culture learned during the early years, often more so than by that learned later. An understanding of the cultural and social class systems and their influence on behaviour is essential to understanding yourself and the person under your care.

# DEFINITIONS

**Culture** *is the sum total of the learned ways of doing, feeling and thinking, past and present, of a social group within a given period of time. These ways are transmitted from one generation to the next or to immigrants who become members of the society.* Culture is a group's design for living, a shared set of socially transmitted assumptions about the nature of the physical and social world, goals in life, attitudes, roles and values. *Culture is a complex integrated system that includes knowledge, beliefs, skills, art, morals, law, customs, and any other acquired habits and capabilities of the human being. All provide a pattern for living together.*

A **subculture** *is a group of persons, without a culture, of the same age, socioeconomic status, ethnic origin, education, or occupation, or with the same goals, who have an identity of their own but are related to the total culture in certain ways.*

*Regional, social class, religious, ethnic and family subcultures also exist.*

**Regional culture** *refers to the local or regional manifestations of the larger culture.* Thus the child learns the sectional variant of the national culture – for example, rural or urban, northern or southern or Midland. Regional culture is influenced by geography, trade and economics; variations may be shown in values, beliefs, housing, food, occupational skills and language.

A social class also has its own culture. A **social class** *is a cultural grouping of persons who, through group consensus and similarity of occupation, wealth and education, have come to have a similar status, lifestyle, interests, feelings, attitudes, language usage, and overt forms of behaviour.* The people belonging to this group meet each other on equal terms and have a consciousness of cohesion. Social class is not only economic in origin; other factors also contribute to superior status, such as age, sex and personal endownment.

The more a class as a group becomes fixed, the more predictable is its patterns of attitudes and behaviour. The child learns the patterns of his/her own class and the class attitude towards another class. The attitude patterns make up a culture's **value system,** *its concept of how people should behave in various situations as well as which goals they should pursue and how.* The value systems of the general culture and of the subculture or social class may conflict at times.

**Religious culture** also influences the person, for a *religion constitutes a way of living and thinking and therefore is a kind of culture.*

**Family culture** *refers to the family life, which is part of the cultural system.* The family is the medium through which the large cultural heritage is transmitted to the child. *Family culture consists of ways of living and thinking that constitute the family and sexual aspects of group life.* These ways include courtship and marriage patterns, sexual mores, husband-wife relationships, status of men and women, parent-child relationships, childrearing, responsibilities to parents, and attitudes toward unmarried women, illegitimate children and divorce.

The family gives the child status. The family name gives the child a social position as well as an identity; the child is assigned the status of the family and the reputation that goes with it. Family status has a great deal to do with health and behaviour throughout life because of its effect on self-concept.

Family rituals are the collective way of working out household routines and using time within the family culture. **Ritual** *is a system of definitely prescribed behaviours and procedures and it provides exactness in daily tasks of living and has a sense of rightness about it.* The more often the behaviour is repeated, the more it comes to be approved and therefore habitual. Thus rituals inevitably develop in family life as a result of the intimacy of relationships and the repetition and continuity of certain interactions. Rituals change from one life cycle to another – for example, at marriage, after childbirth, when children go to school and when children leave home. Rituals are important in child development for the following reasons:

1. They are group habits that communicate ways of doing things and attitudes related to events, including family etiquette, affectionate responses between family members, organization of leisure time, and education for group adjustment.
2. They promote solidarity and continuity by promoting habitual behaviour, unconsciously performed, which brings harmony to family life. Many rituals will continue to the next generation, increasing the person's sense of worth, security and family continuity or identity.
3. They aid in maintaining self-control through disciplinary measures.
4. They promote feelings of euphoria, sentimentality, or wellbeing – for example, through holiday celebrations.
5. They dictate reactions to threat, such as at times of loss, illness or death.

You must consider the person's standard rituals as you plan care.


CHARACTERISTICS OF CULTURE

*Culture as learned*

Culture has three basic characteristics. First, *culture is learned.* People function physiologically in much the same way throughout the world, but their behaviour is learned and therefore relatively diverse. Because of his/her culture, a child is ascribed or acquires a certain **status** *or position of prestige.* The child also learns or assumes certain **roles,** *patterns or related behaviours* *expected by others, and later by him/herself, that define behaviour and adjustment to a given group.* The behaviour, values, attitudes, and beliefs, learned within his/her culture become a matter of tradition, even though the culture allows choices within limits and may even encourage certain kinds of deviancy. The way in which a person experiences the culture and society and what he/she learns during development are of great significance. Culture determines the kinds of experiences the person encounters and the extent to which responses to life situations will be either unhealthy, maladaptive and self-defeating, or healthy, adaptive, constructive and creative. What the person has learned from the culture determines how and what you will be able to teach him/her, as well as your approach during care.

## Culture as stable but changing

The second characteristic of culture is that *it is subject to and capable of change in order to remain viable and adaptive, although it is basically a stable entity.* The culture of a society, like a human body, is dynamic but maintained at a steady state by self-regulating devices. *Stabilizing features are traditions and the ready-made solutions to life's problems* that are provided for the group, enabling the person to anticipate the behaviour of others, predict future events, and regulate his/her life within the culture. Behaviour, carefully defined by the culture, is difficult to change because of group pressure. Norms and customs that persist may have a negative influence on the group. Food taboos during pregnancy, a high-animal-fat diet, or crowding of people into a common dwelling that provides an apt incubator for spread of contagious disease are examples.

*Another stabilizing, limiting aspect of culture is the use of language.* Although language forms vary from culture to culture, the terms for *mother* and *father* sound very much alike across cultural lines, perhaps because certain vocalizations are easy for a child to articulate and learn.

Learning culture and family language is primarily by ear and can affect the child who learns better by sight. In addition, use of language is determined considerably by age and sex – for example, baby talk, child talk, adult talk, girl talk and boy talk. Subcultural groups, particularly the family, differ in conversational mores – that is, permitted topics of conversation; proper situations for discussing certain topics, such as during mealtime or before bedtime; level of vocabulary used; reaction to new words used; number of interruptions permitted; who can be interrupted; and who talks most.

The meeting ground between cultures is in language and **dialect,** *a variety of a language spoken by a distinct group of people in a definite place.*

Analyses of the habits and practices of various peoples show that traditional language and behaviour patterns practised between parent and child within a culture are related to the interactions within that culture between employer and employee, among peers, and between nurse and patient, making for predictability and stability. Stability of culture promotes adaptability and economy of energy.

*Cultures also change*, sometimes imperceptibly, so that norms, the usual rules for living, are modified to meet the group's needs as new life challenges arise. Cultures change primarily in response to technological innovation or by borrowing from another culture. For example, the harnessing of electrical power and the subsequent invention and use of electical appliances and tools changed the way of life in work, recreation, food preservation, communication, education, vocabulary, women's roles, health care, and the entire value system.

Cultures also change for other reasons:

1. Competition among groups for geographical regions in order to meet the members' sustenance and safety needs.
2. Use of deferred gains for members to induce them to work for the good of the culture, such as in communist countries.
3. Change in political leadership, such as in China.
4. Increased scientific and industrial complexity.
5. Increased population.
6. Change in economic practices and standards, such as the change from feudalism to industrialism seen in Africa and Asian countries.
7. Use of behaviour modification techniques by groups in power.
8. Promotion of values, lifestyle and products through mass media programming and advertisements.

Culture is continually shaped by forces and people outside our awareness; some are discussed in *The People Shapers* by Vance Packard. He discusses how we could use our growing knowledge of science and technology to enslave and depersonalize people and thus radically change our culture.[1]

Moving into a postindustrial society poses some problems:

1. The need for more professional knowledge.
2. Greater expectations by the public.
3. More goods considered to be public goods.
4. Lack of measurements to show what is actually needed and thus where money and resources should be directed.
5. A changing demography with more urban concentration.
6. Increased life expectancy.
7. Changing values.

Resulting problems in health care will include: rising costs, maldistribution of health personnel and specialized services, and greater demand by the consumer for professional competence and accountability and more procedures for ensuring it.[2]

Each culture is a whole, but not every culture is integrated in the same way to the same extent. Some cultures are so tightly integrated that any change threatens the whole. Other cultures are characterized by traditional patterns that are easy to manipulate and change.

When significant numbers of people begin to respond other than usual to one or more facets of a culture, this factor may cause others in the society to realize that a particular custom or norm is no longer useful. Such customs might pertain to marriage, burial, childrearing or moral codes. If a group of people (or isolated persons) can consistently adapt while at the same time following the norm imperfectly, they may establish a new norm, which may be gradually adopted by others until it becomes the generally established pattern. Thus the culture and the people in it can be changed in spite of initial resistance. Such changes can have a positive or negative influence on health.

*Cultural components and patterns*

The third characteristic of culture is that *certain components or patterns are present in every culture,* regardless of how 'primitive' or 'advanced' it may be. Understanding them can help you understand yourself, your patient, and the health-care system in which you work.

**A communication system,** which may include only the language itself or the complexities of mass media, computers and satellites, is the basis for interaction and cohesion between persons and a vehicle for the transmission and preservation of culture. In addition to vocabulary and word taboos, gestures, facial expressions and voice qualities – intonation, rhythm, speed, pronunciation – vary among families or groups within a culture and carry specific meanings. Because millions of British residents nightly watch television, it has become the most powerful cultural communication force in the country today. Television could be used more effectively for mass health teaching, just as it is used now for mass advertising.

**Methods and objects are used by a culture to provide for physical welfare.** Methods include getting food; establishing personal care habits; making, using, saving and improving tools; and manufacturing. Objects include instruments and machines used to change land terrain for farming, home building, or industrialization, and equipment used to diagnose and test disease.

**Means or techniques of travel and transportation of goods and services** are particularized to a culture. Whether walking, use of dog or horse, or a complex system of cars, trucks, railways and airplanes, they will affect the person's ability to obtain health care, among other services and goods.

**Exchange of goods and services** may occur through barter, trade, commerce, involve occupational roles, and affect work and payment in a health-care system.

**Forms of property,** real estate and personal, are defined by the culture in terms of their necessity and worth. Respecting the person's property in the hospital or home shows that you respect him/her personally.

**Sexual and family patterns,** which may vary considerably from culture to culture, affect how you care for and teach the person. Such patterns include wedding ceremonies, divorce proceedings, forms of kinships, guardianship roles, inheritance rights, the family's division of labour, and roles assigned to men, women and children.

**Societal controls and the institution of government** include **mores,** *morally binding attitudes, and* **customs,** *long-established practices having the force of unwritten law.* Other controls include public or group opinion, laws, political offices and the organization of government, the regulation of time, and institutionalized forms of conflict within the society or between tribes, states, or nations, such as war. These factors all influence the health-care system in which you work. Increasingly, the nurse must become familiar with the political system and skilled in using it for improving health care.

**Artistic expression** through architecture, painting, sculpture, music, literature and dance is universal, although what is considered art by one culture may not be so considered by another. Knowledge of these factors can be useful in therapy and rehabilitation.

**Recreational and leisure-time interests and activities,** as defined by each cultural group, are essential for health and must be considered in the nursing history and in medical diagnosis.

**Religious and magical ideas and practices** exist in the form of various beliefs, taboos, ethical codes, rituals, mythology, philosophy, or the organized institution of the church and serve to guide the behaviour of a cultural group during health and illness.

**Knowledge basic to survival and expansion of the group** is always present. In developed countries **science,** *systematized knowledge based on observation, study and experimentation,* is basic to technological innovation and improving material living standards. Education has traditionally been considered a bridge that enables the person to move up in socioeconomic status in Britain. In modern Western cultures science is highly valued as a basis for health care. Medical science influences people biologically and socially.

**Cultural structuring of basic human patterns** includes rules for competition, conflict, cooperation, collaboration and games. Also, the intimate habits of daily life, both personally and in groups, the manner in which one's house and body are perceived, and the many 'taken for granted' activities between people are basically structured.

All the foregoing components and patterns influence and are influenced by climate, natural resources, geography, sanitation facilities, diet, group biological and genetic factors, and disease conditions and health practices.

*Cultural values*

Several orientations and value systems may be simultaneously present in a given society or culture, but only one orientation dominates over a given period of time. The following middle-class orientation and values are dominant at present in Britain:

1. Speed, change, progress, activity, punctuality and efficiency.
2. Personal achievement, occupational and financial success, and status consciousness.
3. Youth, beauty, health, self-reliance.
4. Science and the use of machines and various social institutions.
5. Materialism, consumerism, and use of disposable items.
6. Conformity to the group simultaneously with emphasis on rugged individualism and personal pleasure.
7. Competitive and aggressive behaviour and exploitation of others rather than cooperation and contemplation.
8. Social and geographical mobility.
9. Pursuit of recreational activities.
10. Equally of people, but recognition of social differentiation and inequality based on personal abilities, education and opportunity.
11. Future orientation; interest in long-term goals and willingness to defer immediate satisfaction.

In the past (and to some degree still now), the Protestant ethic described by sociologist Max Weber was the prime influence on British culture, even for those Britons who were not Protestants. An **ethic** *is defined as an outlook or view made up of assumptions that are not often noticed and still less often questioned or tested.* These assumptions are blindly and passively accepted because they have been handed down from generation to generation and had their origins in an unimpeachable, but long forgotten, authority. With new knowledge, the assumptions are often found invalid, but assumptions about living undergo a slow process of change. The Protestant ethic encompasses a harsh, pessimistic view of the human race. It upholds the five following assumptions:

1. Man is basically imperfect and must struggle against imperfection.
2. Man was placed on earth to struggle and so struggle must be valued. Any sign of surrender or softness denotes weakness in the person and is bad.
3. Self-sacrifice and aspiring to good conduct are essential to overcome evil and gain personal salvation.
4. Emotions cannot be overtly expressed. Displaying anger is basically un-Christian. One should love one's neighbour, but expressing love openly is suspect, especially if related to sexuality, for sex is considered an animal pleasure and therefore a taboo topic. Even too intense an expression of nonsexual love can be a sign of weakness and one must be strong and self-controlled in order to struggle. Anxiety must be avoided or denied, for it shows that the struggle is not going well.
5. The world is seen as useful to man and should provide for material satisfaction. Thus the exploitation of land, even ruthlessly, is acceptable. Mastery of the environment is emphasized. Conservation of natural resources is secondary, for the resources of the world (which are supposedly inexhaustible) were put there to be used.[3]

Earlier in this century Puritanical values and rigid Christian morality upheld the tenet of fear of God's judgment. A strong conscience was developed in fear of punishment and social disfavour. Society was stable because traditions were adhered to and proverbs were taken seriously. Hard work, plain living, thrift, self-control, responsibility, will-power, honesty and initiative were emphasized. Family and community roles were clearly defined: father was the patriarch; mother was subservient to him; and children were obedient to all. Education also emphasized discipline, order and obedience to authority. People were tradition-bound and hard-working, and they provided stability in society. Your understanding that many elderly and middle-aged persons still live by these values can help you better accept them and plan their care.

You need only look around at what Toffler calls our superindustrial society to realize that the Protestant ethic has lost its hold.[4] Yet parts of this ethic are being revived by some of the growing fundamentalist religious groups.

The value system of the UK is worldly, in spite of its religious roots, for the most highly valued activities involve competitive, practical, secular pursuits rather than contemplation, devotion, cooperation or aesthetic satisfaction. Thus the ideal society, originally the Kingdom of God on earth, has for many people been secularized into a good society with ideals of liberty, justice, general prosperity and equality of opportunity.

Today's young adults have grown up with the ever-present possibility of instantaneous death or permanent maiming by thermonuclear, chemical or biological warfare agents. The threat and fear of violence are therefore constant facts of life. Fear of violence has led to a fascination with violence that further surrounds people with its symptoms. Society is preoccupied with, almost mesmerized by, the violence of organized crime, urban rioting and political assassinations. Violence on television and in the cinema shows the potential for brutality and aggression in all.

People react differently to constant exposure to violence: they may tolerate it, develop disease symptoms, project their own aggression onto others, develop a neurotic preoccupation with it, or act violently themselves in order to discharge rage. We see examples of each reaction in our society in the form of physical, emotional, and social illness.

*Attitudes towards health and illness*

How health is identified, physically and emotionally, varies from culture to culture, as do ideas about the factors related to health and disease. Attitudes in the UK towards health are influenced considerably by society's emphasis on mastery of the environment as opposed to adjustment to it. Illness is seen as a challenge to be met by mobilizing resources: research, science, funds, institutions and people. The British are taxed to finance health and welfare organizations and persons giving time and effort to these organizations are given special status by the community. Because independence is highly valued, the weak are expected to help themselves as much as possible. The strong help the weak as long as their problems are caused by events beyond their control; otherwise the physically, socially or emotionally weak, deformed or unsightly are devalued.

A person is evaluated on productivity or 'doing good'. Because the ability to be productive depends in part on health, individual health is highly valued. Health in the broadest sense is considered necessary for successful interaction with others, educational accomplishment, ability to work, leadership, childrearing, and capacity to use opportunities. Thus development of medical, nursing, and other health sciences and technology is considered important. The physical cause of illness is generally accepted. Only recently have the sociocultural causes of disease also been emphasized.

The importance of health has been accentuated by industrialization, high-level technology, greater social controls, and mass communications, as well as by a high level of responsibility and stress placed on the person. People at times react to the complexities of society by retreating into ill health, physically, emotionally or socially. Levels of pathology that could be tolerated in pre-industrial societies cannot be tolerated in complex modern life. Americans are more likely to interpret a person's difficulty in fulfilling social-role expectations as illness than would some other societies. Thus the person who is ill is less likely to be tolerated or kept in the family. When ill, the person is supposed to leave home, isolate self from the family, and be cared for in a strange place, the hospital, by strange people who are authorities on illness. One's capacity for meeting social-role expectations is developed primarily through family socialization and education, but it is protected and restored through the health-care system. The ill person is expected to want to return to normal roles and to leave behind the feelings of alienation, regression and passivity that are part of the deviance of illness. The impersonal agency of the hospital exerts pressures that discourage staying dependent and ill.

## SOCIAL CLASS SUBCULTURE

Research about social stratification indicates that the person's class position is influenced by economic and social status and political power of the family and affects formation of values, attitudes and lifestyle. Each class tends to have a more or less well-specified set of values and role expectations regarding practically every area of human activity: sex, marriage, male-female and parent-child responsibilities and behaviour, birth, death, education, dress, housing, home furnishings, leisure, reading habits, occupational status, politics, religion and status symbols. Social class includes a group consciousness. Most persons can be objectively placed within a certain class, but they are sometimes accorded a status by others around them that might be different. Furthermore, they may see themselves at yet a different status level, based on race, sex, religion, ancestry, ethnic origin or wealth in material goods. What seems natural and logical in determining status to some people may be rejected by others.

Some occupations, for example, clergymen, lecturers, teachers, have high status value but do not command high salaries. This tends to skew some areas of social classification data.

The social class you are born into not only has a major influence on your health but also the type of disease you may suffer or even die from. This was highlighted in the Black Report (1980) which looked at the regional and social incidence of disease. Black showed that for every male infant in social class I who died in his first year, four died in social class V.[5]

The Robens Report (1972) on Safety and Health at Work stated that half a million people suffer injuries at work in varying degrees every year and that 23 million working days are lost annually on this account alone.[6]

Unemployment also brings hazards to health. It can be argued that lowered income leads directly or indirectly to lowered health. This may be directly through a poorer diet leading to increased vulnerability to disease, or to stress factors and time to indulge in habits adverse to a healthy lifestyle, leading to ill health.

Lifestyles may also affect vulnerability to disease. Cancer and heart disease are often described as diseases of civilization, caused by the life we lead, with smoking and a fatty diet as two key factors.

Despite the National Health Service being available to all, the higher income groups are able to make better use of the health services. They tend to receive earlier attention and more of it. They have more elective surgery and better maternity care than the lower income groups. Wealthier still means healthier. This is probably affected by the fact than the higher social classes are more articulate and know the right questions to ask and will question their health carers. They also tend to visit the doctor earlier in an illness episode.

Perhaps this is the area where we as health promoters and educators are failing, as access to care and information seems to be lacking for those in most need.[7]

INFLUENCES OF CULTURE ON HEALTH

Because every culture is complex, it can be difficult to determine whether health and illness are the result of cultural or other factors, such as physiological or psychological factors. Yet there are numerous accounts of the presence or absence of certain diseases in certain cultural groups and reactions to illness that are culturally determined. Cultural influences may include food availability, dietary taboos, methods of hygiene, and effects of climate – all factors related to culture. Several examples of the influences of culture on health and illness follow. The examples are necessarily limited.

Leaf studied three cultures in which many people live to be very old. These people live in Vilcabamba, Ecuador; in Hunza, located in Pakistani-controlled Kashmir; and in Abkhazia in the Caucasus Mountain region of the Soviet Union. In each of these cultures the old people share in a great deal of the hard labour. Exercise appears to be a major factor in their longevity. In each culture the aged are accorded high social status and occupy a central and privileged position in the extended family. They live with close relatives, are given useful roles, continue daily to perform useful tasks, contribute to the economy of the community, and are sought for counsel and for their wisdom. Sense of family continuity is strong. The elderly are not shunted aside as in Western industrial societies, nor are they forced to retire; instead they remain independent and expect great longevity. Once they lose their useful roles in the community, however, they die quickly.[8]

The influence of other cultural folkways on health has been studied. Race, social class, ethnic group, and religion influence distribution of disease and death. Epidemiological findings suggest that Jewish women have less cancer of the cervix than non-Jewish women and that these results can be related to circumcision of the Jewish male or to abstinence from intercourse as prescribed by Jewish law for a certain period after the menses. Nuns also have low risk for cancer of the cervix. Generally lower-class and black women in the United States, with earlier sexual intercourse and early and more frequent childbirth, run a higher risk than the rest of the population – than Jews, in particular. Prostitutes also have a higher incidence of cancer of the cervix, possibly because of multiple sex partners.[9] Graham was influenced by the etiological theory proposed by Martin that the uncircumcised non-Jewish male is more likely to harbour a carcinogenic virus, although only certain men carry it. Therefore a woman who has sexual intercourse with a greater number of men during her life has a greater chance of being exposed to the virus and hence runs a greater risk of cervical cancer.

Culturally induced belief in magic can cause illness and death. The profound physiological consequences of intense fear, including inability to eat or drink, may be responsible. Yet there may be no physiological changes except in the terminal moments. If the behaviour of friends and relatives – what they say or do – strongly reinforces the person's conviction of imminent death, the victim becomes resigned to fate and soon meets it.

A culture's favoured drink may have implications for health. Health workers in a remote Mexican village found that the only available beverage was an alcoholic drink made from the juice of a local plant. A safe water supply was brought in, but the people did not fare well on it. The local drink was a rich source of essential vitamins and minerals not otherwise present in the local diet. Thus although it may have appeared desirable to change a cultural pattern for certain health reasons, the unanticipated consequences proved detrimental to health in another way.

NURSING IMPLICATIONS

*Importance of cultural concepts for nursing*

If you live or work in a culture different from your own, you may suffer **cultural shock,** *the feelings of bewilderment, confusion, disorganization, frustration and stupidity and the inability to adapt to the differences in language and word meanings, activities, time and customs that are part of the new culture.* An antidote for cultural shock is to look for similarities between your native and new cultures. In order to adapt to a new culture, be interested in the culture and be prepared to ask questions tactfully and to give up some of your own habits. Leininger and Weis give a number of specific suggestions for adapting to another culture.

The United Kingdom is a **pluralistic society** *in which members of diverse ethnic, racial, religious and social groups maintain independent lifestyles and adhere to certain values within the confines of a common civilization.* Knowledge of other cultures helps you examine your own cultural foundations, values and beliefs, which, in turn, promotes increased self-understanding. But avoid **ethnocentricity,** *believing that your own ways of behaviour are best for everyone.* For example, emphasizing daily bathing to a group who has a severely limited water supply is useless, for the water will be needed for survival. Recognize that your patterns of life and language are peculiar to your culture.

Learning about another's cultural background can promote feelings of respect and humility as well as enhance understanding of the person and the family – his/her needs, likes and dislikes, behaviour, attitudes, care and treatment approaches, and sociocultural causes of disease. Cultural differences should be anticipated not only in foreigners and first-generation immigrants but also in persons even further removed in time from their native country and in persons from other regions within your country. The person's behaviour during illness is influenced by cultural definitions of how he/she should act and the meaning of illness. Understanding this situation and seeking reasons for behaviour help to avoid stereotyping and labelling the person as uncooperative and resistant just because the behaviour is different. As you consider alternate reasons for behaviour, care can be individualized. People from different cultural backgrounds classify health problems differently and have certain expectations about how they should be helped. If cultural differences are ignored, your ability to help the patient and his/her ability to progress toward a personally and culturally defined health status may be hampered. You should be able to translate your knowledge of the health-care system into terms that match the concepts of your patients/clients.

All people have some prejudice; it emerges in such expressions as 'Those upper-crust people always ...' or 'Those social security people never ...' Examine your thinking for unconscious prejudice, understand your own class background, and distinguish your values from those held by people under your care. Try to withhold value judgments that interfere with your relationship with the patient and with objective care. There are too many unknown factors in people's lives to set up stereotyped categories. A family may be in the middle class or upper class in terms of income, education and goals, for example, and yet live in an upper-lower-class neighbourhood because they refuse to emphasize material wealth. A farmer, according to our criteria, may be labelled upper-lower-class and yet regard him/herself very much a part of the middle class. A person who lives in an economically depressed section of the country and is poor may have an adequate public education, a middle-class value system, and upper-class graciousness.

If you feel you are stooping by helping lower-class people, you may be labelled a 'do-gooder' and be ineffective. Recognize the behaviour of the lower class not as pathological but as adaptive for their needs. Realize, too, that not only the poor need your help. The upper-class person may need a great deal of help with care, health teaching, or counselling. Having money does not necessarily mean one is knowledgeable about preventive health measures, nutrition and disease processes. Persons of all classes deserve competent care, clear explanations and a helpful attitude.

Knowledge about social classes and cultural groups may help explain late or broken agency appointments that result from fear or inferiority feelings, lack of transportation, or someone to care for the children at home rather than from lack of interest in health. The client from an ethnic minority may not be accustomed to keeping a strict time schedule or appointments if unemployed, for a strict clock-time orientation is not valued as highly as in the industrialized work force. Take time to talk with the person and you will learn of his/her fears, problems, aspirations, and concern for health and family, and his/her human warmth.

To illustrate, a woman in labour who is a product of a parochial background with reliance on lay medical help and suspicious of the impersonal hospital and professional-looking nurses asks to have a knife placed under the bed to help 'cut labour pains'. While implementing scientific health care, you can be more prepared to act on this belief that psychologically helps the patient. Herbs used by various cultural groups are increasingly found to have medicinal value; they are chemically similar to drugs used by scientific practitioners.

The misinterpretation of behaviour typical of a social class does not always go in one direction, from upper to lower. Suppose that you are a nurse with a working-class background whose patient is a 50-year-old company director, admitted for coronary disease, a member of the newly rich class. He seems obsessed with learning when he can resume his professional duties, exactly how many hours he can work daily, and his chances for a recurrence. An understanding of his class position, along with his possible motives, values and status (which he feels must be maintained), will enable you to work with his seeming obsession rather than simply label him an 'impossible patient'.

Try to accept people as they are regardless of culture or social class. Picture the world from the eyes of others – those you care for. In this way, you can maintain your own personal standards without being shocked by theirs.

Your knowledge of cultures will enable you to practise holistic nursing care, including cultural values and norms in the nursing process. Holistic healing practices combine the best of two worlds: the wisdom and sensitivity of the East and the technology and precision of the West. Although holistic practitioners use conventional therapies in many cases, the emphasis remains on the whole person: physical, emotional, intellectual, spiritual and sociocultural background. The focus is on prevention and overall fitness and on the individual taking responsibility for his/her own health and wellbeing. Multiple techniques are used to restore and maintain balance of body energy – the life force. These techniques include exercise, acupuncture, massage, herbal medicine, nutritional changes, manipulation of joints and spine, medications, stress management and counselling. The nurse-client relationship is the key to holistic nursing care, for the person has come to expect a caring interaction from the healer.

As you assess the person, remember that people differ biologically, physically and culturally. (See Table 8.1.) Studies on biological baselines for

*Table 8.1*   Assessment of skin colour

| Characteristic | White or light-skinned person | Dark skinned person |
|---|---|---|
| *Pallor:* Vasoconstriction present | Skin takes on white hue, which is colour of collagen fibres in subcutaneous connective tissue. | Skin loses underlying red tones. Brown-skinned person appears yellow-brown. Black-skinned person appears ashen-grey. Mucous membranes, lips, nailbeds pale or grey. |
| *Erythema,* inflammation: cutaneous vasodilation | Skin is red. | Palpate for increased warmth of skin, edema, tightness, or induration of skin. |
| *Cyanosis:* hypoxia of tissues | Bluish tinges of skin, especially in earlobes, as well as in lips, oral mucosa, and nailbeds. | Lips, tongue, conjunctiva, palms, soles of feet are pale or ashen grey. Apply light pressure to create pallor; in cyanosis tissue colour returns slowly by spreading from periphery to the centre. |
| *Ecchymosis:* deoxygenated blood seeps from broken blood vessel into subcutaneous tissue | Skin changes colour from purple-blue to yellow-green to yellow. | Obtain history of trauma and discomfort. Note swelling and induration. Oral mucous membrane or conjunctiva will show colour changes from purple-blue to yellow-green to yellow. |
| *Petechiae:* intradermal or submucosal bleeding | Round, pinpoint purplish red spots on skin. | Oral mucosa or conjunctiva show purplish-red spots if person has black skin. |
| *Jaundice:* accumulated bilirubin in tissues | Yellow colour in skin, mucous membranes, and sclera of eyes. Light-coloured stools and dark urine often occur. | Sclera of eyes, oral mucous membranes, palms of hand and soles of feet have yellow discoloration. |

growth and development or normal characteristics have usually been done on white populations. These norms may not be applicable to nonwhites. Biological features, such as skin colour, body size and shape, and presence of enzymes, are the result of biological adjustments made by ancestors to the environment in which they lived.[10]

Various physical differences are known to exist. **Mongolian spots,** *the hyperpigmented, bluish discolouration* occasionally seen in Caucasian neonates, are normal for many Asians, American Indians and blacks. Type of ear wax varies and may determine the presence of ear disease in preschoolers. Dry ear wax is recessive and is found primarily in American Indians and Asians. Wet ear wax is found in most blacks and Caucasians. Also, people with dry ear wax have fewer apocrine glands and perspire less; they usually do not have as much body odour. Thus presence of body odour may be indicative of disease. Pelvic shape of the woman, shape of teeth and tongue, fingerprint pattern, blood type, keloid formation and presence of the enzyme lactase vary among groups. Persons with certain blood types are more prone to certain illnesses. The adult who has lactose intolerance is missing lactase, the enzyme for digestion and metabolism of lactose in milk and milk products. The person becomes ill on ingestion of these foods. Symptoms include flatulence, distention, abdominal cramping, diarrhoea, and colitis. Milk intolerance because of enzyme deficiency occurs in over 80 per cent of Chinese, Japanese, and Eskimo adults and in 60 to 80 per cent of native American, black, Jewish, and Mexican-American adults. Only people of northern European Caucasian extraction and members of two African tribes tolerate lactose indefinitely and even some aged Caucasians will have lactose deficiency. Do not automatically teach everyone to drink milk. Calcium can be obtained in other ways: seafoods (cook fish to yield edible bones); leafy vegetables; yogurt, buttermilk or aged cheese (lactose has been changed to lactic acid during aging); or homemade soup (add vinegar to the water when cooking a soupbone to decalcify the bone). Most ethnic groups have adapted ways of cooking to ensure calcium intake from nondairy sources; listen carefully to their dietary descriptions.

Other biological variations exist. Susceptibility to disease varies with blood type. Rh-negative blood type is common in Caucasians, rarer in other groups, and absent in Eskimos. Myopia is more common in Chinese; colour blindness is more common in Europeans and East Indians. Nose size and shape correlate with ancestral homeland. Small noses (seen in Asians or Eskimos) were produced in cold regions, high-bridged noses (common to Iranians and American Indians) were common in dry areas; and the flat, broad noses characteristic of some blacks were adaptive in moist, warm climates.

Branch and Paxton, Brink and Leininger present much specific information in their books that will help you assess and intervene with people from various cultures and subcultures.[11]

If the person does not speak English as a first language, learn key words of his/her language. Use language dictionaries or a card file of key words. Breach the language barrier so that your assessment is more accurate and care measures will be understood by the person.

Learn about the significant religious practices and the everyday patterns of hygiene, eating, types of foods eaten, sleeping, elimination, use of space, and various rituals that are a part of the person's culture. Interference with normal living patterns or practices adds to the stress of being ill. You will encounter and need to adapt patient care to the following customs: drinking tea instead of coffee with meals, eating the main meal at midday instead of in the evening, refusing to undress before a strange person, avoiding use of the bedpan because someone else must handle its contents, maintaining special religious or ethnic customs, refusing to bathe daily, refusing a pelvic examination by a male doctor, moaning loudly when in pain, and showing unreserved demonstrations of grief when a loved one dies.

Respecting the person's need for privacy or need to have others continually around is essential. Understand that some patients or families will not be expressive, emotionally or verbally. Respect this pattern, recognizing that nonverbal behaviour is also significant. Be aware, too, that word meanings may vary considerably from culture to culture so that the person may have difficulty understanding you and vice versa. Be sure the gesture or touch you use conveys the message you intend. If you are unsure, avoid nonverbal behaviour to the extent that you can.

A patient with a strict time orientation must take medicines and receive treatments on time or feel neglected. You are expected to give prompt and efficient, but compassionate, service to the patient and family. Time orientation also affects making appointments for the clinic and plans for medication routine or return to work after discharge and influences the person's ideas about how quickly he/she should get well. The person with little future-time orientation has difficulty planning a future clinic appointment or a long-range medication schedule. This person cannot predict now how he will feel at a later date and thinks that clinic visits or medicines are unnecessary if he/she feels all right at the moment.

For some patients, the hurrying behaviour of the nurse is distressing; it conveys a lack of concern and lack of time to give adequate care. In turn, the patient expresses guilt feelings when it is necessary to ask for help. Although you may look very efficient when scurrying, you are likely to miss many observations, cues, and hidden meanings in what the patient says.

Examine your own attitude about business and leisure in order to help others consider leisure as part of life. The disabled patient, whose inability to work carries a stigma, must develop a positive attitude about leisure and may seek your help.

Relations between the patient and the family may at times seem offensive or disharmonious to you. Differentiate carefully between patterns of behaviour that are culturally induced and expected and those that are unhealthy for the persons involved.

The changing society may cause families to have a variety of problems. Be a supportive listener, validate realistic ideas, prepare the family to adapt to a new or changing environment, and be aware of community agencies or resources that can provide additional help. When a patient has no family nearby and seems alone and friendless, you may provide significant support.

Develop a personal philosophy that promotes a feeling of stability in your life so that you, in turn, can assist the patient and family to explore feelings and to formulate a philosophy for coping with change. Toffler speaks about ways in which the person can learn to cope with rapid change. One important way is to develop some ritual or pattern in your personal life that you can practise regardless of where you are and thus maintain some sense of continuity and stability.

Several authors have written of their successful experiences in adapting care to certain cultural or social class groups. Success has resulted from an accurate assessment and understanding of the person or group, acceptance of differences, and practical suggestions to promote compliance with prescribed health practices while the person or group also maintained culturally preferred treatments.

*Promoting health in other cultures through education*

One way to have a lasting effect on the health practices of a different cultural group is through health teaching that includes a philosophy of prevention. Present-day China compared with China during the 1940s is an example of how public health standards can be effectively raised through an emphasis on prevention. Increasingly your role includes health education; outsiders cannot make decisions for others, but people should be given sufficient knowledge concerning alternate behaviour so that they can make intelligent choices themselves.

Various pressures interfere with attempts at health teaching. Behind poor health habits lie more than ignorance, economic pressure, or selfish desires. Motivation plays a great part in continuing certain practices even though the person has been taught differently by you. Motivation, moreover, is influenced by the person's culture, status, and role in that culture and by social pressures for conformity. Starting programmes of prevention can be difficult when people place a low value on health, cannot recognize cause-and-effect relationships in disease, lack future-time orientation, or are confused about the existence of preventive measures in their culture. Thus preventive programmes or innovations in health care must be shaped to fit the cultural and health profiles of the population. Long-range prevention goals stand a better chance of implementation if combined with measures to meet immediate needs. A mother is more likely to heed your advice about how to prevent further illness in her sick child if you give the child immediate attention.

Be mindful of how people view you. If they cannot understand you, if you threaten their values, or if they view you as an untouchable professional, you will not cross the cultural barrier.

## REFERENCES

1. Packard, Vance, *The People Shapers* (Little, Brown and Company, Boston, 1977).
2. Toffler, Alvin, *Future Shock* (Bantam Books, New York, 1970).
3. Weber, Max, *The Protestant Ethic and Spirit of Capitalism*, transl. by Talcott Parsons (Charles Scribner's Sons, New York, 1930; student edition 1958).
4. Ibid.
5. Black, Sir Douglas, *The Black Report – Inequalities in Health* (DHSS, 1980).
6. Robens, H., *The Robens' Report* (DHSS, 1972).
7. Rodnall, S. and Watt, A., (eds.) *The Politics of Health Education* (Routledge & Kegan Paul, Ltd, London, 1986).
8. Henley, A., *Asian Patients in Hospital and at Home* (Pitman Publishing Ltd, London, 1979).
9. Graham, Saxon, *Cancer, Culture and Social Structure. Patients, Physicians and Illness*, 2nd edition, ed. E. Gartley Jaco (The Free Press, New York, 1972), pp. 31–9.
10. Moore, L.G., P.N. van Arsdale, J.E. Glittenburg and R.A. Aldrich, *The Biocultural Basis of Healthcare* (The C.V. Mosby Company, St Louis, 1980).
11. Leininger, Madelaine, *Nursing and Anthropology, Two Worlds to Blend* (John Wyley and Sons, Inc., New York, 1970).

# 9

# Religious influences on the person

Study of this chapter will enable you to:

1. Define the terms *religious* and *spiritual* and the connotations of each.

2. Contrast the major tenets of Hinduism, Buddhism, Shintoism, Confucianism, Taoism, Islam, Judaism and Christianity.

3. Compare the major tenets of the various branches of Christianity: Roman Catholicism, Eastern Orthodoxy, various Protestant denominations, other Christian sects.

4. Discuss how religious beliefs influence lifestyle and health status in the various religious groups and subgroups.

5. Identify your religious beliefs, or lack of them, and explore how they will influence your nursing practice.

6. Discuss your role in meeting the spiritual needs of client and family.

Until an illness occurs, the person may give no thought to the meaning of his/her life of spiritual beliefs. But when he/she feels vulnerable and fearful of the future, solace is sought. Religion can provide that solace.

A patient sneezes. You say 'God bless you.' Why? Perhaps unconsciously you are coordinating the medical-physical with the religious-spiritual. But you may feel afraid to work professionally with the combination. This fear comes in part from the long-lived schism between science and religion.

The attitude that medical science is superior to religion has affected us all. Yet religion is there as it always has been. Each culture has had some organization or priesthood to sustain the important rituals and myths of its people. Primitive man combined the roles of physician, psychiatrist and priest. The Indian medicine man and the African witch doctor combine magic with religion; with their herbs, psychosuggestion, and appeals to the gods, they realize that man is a biopsychospiritual being.[1]

> I had the cancer patient visualize an army of white blood cells attacking and overcoming the cancer cells. Within two weeks the cancer had diminished and he was rapidly gaining weight. He is alive and well today.[2]

Is this a priest or a faith healer talking? No, this is a prominent tumour specialist talking in the late 1970s. An internationally known neurosurgeon says, 'In a very real sense, medicine is now – as it has always been – faith healing'. Dr Elisabeth Kübler-Ross, internationally known for studies of dying, states that there is definitely life after death. Thus some health workers are trying to reunite the biopsychospiritual being.

The 1980s are showing an increased awareness of the link between health and religion and the subject is being discussed more openly.[3]

## DEFINITIONS

**Religion** is defined on various levels: *a belief in a supernatural or divine force that has power over the universe and commands worship and obedience; a system of beliefs; a comprehensive code of ethics or philosophy; a set of practices that are followed; a church affiliation; the conscious pursuit of any object the person holds as supreme.*

This definition, however, does not portray the constancy and at times the fervency that can underlie religious belief. In every human there seems to be a **spiritual dimension,** *a quality that goes beyond religious affiliation, that strives for inspiration, reverence, awe, meaning and purpose, even in those who do not believe in any good. The spiritual dimension tries to be in harmony with the universe, strives for answers about the infinite,* and comes into focus when the person faces emotional stress, physical illness or death.

In the midst of our specialized health care you have an opportunity to go beyond the dogma to bring together the biopsychospiritual being through the study of the religions and religious symbols of your patients/clients. And those are world religions, not your personal or country's basic religion. Mass media, rapid transportation and cultural exchanges have nullified the provincial approach.

## WORLD RELIGIONS

Studying world religions poses a semantic difficulty in that an expression in the Chinese-based religion of Confucianism may have no equivalent in the

English language. Thus language has dictated what people think, how they act, and how their religious beliefs are carried out.[4]

Concepts, however, are often basically the same but are rephrased in each religion's own linguistic style. The saying 'Love one another as I have loved you' will appear to the Hindu as 'This is the sum of religion, do not unto others what causes pain to you'; to the Taoist as 'Return goodness for hatred'; and to the Muslim as 'No one is a believer unless he desires for his brother what he desires for himself.'

Each religion also has other characteristics in common:

1. Basis of authority or source(s) of power.
2. A portion of scripture or sacred word.
3. An ethical code that defines right and wrong.
4. A psychology and identity so that its adherents fit into a group and the world is defined by the religion.
5. Aspirations or expectations.
6. Some ideas about what follows death.

The major world religions can be divided into categories in an attempt to group characteristics even further.[5] The *alpha* group includes Christianity, Judaism, and Islam. All adhere to a biblical revelation of a supernatural, monotheistic God. People in these religions are 'doers'. They obey because God commands; they make covenants with God for protection; they have a historical fixed scripture that is canonized for public use; and they often proselytize. Into the *gamma* group go Taoism, Confucianism and Shinto-ism. In these religions people believe either that everything is in the being of God or that there is no Godhead (still a definite belief). These people try to be in harmony with the world around them. Their most immediate con-cern is in relationships with others. Scripture is a family affair. They can be characterized as simple in faith, spontaneous, and straightforward in feel-ings of affection for people, flowers and birds. The final grouping is the *beta* group, which includes Buddhism and Hinduism. These religions have their roots in Indian soil and teach that everything is in the being of God. Adhe-rents are interested in 'being' rather than 'doing'. They have a collective literature for private devotion. Control of mind and body is desired, as some of the yoga practices show. The beta and gamma groups do not define God as clearly as the alpha group. The beta and gamma groups look inside themselves for answers: common sense rather than commands from God determines good.

There follows a general outline of some major religions. Remember that the person's culture, family background and personality affect how that person lives out any experience. Thus, a particular Hindu or a certain Ro-man Catholic may be more in agreement religiously that two Protestants. You cannot make generalisations about a religion from knowing a single follower.

# HINDUISM

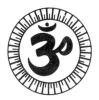

The Hindu tells us that nothing is typically Hindu and that anyone who puts religion in neat packages will have difficulty comprehending his outlook. The history of Hinduism goes back to around 1500 BC when the VEDAS – divine revelations – were written. The main religious texts are the Upanishads, or scriptures, and the Bhagavad-Gita, a summary of the former with additions. The most expressive and universal word of God is OM or AUM as shown on the symbol at the beginning of this section.

A trinity plays a part in Hindu worship. This comprises local and family deities being Brahma, the creator, Vishnu, preserver and god of love and Shiva, the destroyer. Shrines in the house are used for meditation before various pictures of incarnations of the deities, whilst incense burns. The Hindu thinks of Buddha, Mohammed and Jesus as incarnations and sometimes reads from the scriptures inspired by their teachings although they represent other major religions.

In spite of this vast array of deities and the recognition that all religions are valid, Hindus believe in one universal concept – BRAHMAN, the Divine Intelligence, the Supreme Reality. He believes that all paths lead to the understanding that this 'reality' exists as part of all physical beings, especially humans. The entire spiritual quest for the Hindu is directed towards uniting his inner or real self, the atman, with the concept of Brahman. So although he has gone through several stages of desire – for pleasure, power, wealth, fame and humanitarianism – the last stage, his desire for freedom, for touching the infinite is his main goal.

The Hindu is interested in health and illness only as a guide to this goal. He feels that human love for the body is a cause for illness; for example, we overeat – we get stomachache. He views the pain as a warning, in this case to stop overeating. He does not oppose medical treatment if absolutely necessary, but feels that medicine can sometimes dull pain and then the person abuses the body again, thus perpetuating the cause of the problem. Medical or psychiatric help is at best transitory. The cause of the pain must be rooted out.

In order not to dwell on physical concerns the Hindu strives for moderation in eating as well as in other bodily functions. He considers only the atman as real and eternal, the body as unreal and finite. The body is a vehicle, no more. He is a vegetarian, feeling that meat and intoxicants would excite the senses too much. Hindu diet is flexible with no set rules. Sickness is born with resignation as a temporary thing. To him, death and rebirth are nearly synonymous for the atman never changes and always remains pure. If death is imminent, the Hindu believes that body, mind and senses weaken but the atman is ready to enter into a new form of life depending on the person's knowledge, experiences and deeds. Full acceptance of death is encouraged as a friend to be faced bravely, calmly and confidently.

The Hindu, as a devotee of God, may enter into a form of spiritual training called yoga. Various forms of yoga have spread around the world to form various hybrid groups. One branch, hatha yoga, is used as a medical relaxation technique in some areas. Another, bhakti yoga, is embraced by the Hare Krishna movement, formed in the United States in 1965 and now represented throughout the western world.

For the Hindu, religion is not something to be picked up and put down according to schedule or mood. It is a constant and all-pervading aspect of his life and the life of his country.

If you give nursing care to someone with this background, consider how his religious beliefs will influence your approach. Be accepting if the person seems to minimize bodily ills. Keep in mind the view of the body as only a vehicle to carry the atman and the belief that the desire for bodily cure is a low form of prayer. Yoga training, emphasizing self-control and devotion to God through reading and meditation, may cause the person to seek help from inner resources and the literature of Hinduism rather than from medication or consultation with staff. Providing an atmosphere conducive to this practice will be appreciated. Should death seem imminent, remember that death is perceived as a rebirth. The person will want rebirth to have as much dignity as possible.

## BUDDHISM AND SHINTOISM

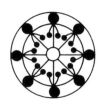

Gautama, shortly after a historic enlightenment experience during which he became the Buddha, preached a sermon to his followers and drew on the earth a wheel representing the continuous round of life and death and rebirth. Later eight spokes were added to illustrate the sermon and to provide the most explicit visual symbol of Buddhism today.

Buddhism states four noble truths:

1. Life is disjointed or out of balance, especially in birth, old age, illness and death.
2. The cause of this imbalance is ignorance of one's own true nature.
3. Removal of this ignorance is attained by reaching NIRVANA, the divine state of release, the perfect knowledge via:
4. The eightfold path.

The eight spokes of the wheel represent the eightfold path used to reach Nirvana. Followers subscribe to right knowledge, right intentions, right speech, right conduct, right means of livelihood, right effort, right mindfulness and concentration. From these concepts has arisen a moral code that, among other things, prohibits intoxicants, lying, and killing of any kind (which explains why Buddhists are often vegetarians). The Mahayana branch of Buddhism took hold in Japan as opposed to the Theravada branch. The **Theravada branch** *emphasizes an intellectual approach through wisdom, man working by himself through meditation and without ritual.* The **Mahayana branch** *emphasizes involvement with mankind, ritual, petitionary prayer, and concern for one's sibling. Most believe in* **Amitabha Buddha,** *a god rather than a historical figure,* who in replacing the austere image of Gautama is a glorious redeemer, one of infinite light. Also, the people worship **Kwannon,** *a goddess of compassion.*

One austere movement within the Mahayana branch is the Zen sect. Taking their example from Gautama's extended contemplation of a flower, Zen followers care little for discourse, books, or other symbolic interpretations and explanations of reality. Hours and years are devoted to meditation, contemplation of word puzzles, and consultation with a Zen master. In seeking absolute honesty and truthfulness through such simple acts as drinking tea or gardening, the Zen student hopes to experience enlightenment. Whilst Buddhism produces a solemnizing effect, Shintoism has an affirmative and joyous effect. Emperor, ancestor, ancient hero, and nature worship form its core. Those who follow Shintoism feel an intense loyalty and devotion to every lake, tree and blossom in Japan as well as to the ancestral spirits abiding there. They also have a great concern for cleanliness, a hangover from early ideas surrounding dread of pollution in the dead. Followers of Shintoism have two god shelves in their home. One contains wooden tablets inscribed with the name of the household's patron deity and a symbolic form of the goddess of rice, as well as other texts and objects of family significance. Here the family performs simple rites, such as offering a prayer or a food gift each day. In a family crisis, perhaps an illness, the family conducts more elaborate rites, such as lighting tapers or offering rice brandy. The other god shelf, in another room, is the Buddha shelf; and if a family member dies, a Buddhist priest, the spiritual leader, performs specified rituals there.

If illness or impending death causes a family member to be hospitalized, another well family member will stay at the hospital to bathe, cook for, and give emotional support to the patient. They feel that recovery largely depends on this family tie. If death occurs, they will be reminded of the Buddhist doctrine teaching that death is a total nonfunction of the physical body and mind and that the life force is displaced and transformed to continue to function in another form. Every birth is a rebirth, much as in the Hindu teaching, and rebirth happens immediately after death, according to some Buddhists. Others believe that rebirth occurs 49 days after death, during which time the person is in an intermediary state. The difference in quality of death, birth, and existence depends on whether the person lived a disciplined or undisciplined life.

Buddhist teachings teach the living how to die well. The elderly, or feeble, are to prepare themselves mentally for a state that would be conducive for a good rebirth. The person is to remain watchful and alert in the face of death, to resist distraction and confusion, to be lucid and calm. Distinct instructions are given in what to expect as life leaves the body, as the person enters an intermediary state, and as Nirvana is about to occur.

In giving care to a person with this type of background, be aware of the varied religious influences on life. The sect's emphasis on the here and now rather than on the long road to Nirvana may place a high value on physical health so that the person can benefit from the joys and beauty of this life. The person may readily voice impatience with the body's dysfunction. You can also respond to the great concern for cleanliness, the desire to have family nearby, and the need for family rites that are offered for the sick member.

## CONFUCIANISM AND TAOISM

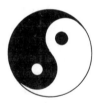

To provide insights into these Chinese modes of thinking, although it is more representative of Taoism, use is made of *yin-yang symbol.* The symbol is a circle, representing **Tao** or *the absolute,* in which two tear shapes fit perfectly into one another, each containing a small dot from the other. Generally yang is light or red, and yin is dark. Ancient Chinese tradition says that everything exists in these two interacting forces. Each represents a group of qualities. Yang is positive or masculine – dry, hot, active, moving and light. Yin is feminine or negative – wet, cold, passive, restful and empty. For example, fire is almost pure yang and water almost pure yin – but not quite. The combination of yin and yang constitutes all the dualisms a person can imagine: day–night, summer–winter, beauty–ugliness, illness–health, life–death. Both qualities are necessary for life in the universe; they are complementary and, if in harmony, good. Yang and yin energy forces are embodied in the body parts and affect food preferences and eating habits. This symbol translates into a relaxed philosophy of life: 'If I am sick, I will get better. Life is like going up and down a mountain; sometimes I feel good and sometimes I feel bad. That's the way it is.'

**Confucius** was *the first saint of the nation.* Although **Lao-tzu,** *the founder of Taoism,* is a semilegendary figure said to have vanished after he wrote the *bible of Taoism,* **Tao-te-ching,** Confucius has a well-documented existence.

Confucius, born in 551 BC, wrote little. His disciples wrote the **Analects,** *short proverbs embodying his teachings.* He is revered as a teacher, not as a god. Followers try to emulate him and his teachings, which she or he has heard since birth. The temple in his memory is a place for studying, not for praying. And on his birthday, a national holiday, people pay respect to their teachers in his memory.

Five important terms in Confucius's teaching are **Jen,** *a striving for goodness within;* **Chun-sui,** *establishing a gentlemanly/womanly approach with others;* **Li,** *knowing how relationships should be conducted and having respect for age;* **Te,** *leading by virtuous character rather than by force;* and **Wen,** *pursuing the arts as an adjunct to moral character.* So strongly did Confucius feel about the family that he gave directives on proper attitudes between father and son, elder brother and junior brother, husband and wife. Concepts of immediate family includes grandparents, uncles, aunts and cousins. Chinese has more words for relationships between relatives than the English language has. Followers feel that in caring for the body one cares for the family, the country and the universe. Essentially, all people are family.

Important in your understanding of a person with this background is the dualism that exists in such thinking. Acceptance of the particular version of mysticism and practicality, and of the yin and yang forces that are seen as operating within self, will help in building a foundation of personalized care.

The person may have more respect for older than younger staff members and may respond well to teaching. There may be a strong desire to attain and maintain wellbeing. These factors are directly related to the religious teaching; you can use them to enhance care.

ISLAM

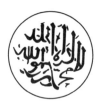

Islam is *the youngest of the major world religions*. This faith, with its Arabic colouring and tenacious monotheistic tradition, serves as a bridge between eastern and western religions. 'There is no God but Allah; Muhammed is His Prophet' provides the key to Moslem belief. He must say this but once in his life as a requirement, but he will repeat it many times as an affirmation.

The founder, Muhammed, was born in approximately AD 571 in Mecca, then a trading point between India and Syria on the Arabian peninsula. Hating polytheism and influenced by Judaism and Christianity, Muhammed wrote *God's revelation to him* in the **Koran** *scriptures* that to Moslems confirm the truths of the Jewish-Christian Bible. He believes in the biblical prophets, but he calls Muhammed the greatest – the Seal of Prophets.

Through the Koran and the **Hadith,** *the traditions,* he has guidelines for his thinking, devotional life and social obligations. He believes he is a unique individual with an eternal soul. He believes in a heaven and hell and while on earth he wants to walk the straight path.

To keep on this path, he prays five times a day: generally on rising, at midday, in the afternoon, in the early evening and before retiring. Articles needed are water and a prayer rug. Because he emphasizes cleanliness of body, he performs a ritual washing before each prayer. Then, facing Mecca, he goes through a series of prescribed bodily motions and repeats various passages in praise and supplication. A Moslem also observes **Ramadan,** *a fast month,* during which time he eats or drinks nothing from sunrise to sunset; after sunset he takes nourishment only in moderation. He explains **fasting** *(abstinence from eating)* as a *discipline aiding him to understand those with little food.* At the end of Ramadan, he enters a festive period with feelings of goodwill and gift exchanges.

A pilgrimage to Mecca is a requirement for all healthy and financially able Moslems. In line with the Koran's teaching the Moslem does not eat pork, gamble or drink intoxicants. He worships no images or pictures of Mohammed, for the prophet is not deified. He gives a portion of his money to the poor, for Islam advocates a responsibility to society.

Parts of the basic Islam faith are used by a United States-based group called the Black Muslims (Nation of Islam). Known to have stringent, seclusionist rules, the Black Muslims have taken some new positions since 1976 and seem to be moving towards more orthodox Islam. Members may now get politically involved; membership is open to whites; dress codes have changed; and some of the myths about the American founder, W.D. Fard, have been erased.

Moslem patients are excused from religious rules, but many will still want to follow them as closely as possible. Even though in a body cast and unable to get out of bed, a patient may want to go through prayers symbolically. The person might also recite the first chapters of the Koran centred on praise to Allah, which are often used in times of crises. Family is a great comfort in illness and praying with a group is strengthening, but the Moslem has no priest. The relationship is directly with God. Some patients may seem completely resigned to death, whereas others, hoping it is God's will that they live, cooperate vigorously with the medical programme. After death, a body must be washed and the hands folded in prayer. Knowledge of these attitudes and traditions can greatly enhance your care. Submission to God's will is the very meaning of Islam.

## JUDAISM

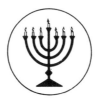

In the Jewish community each member is expected to contribute to others' needs according to his/her ability. Jews have traditionally considered their community as a whole responsible for feeding the hungry, helping the widowed and orphaned, rescuing the captured, and even burying the dead. Jewish retirement homes, senior citizens' centres, and medical centres are witness to this philosophy.

Jews live by the law as given in the **Torah,** *the first five books of the Bible;* and in the **Talmud,** *a commentary and enlargement of the Torah. His spiritual leader is the* **rabbi.** His spiritual symbol is the *menorah. A Jew's entrance into a responsible religious life and manhood* is through the **Bar Mitzvah,** a ceremony which takes place in the synagogue when he is 13. (Girls are also educated to live responsible religious lives, and a few congregations now have a similar ceremony, the **Bas Mitzvah,** for girls.)

Judaism is divided into three groups, orthodox, reform and the conservatives. **Orthodox** *believe God gave the law;* it was written exactly as He gave it; it should be followed precisely. **Reform** *Jews believe the law was written by inspired men* at various times and therefore is subject to reinterpretation. **Conservatives** *are in the middle,* taking some practices from both groups. Overriding any differences in interpretation of ritual and tradition is the fundamental concept expressed in the prayer 'Hear, O Israel, the Lord our God, the Lord is One.' Not only is He one, He loves His creation, wants His people to live justly, and wants to bless their food, drink and celebration. Judaism's double theme might be expressed as 'Enjoy life now, and share it with God.' Understandably, then, religious emphasis isn't on an afterlife, although some Jewish people believe in one. Although Jews have had a history of suffering, the inherent value of suffering or illness isn't stressed. Through their observance of the law, the belief of their historical role as God's chosen people, and their hope for better days, Jews have survived seemingly insurmountable persecution. Although Jewish law can be suspended when a person is ill, the patient will be most comfortable following as many practices as possible.

Every Jew observes the **Sabbath,** *a time for spiritual refreshment, from sundown on Friday to shortly after sundown on Saturday.* During this period Orthodox Jews may refuse freshly cooked food, medicine, treatment, surgery, and use of radio, television and writing equipment lest the direction of their thinking be diverted on this special day. An Orthodox male may want to wear a **yarmulke** *or skullcap* continuously; use a *prayerbook called* **Siddur,** and use **phylacteries,** *leather strips with boxes containing scriptures,* at weekday morning prayer. Also, the ultra-Orthodox male may refuse to use a razor because of the Levitical ban on shaving.

Some Orthodox Jewish women observe the rite of **Mikvah,** an *ancient ritual of family purity.* From marriage to menopause (except when pregnant) these women observe no physical-sexual relations with their husbands from 24 hours before menstruation until 12 days later when a ritual immersion in water renders them ready to meet their husbands again.

Jewish dietary laws have been considered by some scholars as health measures: to enjoy life is to eat properly and in moderation. The Orthodox, however, obey them because God so commanded. Food is called **treyfe** (or treyfah) if it is *unfit* and **kosher** if it is *ritually correct.* Foods forbidden are pig, horse, shrimp, lobster, crab, oyster and fowl that are birds of prey. Meats approved are from those animals that are ruminants and have divided hooves. Fish approved must have both fins and scales. Also, the kosher animals must be healthy and slaughtered in a prescribed manner. Because of the Biblical passage stating not to soak a young goat in its mother's milk, Jews do not eat meat products and milk products together. Neither are the utensils used to cook these products ever intermixed, nor the dishes from which to eat these products.

Guidelines for a satisfactory diet for the Orthodox are as follows:

1. Serve milk products first, meat second. Meat can be eaten a few minutes after milk, but milk cannot be taken for 6 hours after meat.

2. If a person completely refuses meat because of incorrect slaughter, encourage a vegetarian diet with protein supplements, such as fish and eggs, considered neutral unless prepared with milk or meat shortening.

Two important holy days are *Rosh Hashanah* and *Yom Kippur*. **Rosh Hasha-nah,** *the Jewish New Year,* is a time to meet with the family, give thanks to God for good health, and renew traditions. **Yom Kippur,** *the day of atone-ment,* a time for asking forgiveness of family members for wrongs done, occurs 10 days later. On Yom Kippur Jews fast for 24 hours, a symbolic act of self-denial, mourning and petition. **Tisha Bab,** *the day of lamentation,* re-calling the destruction of both Temples of Jerusalem, is another 24-hour fast period. **Pesach** or **Passover** (eight days for Orthodox and Conserva-tive, seven days for Reform) *celebrates the ancient Jew's deliverance from Egyp-tian bondage.* **Matzo,** *an unleavened bread,* replaces leavened bread during this period.

The Jewish person is preoccupied with health. Jews are future-oriented and want to know diagnosis, how a disease will affect business, family life and social life. The Jewish people as a whole are highly educated, and although they respect the doctor, they may get several medical opinions before carrying out a treatment plan.

While family, friends and rabbi may visit the ill, especially on or near holidays, they will also come at other times. Visiting the sick is a religious duty. And although death is final to many Jews except for living on in the memories of others, guidelines exist for this time. When a Jewish person has suffered irreversible brain damage and can no longer say a **bracha,** *a blessing to praise God,* or perform a **mitzvah,** *an act to help a fellow,* he/she is considered a 'vegetable' with nothing to save. Prolonging the life by arti-ficial means would not be recommended. But until then the dying patient must be treated as the complete person he/she always was, capable of con-ducting his/her own affairs and entering into relationships.

Jewish tradition says never to leave the bedside of the dying person, which is of value to the dying and the mourners. The dying soul should leave in the presence of people and the mourner is shielded from guilt of thinking that the patient was alone at death or that more could be done. The bedside vigil also serves as a time to encourage a personal confession by the dying, which is a *rite de passage* to another phase of existence (even though unknown). This type of confessional is said throughout the Jewish life cycle whenever one stage has been completed. Confessional on the deathbed is a recognition that one cycle is ending and that another cycle is beginning. Recitation of the *Shema* in the last moments before death helps the dying to affirm faith in God and focus on the most familiar rituals of life.

Death, being witnessed at the bedside, helps to reinforce the reality of the situation. Immediate burial and specified mourning also move the remain-ing loved ones through the crisis period. (Note, however, that if a Jew dies on the Sabbath, he cannot be moved, except by a non-Jew, until sun-down.) After the burial, the mourners are fed in a meal of replenishment called *se'udat havra'ah*. This step symbolizes the rallying of the community and the sustenance of life for the remaining. Also, Jews follow the custom of sitting *shiva* or visiting with remaining relatives for one week after the death.

Judaism identifies a year of mourning. The first three days are of deep grief; clothes may be torn to symbolize the tearing of a life from others. Seven days of lesser mourning follow, leading to 30 days of gradual readjustment. The remainder of the year calls for remembrance and healing. During that year a prayer called the mourner's *Kaddish* is recited in religious services. It helps convey the feeling of support for the mourner. At the annual anniversary of death, a candle is burned and special prayers said.

So from circumcision of the male infant on the eighth day after birth to his deathbed, and from the days of the original menorah in the sanctuary in the wilderness until the present day, the followers of Judaism re-enact their traditions. Because many of these traditions remain an intrinsic part of the Jew while striving to maintain or regain health, the preceding guidelines offer a foundation for knowledgeable care.

## CHRISTIANITY

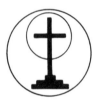

Christianity has many divisions and sects within its beliefs, but all share basic beliefs as follows. Most importantly that Jesus Christ as described in the Bible is God's son. Jesus, born in Palestine, changed 'BC' to 'AD'. The details of His 33 years are few, but His deeds and words recorded in the Bible's New Testament show quiet authority, loving humility, an ability to perform miracles and an affinity with people in varied social positions.

The main symbol of Christianity is the cross, but it signifies more than a wooden structure on which Jesus was crucified. It also symbolizes the finished redemption – Christ rising from the dead and ascending to the Father in order to rule with Him and continuously pervade the personal lives of His followers.

Christians observe **Christmas** *as Christ's birthday;* **Lent** *as a season of penitence and self-examination preceding* **Good Friday,** *Christ's crucifixion day;* and **Easter,** *His Resurrection day.* Christians rely on the New Testament as a guideline for their lives. They believe that Jesus was fully God and fully man at the same time, that their original sin (which they accept as a basic part of themselves) can be forgiven, and that they are acceptable to God because of Jesus Christ's life and death. They believe God is three persons – the Father, the Son, and the Holy Spirit (Holy Ghost), the last providing a spirit of love and truth.

All Christians highly regard their individuality as children of God and hope for life with God after death. They feel responsible for their own **souls,** *the spiritual dimension of themselves,* and for aiding the spiritual needs of others.

Roman Catholicism is a religion based on the dignity of man as a social, intellectual and spiritual being, made in the image of God. The teaching authority of the church is traced through the scriptures.

God sent His Son to provide salvation and redemption from sin. He established the Church to continue His work after ascension into heaven. Jesus chose apostles to preach, teach, and guide. He appointed Saint Peter as the Church's head to preserve unity and to have authority over the apostles. The mission given by Jesus to Saint Peter and the apostles is the same that continues to the present through the Pope and his bishops.

A Catholic believes that the seven Sacraments are grace-giving rites that give a share in Christ's own life and help sustain efforts to follow His example. The Sacraments that are received once in life are Baptism, Confirmation, Holy Orders and, usually, Matrimony.

*Through* **Baptism** *the soul is incorporated into the life of Christ and shares his divinity.* Any infant in danger of death should be baptized, even an aborted foetus. If a priest is not available, you can perform the sacrament by pouring water on the forehead and saying, 'I baptize thee in the name of the Father, of the Son, and of the Holy Spirit.' The healthy baby is baptized some time during the first weeks of life. Adults are also baptized when they convert to Catholicism and join the church.

**Confirmation** *is the sacrament in which the Holy Spirit is imparted in a fuller measure to help strengthen the individual in his/her spiritual life.* **Matrimony** *acknowledges the love and lifelong commitment between a man and a woman.* **Holy Orders** *ordains deacons and priests.*

The Sacraments that may be received more than once are Penance (Confession), the Eucharist (Holy Communion), and the Anointing of the Sick (Sacrament of the Sick). **Penance,** *an acknowledgment and forgiveness of sins in the presence of a priest,* should be received according to individual need even though it is required only once a year by church law. The Mass, often called the **Eucharist,** is the *liturgical celebration* whose core is the sacrament of the Holy Eucharist. Bread and wine are consecrated and become the body and blood of Christ. The body and blood are then received in Holy Communion. The Eucharist is celebrated daily and all Roman Catholics are encouraged to participate as often as possible; they are required by church law to attend on Sundays (or late Saturdays) and specified holy days throughout the year unless prevented by illness or some other serious reason.

The Anointing of the Sick has been modified and broadened. Formerly known as Extreme Unction or the last rites, this sacrament was reserved for those near death. Now **Anointing of the Sick,** *symbolic of Christ's healing love and the concern of the Christian community,* can provide spiritual strength to those less gravely ill. Following anointing with oil, the priest offers prayers for forgiveness of sin and restoration of health. Whenever possible, the family should be present to join in the prayers.

If the patient is dying, extraordinary artificial measures to maintain life are unnecessary. At the hour of death the priest offers communion to the dying person by means of a special formula. This final communion is called *Viaticum.* In sudden deaths the priest should be called and the anointing and *Viaticum* should be administered if possible. If the person is dead when the priest arrives, there is no anointing, but the priest leads the family in prayers for the person who just died.

The Roman Catholic funeral is divided into three phases: the **wake,** *a period of waiting* or vigil during which the body is viewed and the family is sustained through visiting; the **funeral mass,** *a prayer service* incorporated into the celebration of the Mass; and the **burial,** *the final act* of placing the person in the ground. (This procedure may vary somewhat, for some Catholics are now choosing cremation.) The mourners retain the memory of the dead through a Month's Mind Mass, celebrated a month after death, and anniversary masses. Finally, the priest integrates the liturgy for the dead with the whole parish liturgical life.

While in hospital, a Roman Catholic may want to attend Mass, have the priest visit, or receive the Eucharist at bedside. (Fasting an hour before the sacrament is traditional, but in the case of physical illness, fasting is not necessary). Other symbols that might be comforting are a Bible, prayer book, holy water, a lighted candle, crucifix, rosary, and various relics and medals.


## PROTESTANTISM AND OTHER GROUPS OF INTEREST

Practices or beliefs unique to certain groups should be part of every health worker's knowledge.

*Seventh-Day Adventists* rely on Old Testament law more than do other Christian churches. As in Jewish tradition, the Sabbath is from sundown Friday to sundown Saturday. And like the Orthodox Jew, the Seventh-Day Adventist may refuse medical treatment and the use of secular items, such as television, during this period and prefer to read spiritual literature. Diet is also restricted. Pork, fish without both scales and fins, tea and coffee are prohibited. Some Seventh-Day Adventists are **lacto-ovo-vegetarians:** *they eat milk and eggs but no meat.* Tobacco, alcoholic beverages and narcotics are also avoided. Because Adventists view the body as the 'temple of God', health reform is high on their list of priorities and they sponsor health institutes, cooking schools and food-producing organizations. They have pioneered in making foods for vegetarians, including meatlike foods from vegetable sources. Worldwide they operate an extensive system of over 4000 schools and 400 medical institutions and are active medical missionaries. Much of their inspiration comes from Ellen G. White, a nineteenth-century prophetess who gave advice on diet and food and who stressed Christ's return to earth.

*The Church of Jesus Christ of Latter-Day Saints (Mormons)* takes much of its inspiration from the **Book of Mormon,** *translated from golden tablets found by the prophet Joseph Smith.* The Mormons believe that this book and two others supplement the Bible. Every Mormon is an official missionary. There is no official congregational leader, but a **seventy** and a **high priest** *represent successive steps upward in commitment and authority.*

The Articles of Faith of the Church of Jesus Christ of Latter-day Saints, as given by Joseph Smith, include statements of belief:

1. God and His Son, Jesus Christ, and the Holy Ghost.
2. The same organization that existed in the Primitive Church.
3. Worship of God according to personal conscience while obeying the law of the land.
4. People being punished for their own sins and not for Adam's transgression.
5. All people being saved, repentance, and obedience to the laws and ordinances of the Gospel.
6. Being honest, true, chaste, benevolent, virtuous, hopeful, persistent, and doing good to all people.

Specific Mormon beliefs are that the dead can hear the Gospel and can be baptized by proxy. Marriage in the temple seals the relationship for time and eternity. After a special ceremony in the temple, worthy members receive a white garment. This garment, worn under the clothes, has priesthood marks at the navel and at the right knee and is considered a safeguard against danger. The church believes in a whole-being approach and provides education, recreation, and financial aid for its members. A health and conduct code called 'Word of Wisdom' prohibits tobacco, alcohol and hot drinks (interpreted as tea and coffee) and recommends eating, though sparingly and with thankfulness, herbs, fruit, meat, fowl and grain, especially wheat.

The Mormon believes that disease comes both from failure to obey the laws of health and from failure to keep the other commandments of God. However, righteous persons sometimes become ill simply because they have been exposed to microorganisms that cause disease. They also believe that by faith the righteous sometimes escape plagues that are sweeping the land and often, having become sick, the gift of faith restores the obedient to full physical wellbeing.

Statistics indicate that the Mormon population succumbs to cancer and diseases of the major body systems at a much lower rate than the general population in this country. The death rate for patients suffering from cancer is less than 50 per cent that of the general population; 50 per cent less for those with diseases of the nervous, circulatory and digestive systems; 33 per cent less for kidney diseases, and 10 per cent less for those with respiratory diseases. Mental illness occurs only half as often among Mormons as among the general population. An explanation for these differences from the norm might be that the Mormons literally believe that the body is the 'temple of God'. And they have programmes of diet, exercise, family life and work to help that 'temple' function at optimum level.

Although the two groups just discussed – the Seventh-Day Adventists and the Mormons – generally accept and promote modern medical practices, the next two groups hold views that conflict with the medical field. The first group, *Jehovah's Witnesses*, refuses to accept blood transfusions. Their refusal is based on the Levitical commandment, given by God to Moses, declaring that no one in the House of David should eat blood or he would be cut off from his people, and on a New Testament reference (in Acts) prohibiting the tasting of blood.

Every Jehovah's Witness is a minister. Members meet in halls rather than in traditional churches and they produce massive amounts of literature explaining their faith.

The second group, *Church of Christ, Scientist (Christian Scientists)*, turn wholly to spiritual means for healing. Occasionally they allow an orthopaedist to set a bone if no medication is used. Parents do not allow their children to get a physical examination for school; to have eye, ear, or blood-pressure screening; or to receive immunizations. In addition to the Bible, Christian Scientists use as their guide Mary Baker Eddy's *Science and Health with Key to the Scriptures*, originally published in 1875. The title of this work indicates an approach to wholeness and those who follow its precepts think of God as Divine Mind, of spirit as real and eternal, of matter as unreal illusion. Sin, sickness and death are unrealities or erring belief. Christian Scientists do not ignore their erring belief, however, for they have established nursing homes and sanitoriums. These facilities are operated by trained Christian Science nurses who give first-aid measures and spiritual assistance.

A Christian Science graduate nurse must complete a 3-year course of training at one of a number of accredited sanitoriums. The training includes, among other subjects, classes in basic nursing acts, care of the elderly, cooking, bandaging, nursing ethics, care of notifiable diseases, and theory of obstetrical nursing. The training is nonmedical and in the work of a Christian Science nurse no medication is administered. The nurse supports the work of the **practitioner,** *who devotes full time to the public practice of Christian Science healing.* Healing is not thought of as miraculous but as the application of natural spiritual law.

The practitioner helps people apply natural spiritual law. Such a person is not a clergyman and does not necessarily hold special church office. Becoming a practitioner is largely attained through self-conducted study and a short course of intensive study from an authorized teacher of Christian Science, but daily study, prayer, application and spiritual growth are the foundation of practice. The practitioner will treat anyone who comes for help and is supported, like other general practitioners, by patients' payments. A Christian Scientist who is in a medical hospital has undoubtedly tried Christian Science healing first, may have been put there by a non-Scientist relative, or may be at variance with sacred beliefs. If brought in while unconscious, the person would want to be given the minimum emergency care and treatment consistent with hospital policy. The person may also appreciate having a Christian Science practitioner called for treatment through prayer.

Another group of special interest because of their positive personal and health emphasis is the *Society of Friends (Quakers).* While most Roman Catholics acknowledge the earthly spiritual authority of the Pope and most Protestants regard the Bible as their ultimate authority, the Friend's authority resides in direct experience of God within the self. A Friend obeys the **light within,** *the* **inner light** *or the* **divine principle;** *this spiritual quality causes the Friend to esteem self and listen to inner direction.* All Friends are spiritual equals. Without a minister and without any symbols or religious decor, unprogrammed corporate worship consists of silent meditation with each person seeking divine guidance. Towards the end of the meeting, people are free to share their inspiration. The meeting closes with handshaking. Always interested in world peace, Friends have been instrumental in establishing organizations that work towards human brotherhood and economic and social improvements resulting in better health. Friends have staffed hospitals, driven ambulances, and served in medical corps, among numerous other volunteer services.

*Agnosticism and atheism*

This chapter has concentrated so far on worship of God, the divine spirit, with an emphasis on traditional teaching. Some people live by ethical standards, considering themselves either **agnostic,** *incapable of knowing whether God exists,* or **atheistic,** *believing that God does not exist.*

## NURSING IMPLICATIONS

You can use the foregoing – basic beliefs, dietary laws, and ideas of illness, health, body, spirit, mysticism, pragmatism, pain, death, cleanliness and family ties – as a *beginning*. Even more basic than understanding these concepts is respecting your patient as a person with spiritual needs who has a right to have these needs met, whether he/she has formal religious beliefs. No one will respect your spiritual aid if you do not appear competent and thoughtful in your work. You are not expected to be a professional spiritual leader, for which lengthy training and experience would be required. You can, however, aid patients. You are the transition, the key person between the patient and spiritual help. An adolescent or young adult caught up in sorting out various facets of learned idealism and trying to fit them into more realistic daily patterns may temporarily discard religious teaching. He/she may reject the guidance of a spiritual leader because the latter is associated with the parents' beliefs; yet the adolescent is nevertheless searching and needs guidance. An elderly person suffering the grief of a recently lost mate may repeatedly question how a God of love could allow this loss. Some physiologically mature people are not religiously mature; they may expect magic from God. The spiritually maturing individual experiences the fruits of faith in God in behavioural terms of love, trust and security. The external spiritual stimuli of God's word, sacraments, and relationships with other believers create an inner peace and love through which the person experiences God within and then reaches out to others in supporting relationships.

Furthermore, realize that people can use the same religious terms differently: *saved, sanctified, fell out, slain by the spirit,* and *deathbed conversion* all connote religious experiences. You should listen carefully and you may have to ask questions to determine accurately the individual person's meaning.

For too long there has been no communication between the nurse and the chaplain. You can fill that gap. Nurse and chaplain rapport can mean that the *whole* person is served rather than segmented parts. Chaplains are especially helpful to clients, as well as to nurses, when they assist with the expression of anger, death, and the expression of grief. Nurse and chaplain, however, need to know what to expect from each other; there is no substitute for talking about these expectations and agreeing on strategies.

When determining medical background, such as drug or food allergies, you could also ask about religious dietary laws, special rituals, or restrictions that might be an important part of the patient's history. Recording and helping the patient follow beliefs could speed recovery.

The spiritual needs of the patient have become a part of the evolving nursing diagnosis system of classification. Three areas have been pinpointed: spiritual distress related to the need for (a) love and relatedness; (b) forgiveness, and (c) meaning and purpose. As nurses become more attuned to this situation, perhaps meeting the patient's spiritual needs will not be unattached from other care. Perhaps you could share with the chaplain the responsibility for asking some of the following questions as you give patient care. No specific set of questions will be right for every patient.

Be sure to look for the patient's strengths, not weaknesses. And remember that you must not preach or reconstruct. Allow the patient to assume his/her own spiritual stance.

Because your relationship with the patient may be of short duration, be sure to document well the results of this interview. And later, when you or others care for the patient, you should watch for religious needs that may be expressed through nonreligious language. You must again let the patient know what options are open for spiritual help. If you hide behind business and procedures, you may lose a valuable opportunity to aid in health restoration.

Religion influences behaviour and attitudes towards:

1. Work – whether you work to expiate sin, because it's there to do, or because of a conviction that it is a God-given right and responsibility.
2. Money – whether you save money or deny yourself something, do instalment buying, buy health insurance, consider money the root of all evil, or believe that it is to be used for the betterment and development of persons and society.
3. Political behaviour – ideas about the sanctity of the monarchy, effects of Communism, importance of world problems, spending abroad versus spending for national defence, education and union membership.
4. Family – kinds of interaction within the family, honouring of parents or spouse, children, or siblings.
5. Childrearing – interest in the child's present and future, attitudes toward punishment or rewards for behaviour, values of strict obedience as contrasted with independent thinking, or how many children should be born.
6. Right or wrong – what is sin, how wrong is gambling, drinking, birth control, divorce, smoking and abortion.

Ideally, religion provides strength, an inner calm and faith with which to work through life's problems. But you must be prepared to see the negative aspect. To some, religion seems to add guilt, depression and confusion. Some may blame God for making them ill, for letting them suffer, or for not healing them in a prescribed manner. One Protestant felt she had made a contact with God: if she lived the best Christian life she could, God would keep her relatively well and free from tragedy. When an incurable disease was diagnosed, she said, 'What did I do to deserve this?' Another

Protestant, during her illness, took the opposite view of her contract with God. She said 'I wasn't living as well as I should and God knocked me down to let me know I was backsliding.'

Healing, too, has varied meanings. Some will demand that God provide a quick and miraculous recovery whereas others will expect the process to occur through the work of the health team. Still others combine God's touch, the health workers' skill, and their own emotional and physical cooperation. Some will even consider death as the final form of healing.

Sometimes you must deal with your own negative reactions. Your medical background and knowledge may cause you to be dismayed at some religious practices. For instance, how will you react as you watch a postoperative Jehovah's Witness patient die because she has refused blood? How will you react to a Christian Scientist patient who, in your opinion, should have sought medical help a month ago to avoid present complications?

*Intervention*

With all these aspects to consider, a team approach that includes the patient, family, health workers, and chaplain or other spiritual leader is imperative.

Weekends are when most people attend corporate worship, therefore chaplains are not always available, so preparing the patient for chapel service, or seeing that the Sabbath ritual is carried out, puts a special responsibility on you, the nurse.

If a patient is confined to bed you can simply prepare a worship centre or shrine by arranging flowers, prayer book, relics, or whatever other objects have spiritual meaning.

Maintaining a list of available spiritual leaders, knowing when to call them, and knowing how to prepare for their arrival are other important responsibilities. If a patient can't make the request, consult with the family. Sometimes the family needs reassurance and guidance from the chaplain. You can suggest this option.

As you prepare the patient and the setting for a spiritual leader, help create an atmosphere that reflects more than sterile procedure. Privacy has previously been emphasized by drawing curtains and shutting doors. Although acceptable to some, this approach may produce a negative response in others. Perhaps more emphasis should be given to cheerful surroundings: sunshine, flowers, lighted candles, openness, and participation by family and staff in at least an introductory way. Perhaps the patient and spiritual leader could meet outdoors in an adjoining garden.

If the patient is a child on a prolonged hospitalization, a special area might be designated for religious instruction.

Brief the spiritual leader on any points that might provide special insight and be sure that the patient is ready to receive him/her. Prepare any special arrangements, such as having a clean, cloth-covered tray for Communion. Guard against interruption by health workers from other departments who may be unaware of the visit. Finally, incorporate the results of the visit into the patient's record.

Many will benefit from the sacraments, the prayers, Scripture reading, and counselling given by the spiritual leader, but others will want to rely on their own direct communication with God. The Zen Buddhist, Hindu, Moslem, and Friend might be in the latter category. All may wish reading material, however. Most will bring their sacred book with them, but if they express a desire for more literature, offer to get it.

If you feel comfortable doing so, you can at times say a prayer, read a Scripture, or provide a statement of faith helpful to the patient. If you do not feel comfortable in providing this kind of spiritual care, you can still meet the patient's spiritual needs through respectful conversation, listening to the patient talk about beliefs, referral to another staff member, or calling one of the patient's friends who can bolster his/her faith. If spiritual leaders aren't available, you could organize a group of health workers willing to counsel with or make referrals for patients of their own faiths.

The atheist is not to be neglected because he/she does not profess a belief in God. He/she has the same need for respect as anyone else and may need you to listen to fears and doubts. The person doesn't need your judgment.

Moreover, just as health teaching is often omitted for health workers who are patients, so is spiritual guidance often omitted for spiritual leaders who are patients. You must recognize that each person, regardless of religious stand or leadership capacity, may need spiritual help.

Although a hospital setting has been used as a point of reference throughout this chapter, you can improvise in your setting – nursing home, school, industry, clinic, home, or other health centre – in order to provide adequate spiritual assistance.

## REFERENCES

1. Smith, Huston, *The Religions of Man* (Harper & Row Publishers Inc., New York, 1965).
2. 'Doctors Use Psychic Tools for Healing', *St Louis Globe-Democrat*, 30 September 1975, sec. Ap. 12.
3. Neuberger, Julia, *Caring for Dying People of Different Faiths* (Austin Cornish, 1987, for the Lisa Sainsbury Foundation).
4. Ibid.; also, Okamoto, Abraham, 'Religious Barriers to World Peace', *Journal of Religion and Health*, vol. 15 no. 1 (1976) pp. 26–33.
5. Ibid.

# 10

# The family – basic unit for the developing person

Study of this chapter will enable you to:

1. Define *family* and discuss the family as a system and the implications for the developing person.

2. Describe the purposes, tasks, roles, and functions of the family and their relationship to the development and health of its members.

3. List the stages of family life and the developmental tasks for the establishment, expectancy, and parenthood phases.

4. Relate the impact of feelings about the self and childhood experiences on later family interaction patterns.

5. List and describe the variables affecting the relationship between parent and child and general family lifestyle, including single-parent, step-parent and adoptive families.

6. Identify ways in which your family life has influenced your present attitudes about family.

7. Discuss the influence of twentieth-century changes on family life and childrearing practices.

8. Predict how a changing culture may affect the development and health of the family system.

## DEFINITIONS

The **family** *is a social system and primary reference group made up of two or more persons living together who are related by blood, marriage, or adoption or who are living together by agreement over a period of time.* The family unit is *characterized by face-to-face contact, bonds of affection, love, harmony, simultaneous competition and mutual concern, a continuity of past, present and future, shared goals and* *identity, and behaviours and rituals common only to the specific unit.* With the family, the person can usually let down his/her guard and be more himself/ herself than with other people.

The family may be **nuclear** *(mother, father, child),* **extended** *(nuclear plus other relatives of either or both spouses live together),* **patriarchal** *(the man has the main authority and decision-making power),* **matriarchal** *(the woman has the main authority),* or **reconstituted** *(one divorced or widowed adult with all or some of his/her children and a new spouse with all or some of his/her children, so that parents, step-parents, children, and stepchildren live together.)* Or the family may be made up of siblings, especially in middle or late life, homosexuals, friends in a commune, or a male and female living together without being married. The family may be symbolically duplicated in the work setting: a woman may be perceived as a grandmother, mother or sister, or a man may be perceived as a grandfather, father or brother to an employee. The family member who is dead or missing may remain clearly in the other members' memory; they may refer to the person on special occasions. Or the deviant of the family – the alcoholic or runaway – may influence other family members to act in an opposite manner.

The family may also be a series of separate but interrelated families. The middle-aged parents are helping the adolescent and young adult offspring to be emancipated from the home while simultaneously caring for in- creasingly dependent parents and sometimes up to four pairs of grandpa- rents and older aunts and uncles as well. All related family members may not live under the same roof, but the extended family exists psychological- ly – in spirit. Often the responsibility is nearly overwhelming to the middle- agers, who have no time or resources to spend on themselves. The conflict inherent in having to care for a number of relatives and in-laws can contri- bute to marital disharmony as well as poor relationships between the gen- erations.

The elderly person is sometimes aware of such a situation and will try to make minimal demands. Often he/she feels that more attention is deserved and may make extra demands or chastise the middle-aged offspring for not doing more for elder family members.

The mass media present a picture of family life dissolving. Although the divorce rate is high, most divorced people remarry. Because of greater life expectancy and the young age at which people marry, the young couple of today enter and remain in marriage longer than did their grandparents.

## PURPOSES, TASKS, ROLES AND FUNCTIONS OF THE FAMILY

Although the institution of the family is being scrutinized and predictions are made that it is about to pass into oblivion, the family has demonstrated throughout history that it is a virtually indestructible institution. Family structure, roles and responsibilities have always been influenced by technology and the resulting social changes. But technological advances alone do not determine family structure and function. Family systems are a force in themselves endlessly adaptive, and very resistant to outside pressure. In a society where objects are often disposable and people feel uneasy and dispensable, they seek secure relationships.

The family has passed through major transitions. It was once a relatively self-contained, cohesive domestic work unit; it has become a group of persons dispersed among various educational and work settings. Various agencies have absorbed many purposes once handled solely by the family group. Schools educate; hospitals care for the sick; mortuaries prepare the dead for burial; churches give religious training; government and private organizations erect recreational facilities; nursing homes care for the aged; and various manufacturing firms bake, can, or bottle food and make clothes.

When the family changed from a production unit to a consumption unit, it also lost some degree of authority to regulate its members' behaviour. The emphasis is now on democratic sharing, togetherness, the child's potential as an individual, and the fun aspects of parenthood. Enjoyment and relaxation in every human relationship are considered important. Technology is seen as the reason for this view, and the way to attain the happy state, but the person who believes too strongly in what technology can accomplish may have unrealistic expectations about living and thus undergo considerable stress in marriage and childrearing.

Yet the family is still considered responsible for the child's growth and development and behavioural outcomes; indeed, the family is a cornerstone for the child's competency development. Because the family is strongly influenced by its surrounding environment as well as by the child itself, the family should not bear full blame for what the child is or becomes. Few parents deliberately set out to rear a disturbed, handicapped, or delinquent offspring, although many such failures occur.

The family is expected to perform the following tasks:

1. Provide for physical safety and economic needs of its members and obtain enough goods, services and resources to survive.
2. Create a sense of family loyalty and a mentally healthy environment for the family's wellbeing.
3. Help members to develop physically, emotionally, intellectually and spiritually, as well as to develop a personal and family identity.
4. Foster a value system built on spiritual and philosophical beliefs and the cultural and social system that is part of the identity.
5. Teach members to communicate effectively their needs, ideas, feelings, as well as respect for each other.

6. Provide social togetherness simultaneously with division of labour, patterning of sexual roles, and performance of family roles with flexibility and cooperation.
7. Reproduce and socialize the child(ren), inculcating values and appropriate behaviour, providing adult role models, and fostering a positive self-concept and self-esteem in the child(ren).
8. Provide relationships and experience within and without the family that foster security, support, encouragement, motivation, morale and creativity.
9. Help the members to cope with crises and societal demands.
10. Maintain authority and decision making, with the parents representing society to the family as a whole and the family unit to society.
11. Promote integration into society and the ability to use social organizations for special needs when necessary.
12. Release family members into the larger society – school, church, organizations, work and politics.
13. Maintain constructive and responsible ties with the neighbourhood, school, and local and central government.

The family's ability to meet its tasks depends on the maturity of the adult members, the support given by the social system – educational, work, religious, social, welfare, governmental and leisure institutions. The family that is most successful as a unit has a working philosophy and value system that is understood and lived, uses healthy adaptive patterns most of the time, can ask for help and use the community services available, and develops linkages with nonfamily units and organizations.

To remain adaptive, families manoeuvre to secure compliance of all members with the family rules through verbal and nonverbal communication to each other. Usually one member is designated as the one who must maintain a specific pattern of dependent behaviour, sometimes negative or unhealthy, in order to keep all other family members comfortable. If the designated member tries to change behaviour and become more independent, he/she receives no support. The feedback received is that he/she is disrupting the status quo and the other family members are uncomfortable. Thus sick behaviour will be maintained at the expense of the development of the designated person and of the family.

Signs of strained or destructive family relationships include:

1. Lack of understanding and communication between spouses.
2. Each family member alternately acting as if the other didn't exist or harassing through arguments.
3. Lack of family decision making.
4. Parent's possessiveness of the children or the mate.
5. Children's derogatory remarks to parents or vice versa.

6. Extreme closeness between husband and his mother or family or the wife and her mother or family.
7. Parent being domineering about performance of household tasks.
8. Few outside friends for parents or children.
9. Scapegoating or blaming each other for difficulties.
10. High level of anxiety or insecurity present in the home.
11. Lack of creativity.
12. Pattern of immature or regressive behaviour in parents or children.

*Roles of the family*

The family apportions **roles,** *prescribed behaviours in a situation,* in a way similar to society at large. In society there are specialists who enforce laws, teach, practise medicine and fight fires. In the family there are also such performance roles: breadwinner, homemaker, handyman (or handy-woman), the expert, political advisor, chauffeur and gardener. There are also emotional roles: leader, nurturer, sustainer, protector, healer, arbitrator, scapegoat, jester, rebel, dependent, 'sex-pot', and 'black sheep'. Members may fill more than one role. The fewer people there are to fulfil these roles, as in the nuclear family, the greater the number of demands placed on one person. If a member leaves home, someone else takes up his/her role. Any member of the family can satisfactorily fulfil any role in either category unless he or she is uncomfortable in that role. The man who is sure of his masculinity will have no emotional problems changing a baby or cooking a meal. The woman who is sure of her femininity will have no trouble gardening or taking the car for repair.

The emotional response of a person to the role he/she fulfils should be considered. Someone may perform the job competently and yet dread doing it. The man may be a carpenter because his father taught him the trade, although he wants to be a music teacher. Changes in performance roles also necessitate emotional changes – for example, in the man who takes over household duties when his wife becomes incapacitated.

The child learns about emotional response to roles in the family while imitating adults. The child experiments with various roles in play and eventually finds one that is emotionally comfortable. The more pressure put on the child by the parents to respond in a particular way, the more likely that child is to learn only one role and be uncomfortable in others, as evidenced by the athletic champion who may be a social misfit. The child becomes less adaptive socially and even within the family as a result.

Exercising a capacity for a variety of roles, either in actuality or in fantasy, is healthy. The healthy family is the one in which there is opportunity to shift roles intermittently with ease. Through these roles family functions are fulfilled.

*Functions of the family as a social system*

The family is a system. It functions as a unit to fulfil its purposes, roles, tasks. It provides shelter, stability, security, and a setting for nurturing and growth. It is a safe place to experiment with the dynamics and role behaviours required in a system. It has an energy that provides a support system for individual members. As the social system changes, the family system must also adapt if it is to meet individual needs and prepare its members to participate in the social system.

The organization of a family system is hierarchal, although it may not be directly observable. The usual family hierarchies are built on kinship, power, status, and privilege relationships that may be related to individual characteristics of age, sex, education, personality, health, strength or vigour. We can infer a hierarchy by observing each person's behaviour and communication. For instance, who talks first? Last? Longest? Who talks to whom? When? Where? About what? If one family member consistently approaches the staff about the client's health care, he/she probably holds an upper position in the family and has the task of being 'expert' on the client's status. Your attempt to communicate with family members may meet with resistance if the communication inadvertently violates the family communication hierarchy.

Hierarchal relations in the family system determine the role behaviour of family members. These hierarchal role relationships typically have great stability and ordinary family members can be counted on to behave congruently with their roles. When there are differences in behaviour from situation to situation, they are almost inevitably in response to the family's expectations for that particular situation or circumstance. Families develop a system of balanced relationships. When one member leaves the family or experiences a change, such as illness, other family members must adapt as well. Roles and relationships are based on reciprocal interaction, each member of the family contributing to the total unit in a unique and functional way. If a member should fail to meet the expectations of the roles established by his or her position in the hierarchy for the moment, the remaining members of the family generally react by using pressure (for example, persuasion, punishment, argument, being ignored) on the 'deviant' person. Ackerman states that all family functions can be reduced to two basic ones: (a) ensuring the physical survival of the species and (b) transmitting the culture, thereby ensuring essential humanness. The union of mother and father, of parent and child, forms the bonds of identity that are the matrix for the development of this humanness.[1]

**Physical functions** of the family are met by the parents providing food, clothing and shelter, protection against danger, provision for bodily repairs after fatigue or illness, and by reproduction. In 'primitive' societies these physical needs are the dominant concern. In western societies many families take them for granted.

**Affectional functions** are equally important. Although many traditional family functions, such as education, job training and medical care, are being absorbed by other agencies, meeting emotional needs and promoting adaptation and adjustment are still two of the family's major functions. The family is the primary unit in which the child tests emotional reactions. Learning how to reach and maintain emotional equilibrium within the family enables him/her to repeat the pattern in later life situations. The child who feels loved is likely to contract fewer physical illnesses, learn more quickly, and generally have an easier time growing up and adapting to society.

A healthy family has five dominant attitudes:

1. No distinctions are made about worth of people; all members are perceived as equal.
2. All persons are seen as unique and developing.
3. When a disturbing situation arises, members understand that many factors were involved – people were not simply trying to be difficult.
4. Members accept that change is continuous.
5. Members freely share their thoughts and feelings with a minimum of blame and feel good about each other and themselves.

Other important attitudes are as follows:

1. The feeling of unity between man and woman and a separateness from their families of origins so that interfamily interference with the marriage is avoided.
2. An ability to invest in the marriage to a greater degree than in other relationships.
3. A feeling of balance or harmony, for perfect equality is probably impossible.
4. A movement from a romantic 'falling in love' to a warm, loving, companionable, accepting relationship.
5. An ability to maintain variety and frequent interactions with each other.

**Social functions** of the modern family include providing social togetherness, fostering self-esteem and a personal identity tied to family identity, providing opportunities for observing and learning social and sexual roles, accepting responsibility for behaviour, and supporting individual creativity and initiative. The family actually begins the indoctrination of the infant into society when it bestows a name and hence a social position or status in relation to the immediate and kinship-group families. Simultaneously, each family begins to transmit its own version of the cultural heritage of its own family culture to the child. Because the culture is too vast and comprehensive to be transmitted to the child in its entirety and all at once, the family selects what is to be transmitted. In addition, the family interprets and evaluates what is transmitted. Through this process, the child learns to share family's values.

Thus socialization is a primary task of the parents, for they teach the child about the body, peers, family, community and age-appropriate roles as well as language, perceptions, social values and ethics. The family also teaches about the different standards of responsibility society demands from various social groups. For example, the professional person, such as a physician, nurse, or lawyer, those in whom people confide and to whom they entrust their lives and fortunes, are held more accountable than the farmer or day labourer. There is also a difference in the type of contact that society has with a particular group: for example, the post or milk deliverer does not enter the home, but the exterminator is free to enter a home and look into every corner.

The parent generation educates by literal instruction and by serving as models. Thus the child's **personality,** *a product of all the influences that have and are impinging on him/her,* is greatly influenced by the parents. The types and importance of family interactions in carrying out these functions in each life era are further discussed by Murray and Zentner.[2]

## STAGES OF FAMILY DEVELOPMENT

Like an individual, the family has a developmental history marked by predictable crises. The developmental crises are normal, but they are also disturbing or frightening because each life stage is a new experience. The natural history of the family is on a continuum: from marriage or cohabitation; choosing whether to have children; rearing biological or adoptive offspring, if any; and releasing children into society to establish homes of their own. In later life the aging parents or grandparents are a couple once again, barring divorce or death. The nurturing of spouse or children goes on simultaneously with a multitude of other activities: work at a job or profession, managing a household, participation in church and community groups, pursuit of leisure and hobbies, maintaining friendships and family ties. Or the person may decide to remain single but live with a person of the same or opposite sex; then the purposes, tasks, and roles of family life must also be worked out.

### Initial or establishment stage

When the couple establish a home of their own, their main psychological tie is no longer with family of orientation (parental family). They commit themselves to living together, usually through marriage. They must work out patterns of communication, daily living, sexual relations, a budget and a philosophy of life. Often this work begins during courtship. Relationships with family and friends are also different after marriage and must be worked out.

Today families may choose to have no children, one child and adopt, or one, two, or three children instead of a larger family. Some women feel that motherhood is not necessary for fulfilment. Certainly the man's chief fulfilment is not necessarily from fatherhood. Some people are wise enough to know that children do not automatically bring happiness to a marriage. Children bring happiness to parents who want them and who are selfless enough to become involved in the adventure of rearing them. Children bring trauma to a troubled marriage.

Limitation of family size and birth spacing yield substantial family health benefits. Certain associations in death, disease and disability are apparent. Maternal deaths increase when maternal age is below 20 or above 40 years and after a third pregnancy for women of all age groups except those over 40. Increased maternal disease, obstetric complications, maternal deaths, and postnatal mortality occur with six or more pregnancies. Unwanted pregnancy increases maternal disease and death, especially if the pregnancy is terminated by illegal abortion that results in infection or haemorrhage. Other effects of unwanted pregnancy include excessive nausea and vomiting, spontaneous abortion, toxaemias, complications of labour and delivery, emotional illness prenatally or postnatally, marital friction and divorce. Infant mortality rate increases for birth order above three in the lower social class and rises among women under 17 years of age. The safest years for a normal delivery are between ages 20 and 29. Infants of youngest mothers of highest parity are at greatest risk for disease and death regardless of social class. Mothers are less likely to have premature or low-birthweight, and therefore healthier, infants when spacing is greater than 2 years but less than 6 years.

The number of children in a family is related to the quality of care provided by the mother. A long-term follow-up study of 13,000 British infants revealed that the smaller the family size, the better the quality of infant care and management, use of medical services, interest in the child's school progress, and the less the tendency for child abuse. Additionally, the child of the smaller family does better in school and finishes more schooling than does the child from a large family. Incidence of infectious diseases, such as gastroenteritis and respiratory infections, are greater in larger-sized families. Children in large families are smaller in physical size, and first-born children with one or more siblings do not reach the height and weight obtained by those who remain only children. Intellectual development in children is affected negatively by large family size.

The establishment phase ends when the woman becomes pregnant or when the couple work out their living patterns and philosophy of life (which may include a decision not to have children).

### The expectant stage

During pregnancy, which is a development crisis, many domestic and social adjustments must be made. The couple are learning new roles and gaining new status in the community. Attitudes toward pregnancy and the physical and emotional status of both partners will affect parenting abilities. Now the couple think in terms of family instead of a pair. They explore beliefs about childrearing and plan for the expanded family in terms of space, budget and necessary supplies.

The woman may initially dislike being pregnant because it interferes with her personal plans or she may feel proud and fulfilled. Sexual desire may either increase or decrease. She may be more or less interested in her surroundings. Usually she is more preoccupied with herself, her new feelings, and changing body image, and she experiences fantasies and fears regarding the baby and the childbirth experiences.

The man experiences a variety of feelings on learning of the pregnancy, feelings that change during the pregnancy. The reality of the pregnancy increases with time. One study showed that 70 per cent of the men experienced ambivalent feelings initially, but fatherly feelings developed. The men also felt guilty about the wife's pregnancy and her physical symptoms, anxious and depressed about their own adequacy, proud of their virility, and fearful of approaching the wife sexually. Concerns identified by fathers may include: caring for the infant, adequacy as a father, financial security and concern related to the baby's effect on the marital dyad. Early and thorough prenatal care for the woman is essential. Both the woman and the man may experience similar physical and emotional symptoms, such as nausea, indigestion, backache, distention, irritability and depression. Symptoms may result from hormonal changes or feelings about the pregnancy in the woman. In the man they are part of the **couvade syndrome,** *which may be a reaction based on identification with or sympathy for the woman, ambivalence or hostility toward the pregnancy, or envy of the woman's childbearing ability.*

Major decisions for the couple are whether to attend childbirth preparation classes and whether the man should be present in the labour and delivery rooms. The woman may feel eager to have the man with her or she may fear that he will think of her as sexually unattractive or be repulsed. The man may be curious about what is happening and want to attend his child's birth, or he may feel guilty about not wanting to when he feels others expect him to be there. He may be embarrassed about his wife's behaviour and appearance during labour and delivery, or he may fear that he cannot cope with the childbirth event if present. Sexual fantasies triggered by labour and delivery may threaten the man who has tenuous emotional equilibrium. If the man has considerable unconscious conflicts or a weak self-image as a man, he may wish not to be involved in childbirth preparation, labour, or delivery. Some men and women cannot participate in childbirth preparation classes and should not be made to feel guilty about their decision. Participation may not enhance the couple's self-esteem and may create additional emotional crisis. Participation in classes and childbirth does not change the woman's perception of her partner as ideal man, husband, or father, but it does improve her self-image as ideal woman, wife and mother. In addition, the woman is more likely to be in good physical condition for labour if she has had preparation.

Although the woman needs extra 'mothering' from the partner during pregnancy, the man also needs extra attention and nurturing or he may be unable to continue to support the mother-to-be emotionally. You can listen to the woman's and man's concerns and help them understand that what they are experiencing is normal. Various teaching aids explaining pregnancy and what to expect during the birth experience are also useful. Your care should be family centred, directed toward both parents-to-be. You can help the woman to gain maternal feelings and the man to see the importance of his role as provider as well as nurturer.

The man must be prepared for fathering just as the woman is for mothering.

*Parenthood phase*

With the birth of a child, the couple assume a status that they will never lose as long as each has memory and life – that of parent. The following are the stages of parenthood:

1. Anticipatory stage. The woman is pregnant and the couple are learning the new roles and perceptions associated with pregnancy discussed earlier.
2. Honeymoon stage. The time following birth when the parents feel excited about the new relationship but also uncertain about the meaning of parental love. A parent-child attachment is being formed. During this time difficult adjustments need to be made. Because the parents lose sleep, husband-wife intimacy diminishes and there is less freedom for the couple to follow their own interests.
3. Plateau stage. The years during the child's development when the parents are active in the role of mother and father. During this time the parents deal with problems in the family, community, church, school and immediate social sphere. They are concerned with family planning,

socialization and education of the child, and participating in community organizations.

4. Disengagement stage. The termination of the parent-child family unit that occurs when the last child marries or leaves home permanently and the parents let go of their major childrearing responsibilities to allow the offspring to be autonomous.

Western society values creativity and individuality; thus no set patterns of parenthood exist. Parents rely on their own uniqueness, wisdom and skills, how their parents raised them, or on books. Youth are poorly prepared to make the transition to parenthood. Yet how parents treat a child is the single most important influence on the child's physical, emotional, and cognitive development and health.

The couple may accept the idea of parenthood but reject a particular child because of the child's sex, appearance, time of the birth in their life cycle, or the child's threatening helplessness. Or the couple may reject the idea of parenthood but genuinely love the baby who was unplanned. Often parents have difficulty because pregnancy, childbirth and parenting are romanticized in our society, and the romantic ideal differs considerably from the reality of 24-hour responsibility and submersion of their personal desires for many years to come.

How the parents care for and discipline the child are influenced considerably by the parents' own maturity; how they were cared for as children (as shown by studies on child abuse); their feelings about self; culture, social class, and religion; their relationship with each other; their perceptions of and experiences with children and other adults; their values and philosophy of life; and life stresses that arise. Moreover, the historical eras in which the parents were reared and are now living in and the prominent social values of each era subtly influence parental behaviour.

Each critical period in the child's development reactivates a critical period in the parent. Demands made on the parent vary with the age of the child. The infant needs almost total and constant nurturing. Some parents thrive during this period and depend on each other for support. Other parents feel overwhelmed by the infant's dependency because their own dependent needs are stimulated but unmet. The baby's cry and behaviour evoke feelings of helplessness, dependency and anger associated with their unacceptable dependency needs and feelings, and then guilt and fatigue. The toddler struggles with individuality and autonomy, exploring and vacillating between dependency and independency. At this stage the child is intense and often unreasonable in demands and refusal to obey commands. The parents may enjoy this explorative, independent behaviour of the child, even though the toddler leaves the parent feeling tired and frustrated. Or the primitive behaviour of the child may stimulate primitive impulses in the parent, who may feel threatened by the will of the toddler.

The parent who has difficulty controlling angry impulses may find the toddler's temper outbursts totally unacceptable. Parents who have difficulty caring for the dependent infant may do very well with the independent preschooler or adolescent or the reverse may be true. The parent may be able to resolve personal conflicts and move to a more advanced level of integration as he/she works with the developing child or the parent may be unable to cope with the aroused feelings.

Some parents feel that they must possess a child and will try to fit that child into a mould – their image. Other parents see their task of parenthood as stewards – to be a guide, helping friend, standard setter for the child. They invest themselves in the creative potentialities of their young – nurturing, educating, and protecting the child. They love but do not smother; guide but do not control; discipline but do not punish; offer freedom but do not abandon. They see the child as a lamp to be lit rather than a vessel to be filled.

Parents who possess their children feel that they have the right to dictate the terms of their child's life. Then the child has only half a life; parental need to control is greater than real love for child. Too much pressure is placed on the growing child, disturbing his/her emotional development.

Just as detrimental are the parents who abandon the child to rear itself, parents who spend too little time with and give too little affection to the child. Such children spend considerable time with television and peers; they learn that the adult world doesn't want them. In one study children who spent most of their time with peers were more influenced by the lack of the parents' presence, attention, and concern than by the attractiveness of the peer group.

Parents should rethink their priorities when they have children. Parents need to invest time in such a way that it brings quality to their relationship with the child. Children need the encouragement of doing things and talking through things with adults.

Developmental tasks for the couple, which are reworked with the birth of each child, include to:

1. Provide for the physical and emotional needs of the child, conveying love and security freely regardless of the child's appearance or temperament.
2. Reconcile conflicting roles – wife–mother, husband–father, worker–homemaker or family man, and parent–citizen.
3. Accept and adjust to the demands and stresses of parenthood, learning or relearning basics of child care, adjusting personal routines and needs to meet the child's needs, and trying to meet the spouse's needs as well.
4. Provide opportunities for the child to master competencies expected for each developmental stage, to allow the child to make mistakes and learn from them, to restrict the child reasonably and consistently for safety, and to attain the emotional developmental tasks.

5. Share responsibilities of parenthood and together make necessary adjustments in space, finances, housing, lifestyle, and daily routines that are healthy for the family (meals, sleep).
6. Maintain a satisfying relationship with spouse – emotionally, sexually, intellectually, spiritually and recreationally – while maintaining a personal sense of autonomy and identity.
7. Feel satisfaction from being competent parents and the parenting experience but maintain contacts with relatives and the community.
8. Provide socialization experiences to help the child make the emotional shift from family to peers and society so that the child can become a functioning citizen.
9. Refine the communication system and relationships with spouse, children and others and permit offspring to be autonomous after leaving home.

As the children mature and leave home, the parents must rework their self-concepts as parents and people in order to take on new roles, responsibilities and leisure activities so that the last stage of parenthood, disengagement, can be accomplished.

*Disengagement stage of parenthood*

Sometimes the last stage, disengagement, does not last too long. The young adult who is unemployed, a college dropout, or divorced may return home to live. The aged parents or other relatives may be unable to continue to live independently and then are included in the household of middle-aged offspring. Consequently, the tasks, functions, roles and hierarchical relationships of the family must be reworked. Space and other resources must be reallocated. Time schedules for daily activities may be reworked. Privacy in communication, use of possessions, and emotional space must be ensured. Old parent–child conflicts, ideas about who is boss and how rules are set and discipline accomplished may resurface and should be discussed and worked through. These families can benefit from counselling; your guidance may be crucial.

The following suggestions to adult children and their parents may make living together more harmonious:

1. Remember what it was like when a new baby came home. No matter how beloved the child, disruptions are bound to occur. Realize that another relative's homecoming will be the same.
2. Everyone involved should remember whose house it is.
3. Realize that no matter how many years sons and daughters have been away, family procedures don't change. Mum may still be critical. Dad may be the constant advice-giver. Expect it.

4. Talk about resentments. Discuss problems if you think it will help.
5. Parents may say offspring are grown up. But that doesn't mean they believe it. Still, they can't exert the same authority with a 30- or 40-year-old as with a youngster.
6. Offspring and elderly parents need to be flexible. It's unfair to expect the middleagers who are the 'hosts' to change their household and life routines too much.
7. Even if parents refuse money, adult offspring should insist on paying something, no matter how minimal. Otherwise the offspring are reinforcing the idea that parents are taking care of them. Elderly parents can also contribute financially most of the time.
8. When grandchildren are involved, set rules about who's in charge. To decrease dependency, babysitters should be hired when possible. Then family members don't feel obligated or constrained.
9. Determine length of the adult offspring's stay. It need not be a precise date, but future plans about leaving the home should be explicitly stated.
10. Both adult offspring and older relatives should share responsibilities if possible. But don't upstage Mum or Dad; for example, if Mum loves cooking, don't make her feel useless by taking over in the kitchen.
11. Space permitting, privacy is important. The relative who has lived on his or her own is probably used to time and space alone.
12. Middleagers should resist meddling in the affairs of either offspring or parents. They can advise. But grown offspring need to think for themselves and older relatives expect to make their own decisions.
13. Realize that the living situation may be temporary. Living together may not be ideal for anyone. But some parents and offspring or middleagers and their parents become closer during such periods.

## FAMILY INTERACTION

**Family interaction** *is a unique form of social interaction based on a set of intimate and continuing relationships. It is the sum total of all the family roles being played within a family at a given time.* Families function and carry out their tasks and lifestyles through this process.

Family therapists, psychiatrists and nurses are giving increased attention to the emotional balance in family **dyads** *or paired role positions,* such as husband and wife or mother and child. They have noted that a shift in the balance of one member of the pair (or of one pair) alters the balance of the other member (or pair). The birth of a child is the classic example. Dyads and emotional balance also shift in single-parent and step-parent families.

Interaction of the husband and wife, or of the adult members living under one roof, is basic to the mental, and sometimes physical, health of the adults as well as to the eventual health of the children. Two factors strongly influence this interaction: (a) the sense of self-esteem or self-love of each family member and (b) the different socialization processes for boys and girls.

## Importance of self-esteem

The most important life task for each person – to feel a sense of self-esteem, to love and have a positive self-image – evolves through interaction with the parents from the time of birth onward and, in turn, affects how the person interacts in later life with others, including spouse and offspring.

The adult in the family who lacks self-acceptance and self-respect is not likely to be a loving spouse or parent. Behaviour will betray feelings about self and others because he/she will perceive no automatic acceptance and little love from others in the family. Because perception of an event is the person's reality, such a person, in turn reacts in ways designed to defend self from the rejection that he/she *thinks* will be received: he/she may criticize, get angry, brag, demand perfection from others, or withdraw. In this way, he/she builds up self, the emotional reasoning being: 'I may not be much, but others are worse.' Such behaviour is corrosive to any relationship but particularly one as intimate as the family's. Because of overt behaviour, those intimate with him/her are not likely to appreciate or respond to the basic needs for love, acceptance and respect. Indeed, the common responses to such behaviour are counterattack or withdrawal, which, in turn, perpetuate the other's negative behaviour. To remain open and giving in such situations is difficult for the mate but may be the only way to elevate the other's self-esteem. Perhaps only then can he/she reciprocate loving behaviour. You can help family members realize the importance of respecting and loving one another and help them work through problems stemming from the low self-esteem of a family member.

## Influence of childhood socialization

The second crucial influence on interaction between adults in the family is the difference in socialization processes for boys and girls. These differences are so embedded in the social matrix that until recently they had gone nearly unnoticed. There is a different social source for self-love in boys and girls. The girl is loved simply because she exists and can attract, as shown by the admiration pretty little girls receive. The girl is also taught to be subtle, for such behaviour is part of her attraction. The boy is loved for what he can do and become; he must prove himself. Boys, especially from school age on, are given less recognition than girls for good looks and much recognition for what they can do. A boy learns to be direct, to brush aside distractions (sometimes including a woman's voice, for most disciplining will come from the mother and female schoolteachers and can be perceived as nagging after a while), and to get to the essence of things.

These concepts of what is appropriate boy and girl behaviour are taught early and continue to affect heterosexual interactions throughout life. In traditional courtship, for example, the boy is expected to be in charge, to be dominant, to prove himself; the girl is expected to attract, to be passive. In marriage, however, these expectations cause problems, for the man is proving himself largely through his work, and this aspect of his earlier courtship behaviour is now less visible to his wife. If the woman does not understand the dynamics of his behaviour, she is likely to feel rejected and unloved, thinking she can no longer attract him. If the wife is also working, the husband may think of her as a competitor and work harder to keep his self-esteem. His physical self, including his involvement in lovemaking, is very much intertwined with his social, professional and financial self, and failure in one is likely to cause feelings of failure in the total self, affecting his sense of masculinity, sexuality and personhood.

All these facts are compounded by the shift in balance between the man and woman found in modern marriage, especially with the advent of the women's liberation movement. The husband often labours under the illusion that he enjoys the rights and responsibilities inherent in a patriarchal family system. Yet he must recognize the qualifications and drive for independence, the basic humanness, of his wife. You can help the couple to recognize the effect of their early socialization on their behaviour and expectations and to work through misunderstandings. Help parents to overcome sexual stereotypes so that they do not inflict them on their children.

*Variables affecting interaction between the child and adult*

Long before the child learns to speak, sensory, emotional, and intellectual exchanges are made between the child and other family members. Through such exchanges, and later with words, the child receives and tests instructions on how to consider the rights of others and how to respond to authority. The child also learns how to use language as a symbol, how to carry out certain routines necessary for health, how to compete, and what goals to seek. The games and toys purchased for and played with the child, the books selected and read, and the television programmes allowed can provide key learning techniques.

The child's spontaneity can evoke in the adult fresh ways of looking at life long buried under habit and routine. The child says 'It's too loud, but my earlids won't stay down' or 'I want one of those little red olives with the green around' or 'Give me that rubber with the handle.' The child can also recreate for the adult the difficulty of the learning process: 'Is it today, tomorrow, or yesterday? You said when I woke up it would be tomorrow, but now you call it "today".'

Family interaction for the child and adult is also affected by the ordinal position and sex of the children, as well as by the presence of an only child or of multiple births, such as twins.

Parents tend to identify with their children and to treat them according to how they were treated as siblings. A parent can identify best with the child who matches his/her own sibling position. A man from a family of boys may not know how to interact with a daughter and may not empathize with her. In the process of identifying with the parent, the child picks up many of the parent's characteristics, especially if the child is the oldest or lone child. For example, the oldest boy may be dependent instead of independent if his father was the youngest sibling and retained his dependent behaviour into adulthood. Using family constellation theory, **the ordinal position of the child** is important to development. Siblings have an important influence on each other. The firstborn, who is an only child until the second one comes along, may enjoy some advantages in achievement of intellectual superiority and perspective about life, including a greater sense of responsibility. He/she has more contact with adults and is the sole recipient of attention for a time. He/she becomes dominant over young siblings. Secondborn boys with an older sister are more feminine than those with an older brother. The younger children benefit from the parents' experience with childraising and from having older siblings to imitate. Lastborns are also more sociable, possibly to ensure acceptance by older siblings or to gain parental attention. The lastborn may be more dependent. The middle child is likely to become caught between the jealousy of the older child and the envy of the younger, who may form a coalition against him/her. But he/she learns double or triple roles and is prepared for more kinds of relationships in adulthood. If two siblings are more than 6 years apart, they tend to grow up like only children.

**The only child** may feel more loneliness but develops more rapidly and may seem older and more serious than peers who have siblings. He/she lacks the opportunities siblings could provide. Thus he/she usually does not share feelings and experiences with someone close, or cope with jealousy and envy from rivals in the home, or learn intimately about ways of the opposite- or same-sexed peers. He/she learns less about compromising with peers, sharing adult attention, and erecting strong defences against the feelings displaced on him/her by adults and peers.

Children are the logical targets for fulfilling many of the parents' frustrated ambitions and needs. In a large family these yearnings and aspirations can be parcelled out among a number of children, but when there is only one child, this child can sense the parents' manipulation and expectations. Thus the only child tends to be a peacemaker if he/she and the parents are the only household members. He/she is inadvertently brought into the parents's conflicts and is forced to help maintain harmony and preserve equilibrium in the household. In a family with only one child, there are few people to fulfil the many roles of a family; thus more is demanded of each member. The only child may be forced prematurely to assume roles for which he/she is ill equipped. The child may become deft at performing adult tasks and roles, but self-confidence in the capacity to do so may be uncertain.

The only child sometimes has special problems on becoming a parent, seeing in the child a longed-for brother or sister. The danger in the situation is that the child is also a rival for the spouse's attention. On reaching adolescence, the offspring may then pose a threat to the parent's own adult roles, and the parent may unconsciously become overly competitive. Yet the only child is now regarded as an answer for the parents who want the parenting experience but who also want time to fulfil their own careers.

Certainly the only child can develop into a wholesome, well-adjusted person. The qualities of being more serious, assertive, responsible, independent, curious and able to entertain self, and find satisfaction in personal pursuits frequently develop because of parental and home demands. These demands can enhance abilities to be a mature, capable adult. The greater opportunities available for adult contact, beginning at home, develop the only child's creativity, language skills, planning abilities and intellectual potential. He/she has a high need to achieve and prefers the novel or complex. Firstborn and only children, such as Isaac Newton, Franklin Roosevelt, Emile Zola, Herbert Spencer, Rainer Maria Rilke, and some of the American astronauts, rank high on the roster of outstanding leaders, artists and scientists. As you counsel parents who plan for or have only one child, emphasize the need for peer activity and the danger of too much early responsibility and pressure.

**Multiple births,** such as twins, have considerable impact on family interaction. If ovulation has been inhibited with contraceptive pills, multiple births are more likely once this method stops being used. The needs and tasks of these parents will differ from the parents who have a single birth. Your suggestions and support can influence how well the parents cope with their responsibility.

Because multiple births are often premature, the first four or five months are very demanding on the parents in terms of the amount of energy and time spent in child care; this means that the parents have less energy and time for each other or other children. The mother should have help for several months if possible – from the husband, a relative, friend, or neighbour. Financial worries and concern about space and material needs may also intrude on normal husband-wife relationships or on relationships with other children.

Although books discourage the mother of twins from breast-feeding or using alternate breast and bottle, the mother may be able to breast-feed both twins successfully, by alternating breast- with bottle-feedings. The babies will not necessarily be poor breast-feeders with this arrangement.

You can suggest shortcuts in, or realities about, care that will not be detrimental to twin babies and that will give the parents more time to enjoy them.

The parents should not be made to feel guilty if they are not as conscientious with two babies as they would be with one. Each can be given a total bath every other day instead of daily. Heating bottles before feeding is not necessary. The parents should try to avoid getting so wrapped up in meeting the babies' physical needs that resentment, anger, or excessive fatigue creep in. Multiple offspring should be fun as well as work.

Encourage the parents of twins (or multiple offspring) to perceive the babies as individuals and to consider the long-term consequences of giving them similar-sounding names, dressing them alike, having doubles of everything, and expecting them to behave alike.

Multiple-birth children are likely to be closer than ordinary siblings. They soon learn about the extra attention resulting from their birth status and may take advantage of the situation. Interaction between them is often complementary; for example, one twin may be dominant and the other submissive. Each learns from reinforcement of his/her experiences about the advantages of the particular role chosen. Twins may each receive less parental affection and communication because parents have less time to devote to each child. Thus twins are often slower to talk and many have a slower intellectual growth unless parents work to prevent it.

**The gender of the child** also influences development within the family. In most cultures a higher value is placed on male than on female children. Actually, in some cultures only a boy's birth is welcomed or celebrated and the family's status is partially measured by the number of sons. Or a family with several girls and no boys may perceive another baby girl as a disappointment. The girl may discover this attitude in later years from overhearing adult conversations and she may try to compensate for her sex and gain parental affection and esteem by engaging in tomboy behaviour and later assuming masculine roles.

If a boy arrives in a family that hoped for a girl, he may receive pressure to be feminine. He may even be dressed and socialized in a feminine manner. If the boy arrives after a family has two or three girls, he will receive much attention but also the jealousy of his sisters. He will grow up with three or four 'mothering' figures (some may be unkind) and in a family more attuned to feminine than to masculine behaviour. Developing a masculine identity may be more difficult for him, especially if there is no male nearby with whom to relate. In spite of being pampered, he will be expected by his family to be manly. The boy may feel envious of his sisters' position and their freedom from such great expectations.

The girl who arrives in a family with a number of boys may also receive considerable attention, but she may have to become tomboyish in order to compete with her brothers and receive their esteem. Feminine identity may be difficult for her. You can help parents understand how their attitude toward their own sexuality and their evaluation of boys and girls influence their relationship with their children. Emphasize the importance of encouraging the child's unique identity to develop.

**The adopted child** may suffer some problems of the only child. In addition, the adopted child may have to work through feelings about rejection and abandonment by the biological parents versus being wanted and loved by the adoptive parents. The child should be told that he/she is adopted as early as the idea can be comprehended. Usually by the preschool years he/she can incorporate the idea of being a wanted child.

Social and legal changes have affected the kinds of children in need of adoption. Earlier adoption agencies served mainly white unmarried mothers who saw adoption as the only alternative for their babies. Today fewer infants are available because there is greater social acceptance of out-of-wedlock births; more unmarried mothers keep their babies. Contraceptives and abortions have also reduced the number of unwanted infants. A different category of adoptable children has grown in size, however. These children with 'special needs' have at least one of the following characteristics: over age 5; black, biracial; or physically, emotionally or cognitively handicapped.

Definition of 'suitable' adoptive parents has been liberalized. Adoption agency requirements of age, marital status, race, and mother's employment status are more flexible.

Additionally, today's couples consider adoption even if they have their own children. Some believe they have a responsibility and enough love to provide a home for an existing child rather than add to the total population. Others are single persons who want to offer love and security to a child.

In spite of more liberal definitions of adoptability, the number of people applying to adopt a child, homes approved, placements made and adoptions completed declined compared to the number of available children. Thus an increasing number of older children need permanent placement. You may have an opportunity to educate adults about the opportunity for adopting an older child with special needs or to work with adoptive parents, who also have needs.

Adoption of a child with special needs involves four phases: (a) commitment of adults and child; (b) honeymoon or placement period; (c) storm period, and (d) adaptation and adjustment. The phases do not abruptly begin and end; each phase builds on the preceding phase and sometimes reversals occur. The phases, along with thoughts, emotions, and activities accompanying each phase, are summarized in Table 10.1. The adoptive process can terminate at any point. If termination is necessary, both sides – the family and child – need help to understand what happened and to understand that no *one person* is responsible. Future adoption procedures are enhanced if proper guidance is given with the first failure.

*Table 10.1* The adoptive process

| Phases | Thoughts and emotions | Activities |
|---|---|---|
| 1. Commitment of adult(s) and child(ren) 'Courting stage' | *Adult(s)* make general decision to adopt (stage 1), leading to decision to adopt specific child(ren) (stage 2). | *Adult(s)* prepare for adoption through dialogue with helpful people/agencies, and sometimes attend sessions on adoption given by adoption agency. |
|  | *Child(ren)* express desire for adoption (stage 1), leading to decision on specific family (stage 2). | *Child(ren)* are counselled for potential adjustment by adoption agency staff. Visits are arranged and made between potential family-child(ren). All members involved (including existing children in family) get to know each other. |
| 2. Placement 'Honeymoon period' | *Parent(s)* are on an 'emotional high'; excitement. | Household routines are altered to accommodate child(ren). Limit-setting is minimal. Parent(s) meet child(ren)'s whims. |
| (Child(ren) come to live with parent(s)) | *Child(ren)* are excited but somewhat scared. 'Can I trust these people?' 'Will they send me away if I don't act my best?' | *Child(ren)* put on best behaviour. Sometimes *parent(s)'* show of affection for child(ren) is not accepted because of child(ren)s' past negative parenting. |
| 3. 'Storm period' | *Parent(s)* are tired of permanent house guest(s), feel anger, disappointment, guilt, and displace these feelings on each other and the child. They may wish the child would leave. | *Parent(s)* treat child(ren) or other family members with decreasing tolerance for behaviour not in family norm. |
|  | *Child(ren)* can no longer keep up good behaviour but want to be loved and accepted. | *Child(ren)* may have tantrums, run away, try to reject parents before they reject him/her. |

|   |   |   |
|---|---|---|
| | *Parent(s)* may feel sense of failure. They may have expected too much of themselves and child(ren), and now may strike out at each other and other family members. Spouse may be jealous of time and energy mate gives to child(ren). | If the outcome is positive, the *parent(s)* will use problem solving, limit-setting with flexibility, sense of humour, ongoing empathy and caring, supportive others, and community resources. |
| | *Child(ren)* may think, 'They don't want me. What's going to happen to me?' and may live with anticipatory grief, fears of rejection, and insecurity based on past hurts. Parent(s) and child(ren) test each other. | |
| 4. Adaptation and adjustment phase (equilibrium occurs) | *All* feel they can live and work together; mutual trust is growing; family feels fused as a unit and able to handle frustrations and crises.<br><br>Child(ren) feel good about self, feel love and acceptance. | Parent(s) are consistent with child(ren). *Parent(s)* and *child(ren)* can attend to outside interests without threatening family status. |

**The stepchild** grieves and mourns the loss of a biological parent from death or divorce and must also deal with problems associated with integration into a new family unit. The stepchild may have conflicting feelings of loyalty to the natural parent and to the step-parent, thinking that acceptance of the step-parent is rejection of the natural parent. The stepchild may also feel rejected by his/her remarried natural parent, seeing the step-parent as a rival for the parent's attention. More on the step-parent family follows in the next session.

## FAMILY LIFESTYLES AND CHILDREARING PRACTICES

There is no single type of contemporary UK family, but the lifestyles of many correspond to the factors discussed in this section, including family structure, family cultural pattern, and the impact of the twentieth century. These factors, in addition to those already discussed, influence family interaction and so understanding them will assist you in family care.

*Family structure*

Childrearing and family relationships are influenced primarily by family structure. The biological and reproductive unit most commonly found is the mother-father-child group. Ordinarily the parents are married, have established a residence of their own, are viewed (along with their children) as an integral social unit, and live in an intimate, monogamous relationship. Emphasis in marriage is on pursuit of love in a romanticized way and on individual happiness rather than on family bonds, as in many other cultures. Yet kinship ties are usually recognized on both sides of the family.

In many situations, however, a child may grow up in a family that differs from the typical one. An aunt, uncle, or grandparent may be a continuing member of the household unit; one or the other parent may be absent because of death, divorce, illegitimacy, military service, or occupation involving travel.

*Families in which only one parent is living full time with offspring are called* **single-parent families.** Although death and illegitimacy may cause the family to have only one parent, divorce of the natural parents is the most common reason. In most cases, these families have undergone a major change in lifestyle. A parent may have died either suddenly or after a long illness. If the parents are divorced, the family may have experienced considerable disruption prior to the breakup. These families – and society – may ignore the changed family structure, for they do not fit the traditional social norm, thereby putting even more stress on people attempting to deal with the situation.

In the single-parent family the children may experience grief for the absent parent, guilt for their real or imagined part in the loss, shame for the change in their family structure, and fear about what changes the future may bring. Roles are changed. Each person may need to assume additional responsibilities and tasks. Parents may change their lifestyles. Mother may go to work or school, for instance; father may move into an apartment; or both parents may begin dating. An adolescent may serve as a parent substitute to younger siblings, or other children may assume new household tasks. The initial task of this family is to accept its family structure as a workable option for family living. Often an open discussion of the changed lifestyle along with support from relatives, friends, and other single-parent families, enhances the problem-solving abilities of these persons. Occasionally some family members may need professional help if they exhibit symptoms of more extreme dysfunction, grieving, or prolonged 'acting-out' behaviours.

The *remarriage of a divorced or widowed parent with children may form a composite family unit known as the* **'reconstituted', 'blended',** or **step-parent family.** The 'wicked stepmother' myth pervades our culture; in addition, the common usage of the word 'stepchild' denotes inferior status. These families may be formed in a variety of ways: a mother with children may remarry; a father whose children visit may remarry; either of the new partners may have an ex-spouse or children from a previous marriage (children and stepsiblings) and, to complicate this family even more, the remarried couple may decide to have children of their own. In-laws and several sets of grandparents complete the picture. This family is now a far cry from the typical nuclear family and the interaction becomes increasingly complex.

When a couple marries for the second time and either or both have children from a previous marriage, the new husband and/or wife becomes an instant step-parent. This addition of children to a couple's life differs from the situation of first-marriage couples, whose children are added at a slower pace. Additionally, the myth that familial love occurs via the marriage ceremony is common.

Adjustment to a new, unique family unit is the major task of the stepfamily. New members cannot be assimilated with an existing family; instead a new family unit is formed. New rules, customs and activities must be developed.

All members of this new family bring a history of life experiences, relationships, and expectations to the stepfamily. Conflict often occurs when the values and rules of individuals or the former single-parent family differ from those of the second.

In time family members develop agreement about what is 'right'. Such agreement may include the 'correct' church to attend, the 'right' time for dinner, and how birthdays are to be celebrated. Open communication between members is essential if decisions that are livable for all members are to be made.

In addition to adjusting in the family, stepfamilies must adjust to expectations of the outside world. Often differences in the reconstituted family are ignored because the family appears to be intact. Feelings of frustration, inadequacy, and isolation in family members stem from expectations that they feel as close to one another as blood relatives are expected to. The absent parent may still be an active influence in the original family. For instance, a divorced father may still contribute to his children's support and spend time with them on a regular basis, but they may be living with a stepfather. Even a deceased parent is remembered, not always accurately, and sometimes the step-parent is compared to the memory.

The child's ability to work through these feelings is influenced by age, sex, level of development, adaptive capabilities, and the understanding and support received from significant adults. He/she may need professional help to work through the difficulties of integration into a new family structure.

The stepfamily, like the single-parent family, needs to accept and be accepted as a combination of persons living together in a unique family unit. It is a potentially stressful situation that requires flexibility and adaptability of its members. Yet this family offers many opportunities for growth and friendship through the differing experiences of its members.

*Family size*

Family size is related to distinctive patterns of family life and child development. Most children in Britain are members of a small family system – that is, one with three children or less.

Common features observable in the small family system are that (a) emphasis is on planning (the number and the frequency of births, the objectives of childrearing, and educational possibilities); (b) parenthood is intensive rather than extensive (great concern is evidenced from pregnancy through every phase of childrearing for each child); (c) group actions are usually more democratic; and (d) greater freedom is allowed individual members. The child or children in the small family usually enjoy advantages beyond those available to children in large families of corresponding economic and social level, including more individual attention. On the other hand, these children may retain emotional dependence on their parents, grow up with extreme pressure for performance, and retain an exaggerated notion of self-importance.

The large family, generally thought of as one with six or more children, is not a planned family as a rule. Parenthood is commonly extensive rather than intensive, not because of less love or concern but simply because parents must divide their attention more ways. In the large family emphasis is on the group rather than on the individual member. Conformity and cooperation are valued above self-expression. Discipline in the form of numerous and stringent rules is frequently stressed and there is a high degree of organization in the activities of daily living. Or if parents lack initiative and use their resources unwisely, disorganization may exist.

A family may be small in size either because the parents wanted a small family or because they failed to achieve a large family. In either case, there is a low probability of unwanted children and they may take great interest in their children. In contrast, a large family is large either because the parents achieved the size they desired or because they have more children than they wanted. Large families therefore have a higher probability than small families of including unwanted and unloved children. Adolescents in small families, for example, have better relations with their parents than adolescents in large families, and mothers of large families are more restrictive towards their children than mothers of small families. Thus, lastborn children may be less wanted than the firstborn or middleborn children, especially in large families. This is consistent with what is known of abortion patterns among married women who typically resort to abortion only when they have achieved the number of children they want or feel they can afford to have. Yet only a small percentage of women faced with such unwanted pregnancies actually resorts to abortion, although these women may not be happy with the child later. Most parents are aware of greater parental skills and confidence with lastborn than with firstborn children. But it does not mean that the attitude of the parent is more positive towards the last child than the first. There is no necessary correlation between skills in and enjoyment of a role. Older homemakers are more skilful in domestic tasks, but they may experience less enjoyment than younger homemakers. Older people rate their marriages as 'very happy' less often than younger people. Women may find less enjoyment in the maternal role with the passsage of time, although women know the difference between the romantic expectation concerning the first baby and the more realistic expectation and sharper assessment of their own ability to do an adequate job of mothering as they face a second or third pregnancy.

### Family cultural pattern

*The ways of living and thinking that constitute the intimate aspects of family group life are the* **family cultural pattern.** The family transmits the cultural pattern of its own ethnic background and class to the child, together with the parents' attitudes toward other classes.

Thus how families rear their children will depend on ethnic group and class region, nation and historical period.

### Influence of twentieth-century changes

The shift in this century from an agrarian to a complex technological society has produced dramatic changes for the family. A greater percentage of children now survives childhood than in 1900 and a higher percentage of mothers survives childbirth. Marriage, on the average, occurs at an earlier age than in former generations. Fewer children are born to most parents and they are spaced closer together. Middle-aged couples now have more time together after their children are grown and leave home. And because of an increased life expectancy, families now have more living relatives than formerly, especially elderly relatives.

There are other trends related to living in a complex industrial society. Families live primarily in urban areas. More women work outside the home. The woman who formerly stayed home and was the 'homemaker' has also gone through several changes. Once homemaking took a good deal of time. Now modern conveniences make tasks easier. The woman who stays home today concentrates more on 'mothering'. Her outside activities may include volunteer work, so she can control her hours, feel she has prime time at home but yet is contributing outside the family unit. Family members are becoming better educated. Family incomes are increasing and acquisition of personal housing and equipment comes earlier in the marriage. Greater individual freedom exists. Sexual mores are changing, with trial and serial marriages.

The emphasis on the family-kinship group has been replaced by acceptance of the nuclear family. Because people are so mobile and are increasingly living in smaller homes or in flats, many ties with kin other than the immediate family are loosened or at least geographically extended. Sometimes close friends become 'the family'. Yet many strengthen kinship ties through letters, telephone calls, and holiday and vacation visits. Religious influences affect family ties. Jews, with their many family traditions, are generally more embedded in a network of relatives than others.

Rapid change is a fact that families must acknowledge. Medical, pharmacological, and scientific advances in birth technology and all areas of health, the increased number of single-parent families, the growing emphasis on the civil and economic rights of minority groups, and the women's liberation movement are only a part of the cultural expansion of this century. As people live longer, more older people will divorce, remarry or cohabitate. Those who lack healthy emotional roots within their nuclear families, who have few or no kinship ties, who cannot adjust to rapid change, and who have little identity except as defined by job and income are more likely to become depressed, alcoholic, unfaithful to mate, or divorced.

**Childrearing practices** have no one traditional national pattern, only the general concern that children develop 'normally'. Parents are encouraged through culture, education and the mass media to use whatever the dominant childrearing theory is at the time. At the turn of the century the dominant theory reflected the prevailing scientific belief in the primacy of heredity in determining behaviour. In the early 1900s child care emphasized the importance of environment, and by the mid-thirties. Freudian psychoanalytic theory had gained ascendency. Today neobehaviouristic theories are prominent. With each new wave of 'knowledge', parents are bombarded by conflicting reports and condemnation of previous practices. Often the change in theory application occurs during the same parental generation so that parents do not trust their own judgment and considerable inconsistency results. The inconsistency, rather than the theory, probably creates the main problems in childrearing. Sometimes parents strive to avoid rearing their children as they were reared, but nevertheless do so unwittingly because of the permanency of enculturation. Children are often given approval and disapproval for their behaviour and told they are 'good' or 'bad'. This practice, along with inconsistency and other factors, contributes to competition and sibling rivalry.

The importance of the father's role is being reconsidered and he is more active in child care. Still, the mother is primarily responsible for the crying baby and young child care. The infant is often unconsciously trained in privacy, individualism, and independence by being left alone in the crib or playpen much of the time. There is still, unfortunately, the fear of 'spoiling' the infant if he/she is held too much or responded to spontaneously. Thus the infant may develop behaviour extremes in order to get needs met. He/she is being given the foundation to later stand out, push forward, to compete and achieve.

Then when the children are old enough to be out of the home, parents often strive to do things for their children and centre their activities around their children's activities. Work responsibilities are not necessary demanded, but there is subtle pressure for the children to repay by pleasing the parents through use of talents, organizational achievements, or honours won. Because of the small size of the nuclear family, the school-age child or adolescent may spend more time with peers than with family members. And because of the youth idealization of our culture, seniority does not invoke special respect for the older person (parent). The childrearing parent must offer more than age if he/she wants to maintain control.

A growing trend is for children to be cared for by day-care centres or babysitters who are usually not relatives. What happens if the mother and parent-surrogate differ greatly about childrearing practices? The child generally acknowledges the authority of parents, or at least the mother, but parent-surrogates affect him/her nevertheless. Any adult who is with the child reinforces behaviour in the child that conforms to the adult's own standard of behaviour. The child conforms to the adult's desires in order to gain approval. If the parent-surrogate acts in a way contrary to the values of the parents, both parents and child are likely to be distressed.

NURSING IMPLICATIONS

The family as the basic unit for the developing person cannot be taken for granted. Although family forms have changed and will continue to change, each person, in order to develop healthily, needs some intimate surroundings of human concern. 'No man is an island.'

You will frequently encounter the entire family as your client in the health-care system, regardless of the setting. Rapid change, increasing demands on the person, technological progress, and other trends mentioned seem to isolate people. More than ever, they need one place in their living where they can act without self-consciousness, where the pretences and roles demanded in jobs, school, or social situations can be put aside. The living centre should be a place where communication takes place with ease; where each knows what to expect from the other; where a cohesiveness exists that is based on nonverbal messages more than verbal; and where a person is accepted for what he/she is.

In doing a family assessment, ask questions related to achieving the developmental tasks that were described earlier. Also, determine communication patterns and relationships, family health, access to health care, occupational demands and hazards, religious beliefs and practices, child-rearing practices, participation in the community, and support systems.

You can help families understand some processes and dynamics underlying interaction so that they, in turn, learn to respect the uniqueness of the self and of each other. Certainly members in the family need not always agree with each other. Instead they can learn to listen to the other person, about how he/she feels and why, accepting each person's impression as real for self. This attitude becomes the basis for mutual respect, honest communication, encouragement of individual fulfilment, and freedom to be. There is then no need to prove or defend the self.

Once the attitude 'We are all important people in this family' is established, conflicts can be dealt with openly and constructively. Name calling and belittling are out of place. Families need to structure time together; otherwise individual schedules will allow them less and less time to meet. Parents need to send consistent messages to their children. To say 'Don't smoke' while immediately lighting a cigarette is hardly effective.

Times of communication are especially necessary when children are feeling peer pressure; children, moreover, should be praised for what they do right rather than reprimanded for what they do wrong. Children need structure but should be told the reason for the structure if old enough to comprehend. As you help the family achieve positive feelings towards the interaction with one another, you are also helping them to fulfil their tasks, roles, and functions.

The person's health problems, especially emotional ones, may well be the result of the interaction patterns in childhood or present family. Knowledge of the variables influencing family interaction – parents' self-esteem and upbringing, number of siblings, the person's ordinal position in the family, cultural norms, family rituals – all will help you assist the person in talking through feelings related to past and present conflicts. Sometimes helping the person understand these variables in relation to the spouse's upbringing and behaviour can be the first step in overcoming current marital problems.

You are a nurse, not a specialized family counsellor, although with advanced preparation you could do family therapy. But you can often sense lack of communication in a family. Through use of an empathic relationship and effective communication, teaching, and crisis therapy, you can encourage family members to talk about their feelings with one another and assist in the resolution to their conflicts. Help them become aware of the need to work for family cohesiveness just as they would work at a job or important project. Refer them to a family counselling service if the problems are beyond your scope. Your work with them should also help them better use other community resources, such as private family or psychiatric counselling or family and children's services.

One liability in working with families of various social classes and cultures may be *you*. For example, if you come from a middle-class background, that fact will affect your opinions about what constitutes family life. Your attitude toward nonconforming families or unconventional living arrangements may interfere with your objectivity and thus with your ability to assist some families. You will need to go through your own maturation process of learning that your way is not always the best or only way. The process is difficult.

*Role of the nurse in well-baby care*

You may care for well babies and mothers in a variety of settings – the clinic, hospital, home, or doctor's surgery. Your actions contribute significantly to their health.

*Prenatal care* to the mother and her partner may include physical assessment, teaching healthy practices for mother and baby, listening to mother vent frustrations or share fears, counselling her during periods of depression or uncertainty, and sharing her happy feelings about becoming a mother. You may conduct childbirth classes for mother and father so that they can better understand changes occurring in the mother as well as the nutrition and hygiene necessary during pregnancy; know what to expect during labour, delivery, and postpartum; and prepare for an active role during birth. An obstetric nursing book will give adequate detail to help you do prenatal assessment and care as well as intrapartal and postpartal assessment and intervention.

If the mother-to-be is unwed, you may also try to work with the father-to-be if both are willing. The father-to-be needs help in talking about his feelings and needs to support her, if they are compatible. He may also seek sex education.

To help the unwed parents, as well as break the cycle for future generations, we must gain a better understanding of the unwed father. Do not perceive him as irresponsible or having taken advantage of an innocent girl. The relationship between the unwed mother and the father is not necessarily a hit-and-miss affair but often meaningful to both. If the parents-to-be are adolescents, they realize that a new life has been created as a result of their actions. They want to act in a responsible way. They are concerned about the child's wellbeing.

The unwed father can be encouraged to stand by the unmarried mother. Often he feels proud of fathering; he has proven his masculinity. The long-term consequences of having a child are such, however, that alternative solutions regarding the future of the child should be thoroughly explored with and by both partners. Alternatives include marriage, placing the child for adoption, or assumption by either parent or the grandparents of the responsibility for caring for and rearing the child. The man needs help in understanding how and why he became a father and the serious implications for the mother, the child and himself.

Adolescents may admit that their sexual experiences were unsatisfactory, leaving them depressed, guilty and scared. The good relationship with the girlfriend may have begun to deteriorate when sexual relations were started. Pregnancy comes as a shock to both. They know about contraceptives, but their use may have been sporadic, if at all, for some people believe that the spontaneity and sincerity of the sexual act are lessened when prepared for.

Sex education must relate to the values of interpersonal relations and concern for others if it is to be successful. The implications and responsibilities of sexual behaviour need to be discussed with the teenagers. The difference between teenage love and a more mature relationship between people who are ready to meet the problems and responsibilities of adulthood should be discussed.

Parents of the unwed father must be involved in helping their son; communication between the boy and parents should be reestablished. In addition, parents should assert themselves in helping the boy take responsibility for his actions and assist the boy in the case of marriage.

Efforts to prevent unwed pregnancies must be directed to improving and strengthening family life and developing a better respect for the father's role in the family. Many unwed fathers come from female-dominanted homes or from homes in which the father is absent or inadequate in his role.

Fathers can help adolescent sons by talking with and listening to them, by being slow to judge, by taking them to work so the youth can see how the father earns a living, by being a role model in relating maturely to the spouse and other women. Fathers can create an atmosphere in which the sons will want to talk about emerging sexual feelings and experiences. If the adolescent son comes from a home where no father is present, the mother can work at listening to and discussing problems and feelings with the son. She may also be able to foster a bond between the son and another male member of the family.

*If you conduct childbirth education classes,* try to interview each couple in their home early in the pregnancy, by the fourth month if possible, to observe their relationship and determine their response to pregnancy. Their response may be different and more honest in their own home than in class. During the class include opportunities for men, as well as women, to talk about the problems they feel are uniquely theirs, their feelings.

Avoid pushing the father into participation and provide support for him. Focus childbirth education on the known benefits to the baby and parents and not on overromanticized and dramatic statements about improved marital relationships. Educate both partners about family planning so that future pregnancies can be mutually planned. Refer either partner, or both, to psychological counselling when necessary, especially if antisocial behaviour is seen or if there has been foetal loss.

*During labour* you do necessary physical care, but you may also act as a coach for the mother, or you may support the father as he assists his wife. Flexibility in hospital routines for obstetrical patients is usually possible and contributes to the parents' sense of control. In fact, negative feelings about traditional hospital deliveries have become so widespread that home deliveries are increasing in many cities.

The physician and nurse or nurse-midwife can work as a team with the expectant couple. In some facilities the nurse-midwife assumes primary responsibility for the family unit. Whenever a mother delivers, she has the right to capable, safe care by qualified caretakers. Home deliveries can be carefully planned and safe. And hospital deliveries can be more homelike. Maternity centres could provide families anticipating a normal childbearing experience with antepartum care that is educational in nature; labour and delivery in a homelike setting (but with adequate equipment) with discharge to home whenever it is safe for mother and baby, probably within 12 hours after delivery; and follow-up care in the home during the postpartum course. The labour-delivery rooms can be designed to accommodate the presence of the father or family during delivery and be less traumatic (cold, with intense lights) for the newborn. Following birth, the infant can remain with the mother; the newborn's physical examination can be done in her presence with the father present as well. Childbirth should be a positive, maturing experience for the couple. Expectant parents have the right and responsibility to be involved in planning their care with the health team and to know what is happening. Cultural beliefs should be recognized, respected, and accommodated whenever possible. A positive childbearing experience contributes to a healthy family unit.

*Delivery methods* are changing in some centres as doctors and midwives follow the trend set by Dr Leboyer in France. The delivery room lights are dimmed; people speak softly or whisper; the infant is placed on the mother's abdomen in order to maintain body temperature and the prebirth curved position in the spine; the baby is massaged by mother and doctor; and the cord is not cut immediately. The baby is placed in warm water. Precautions are taken when necessary, but apparently delivery does not have to be so traumatic for the baby.[3]

In the antenatal period the health visitor is the primary care worker giving way to the midwife, as an independent practitioner for labour and de-livery. The midwife continues to be responsible for ten days after the birth.

*In the early postpartum period* assess mother and baby and give the mother physical care and assist her as necessary even if she looks well and able. 'Mother' the mother. Arrange the environment and hospital routines to enhance bonding between mother and baby. Listen to the mother's concerns; answer her questions; support her maternal behaviour. In a non-threatening way, teach the mother how to handle her baby. Help her begin to unlearn the preconceived ideas about the baby and herself and perceive herself and the baby positively. Give her special assistance if she is breast-feeding. After the initial 'taking-in' period of having received special care and attention, the mother moves to the 'taking hold' stage, where she is able to care for the child.

The interaction between the infant and primary caretaker is crucial. The mothering person helps the baby feel secure and loved, fosters a sense of trust, provides stimulation, reinforces certain behaviour, acts as a model for language development, and trains the baby in basic learning strategies. In turn, maternal behaviour is influenced by baby's cries, coos, smiles, activity and gazes, as well as by how well baby's behaviour meets the mother's expectations.

Your significant contribution to the family unit is to promote attachment between parents and baby, encourage continuing contacts between the family and health professionals so that adequate health and illness care are received, and encourage parents to meet the baby's needs adequately. You can help the parents feel good about themselves and the baby.

You can be instrumental in initiating new trends in care to make the hospital or clinic environment more homelike while providing safe, modern care.

*Continued care in the fourth trimester*

During the fourth trimester, the 6 or 8 weeks after delivery, the mother needs assistance with child care and an opportunity to regain her former self physically and emotionally. Father also needs support as he becomes involved in child-care responsibilities. In the nuclear or single-parent family the parent(s) may struggle alone. Visits by a health visitor will be useful. Some communities have a crisis line for new parents. You may be able to suggest services or help the parent(s) think of people who could be helpful.

As you assess the mother's functioning, consider her physical and emotional energy, support systems, and current level of parenting activity. If she does not appear to be caring adequately for the child, assess for anaemia, pain, bleeding, infections, lack of food or sleep, drug use, or other medical conditions that would interfere with her activity level and feelings of caring. Depression and postpartum blues are difficult to differentiate. In depression the mother is immobilized and forgets basic care, but with postpartum blues she may cry but care for the baby's physical needs.

The new mother usually has enough energy to do only top-priority tasks – eating, sleeping, baby care, and essentials for other family members. A house that is too clean is a danger signal that she is neglecting the baby, herself or both.

The mother's support system is crucial for her energy maintenance, physical as well as emotional. She needs direct support and assistance with daily tasks, plus moral support, a listener, a confidant. Support comes from personal and professional sources – the partner, parents, friends, other relatives, and the nurse, doctor, social worker, or pastor. Negative attitudes from others can drain emotional energy. Actual parenting skills can be manifested in various ways. Touching and cuddling are important, but love can also be shown by a tender, soft voice tone and loving gazes. Ability to obtain adequate medical care is typical of the caring parent; lack of use of medical services for the baby indicates a poor mother-child relationship. Other indications of warm parenting feelings include:

1. Calling the baby by name.
2. Expressing enjoyment of the baby and indicating that the baby is attractive or has other positive characteristics.
3. Looking at the baby and into the eyes.
4. Talking to the baby in a loving voice.
5. Taking safety precautions for the baby.
6. Responding to the baby's cues for attention or physical care.

If the baby is progressing in normal fashion, focus on the mother's needs and concerns. Help her find nonprofessional support systems that can assist her when the professional is unavailable or that can help with child care. In addition to concern over the child care, we must help the mother grow developmentally. Helping her stay in good physical and emotional health ensures better parenting.

Here are some signs of poor parental adaptation to baby on the part of the mother:

1. Sees baby as unattractive.
2. Perceives aspects of care, such as nappy changing, as revolting.
3. Gets upset when baby's secretions or body fluids touch the self.
4. Lets head dangle without support.
5. Picks up baby without warning touch or speech, or at times to meet her own needs.
6. Plays roughly with baby, including after eating, even if baby vomits.
7. Does not coo or talk to baby.
8. Avoids eye contact.
9. Thinks baby does not love the parent.
10. Expresses fears that infant might die with minor illness.

11. Is convinced baby has a defect or is behaving unnaturally when there is no sign of either.
12. Does not speak positively of self or find in baby any attribute that is valued in self.
13. Gives inappropriate responses to baby's needs, such as over- or under-feeding, over- or underhandling or talking to.

Deterrents to adequate mothering include personal immaturity; stress situations, such as loss of loved object; serious disappointments; fear of or rejection from own or partner's parents or other relatives; financial worries; partner punishing her because of his dependency needs; loss of job for partner; having received depersonalized care in hospital; and discharge from hospital soon after delivery without help at home. Assess for these deterrents; your nurturing of the mother and helping her seek additional help may offset the negative impact of these factors.

You may also work with families whose child was born prematurely or with a defect. Prematurity accounts for 50 per cent of neonatal mortality and premature infants who survive contribute significantly to the number of physically, intellectually and emotionally handicapped children. Complications of prematurity include major and minor physical abnormalities, general motor incoordination, short attention span, distractibility and hyperactivity, difficulty separating from parents, preoccupation with the body, and scholastic underachievement.

The last complications may be more related to an early disturbed mother-child relationship than to the prematurity, perinatal complications, or the child's birth defects. Typically the infant is rushed to the nursery after birth, thereby preventing physical or eye contact between mother and baby. The mother is often isolated from other mothers; professionals and family may avoid conversation about the baby. Mother often sees the baby in the premature or intensive care nursery at a distance and only indistinctly; or the baby may have been transported to a children's hospital at some distance so that visiting the baby after her discharge is difficult. The mother may have no opportunity to form any attachment feelings unless nursing staff foster the involvement in child care to the extent possible and keep her informed of baby's condition and progress. The baby who finally comes home to the parents may be a stranger for whom the mother has no maternal response or commitment. Additionally, the mother has developed little confidence in her mothering abilities and no caretaking regimen.

Behaviour patterns that strongly suggest a disturbed parent-child relationship and future problems in parenting include parents who:

1. Are unable to talk about guilt feelings, fears, and their sense of responsibility for the child's early arrival, with each other or others.
2. Demonstrate no visible anxiety about the baby's condition, deny the reality, or displace anxiety onto less threatening matters.

3. Make little effort to secure information about the baby's condition.
4. Consistently misinterpret or exaggerate either positive or negative information about the baby and display no signs of hope as baby's condition improves.
5. Receive no practical support or help from family or friends, and community resources are lacking.
6. Are unable to accept and use help offered.

As a midwife you may be instrumental in promoting certain procedures that can be used by hospital personnel to promote mother-child relationship:

1. Permit the mother to see and touch the baby as soon as possible, preferably in the delivery room. Or transfer the baby to the mother's room in a portable incubator if the baby remains in the same hospital.
2. Permit the mother to become involved in baby's care as soon as possible. Take the mother to the premature care unit, teaching her to use the necessary aseptic technique in order to touch, care for, and visit with the baby.
3. Provide an atmosphere that encourages questions.
4. Encourage parents to talk with each other, family members and friends – using others for support.
5. Recognize that parents' excessive questions, demands and criticisms are a reaction to stress and not personal attacks on the professional worker or hospital.
6. Do not offer reassuring clichés or comforting statements too quickly. Encourage parents to cry, to face the reality of the situation.
7. Do not pressure parents to talk about their feelings all at once, but avoid using the excuse of 'not wanting to probe' to avoid talking with them.
8. Encourage the mother to express breast milk if she wishes; the breast milk can be taken to a breast-milk bank and used for the infant. When the baby is sucking well, the mother can help bottle-feed the baby until the baby is strong enough to breast-feed.
9. Arrange for father to visit the baby prior to discharge, calling him about baby's progress at intervals when he is unable to visit.
10. Encourage the parents to handle the baby and do baby's care prior to discharge; teach about baby care as necessary while the parents are engaged in care of their baby.

*Parent education*

To combat the problems associated with the high adolescent birthrate, some secondary schools are establishing creative programmes in parenthood education. Some hospitals and health clinics are initiating specialized prenatal and postnatal services for the adolescent mother and her at-risk infant. You can initiate nontraditional programmes in your own community.

The adolescent mother who decides to keep her baby needs all the family and outside help she can get. She fears that whatever personal ambitions she has will be thwarted by the baby. Unmarried and unprepared for employment, she finds it almost impossible to make her own way in the world. Anger, frustration, and ignorance hamper her ability to attach to and appropriately care for the baby. Repeated pregnancies, child neglect and abuse, and welfare dependency often occur.

Your work with the mother may prevent maternal deprivation, insufficient interaction between mother and child, conditions under which the deprivation or even abuse develops, as well as negative effects on the child's development.

### Work with adoptive families

You can help the adoptive parents in their adjustment. Assure them that attachment develops over time. Help them think through how and when to tell the child that he/she is adopted so that the child understands and is not traumatized. Help the parents anticipate how they will help the child cope when the child is taunted by peers about being adopted. Help them realize that the adopted child will probably seek answers to many questions when he/she gets older. Who were the parents? Their cultural, racial, or ethnic background? Their ages, occupations, interests, appearance? Why was he/she relinquished? What are the medical facts surrounding heredity and birth? Help parents realize that these questions do not mean that the child does not love them.

### Work with single-parent or reconstituted families

The guidelines already discussed will be useful to you as you help the single-parent or reconstituted family adjust to its situation. Do not rush in with answers for these families until you have heard their unique problems. Acknowledge their strengths; help them formulate their own solutions. Often a few sessions of crisis therapy will be sufficient.

### Family care throughout the life cycle

You may be called on to assist families as they meet various developmental crises throughout the life cycle: school entry of the child, the adolescent period, children leaving home, divorce, retirement, death of a member.

Your goal is health promotion and primary prevention. Your intervention early in the family life cycle may help establish a positive health trend in place of its negative counterpart. The care you give to young parents lays the foundation for their children's health.

Remember you are part of a health-care team. Do not work in isolation.

## REFERENCES

1. Ackerman, Nathan, *Psychodynamics of Family Life* (Basic Books, Inc., New York, 1958).
2. Murray, Ruth and Judith Zentner, *Nursing Assessment and Health Pomotion Through the Life Span*, 3rd edition (Prentice Hall Inc., Englewood Cliffs, NJ, 1975).
3. 'Le Boyer's Babies', *Science News*, 22 January 1977.

# Selected bibliography

Bell, Robert, *Marriage and Family Interaction* (Dorsey Press, Homewood, 1963).

Bossard, James and Gertrude Blanch, *Marriage and Personal Development* (Columbia University Press, New York, 1968).

Bossard, James and E. Boll, *The Sociology of Child Development* (Harper & Row Publishers Inc., fourth edition, New York, 1966).

Branch, Marie and Phyllis Paxton, *Providing Safe Nursing Care for Ethnic People of Colour* (Appleton-Century-Crofts, New York, 1976).

Brink, Pamela ed. *Transcultural Nursing* (Prentice Hall Inc., Englewood Cliffs, NJ, 1976).

Brubaker, Sterling, *To Live on Earth* (New American Library, New York, 1972).

Burgess, Ann, and Lynda Holmstrom, 'The Rape Victim in the Emergency Ward', *American Journal of Nursing*, vol. 73, no. 10 (1973), pp. 1740–5.

Burgess, Ann, and Lynda Holmstrom, 'Rape Trauma Syndrome', *American Journal of Psychiatry*, vol. 131, no. 9 (1974), pp. 981–6.

Burgess, Ann, and Lynda Holmstrom, *Rape: Victims of Crisis* (Robert J. Brady Company, Bowie, MD, 1974).

Burgess, Ann, and Lynda Holmstrom, *Rape: Crisis and Recovery* (Robert J. Brady Company, Bowie, MD, 1974).

Carmichael, Carrie, *Non-sexist Childraising* (Beacon Press, Boston, 1977).

Clemen, Susan, Diane Eigsti and Sandra Maguire, *Comprehensive Family and Community Health Visiting* (McGraw-Hill Book Co., New York, 1981).

Craig, Grace, *Human Development* (Prentice Hall Inc., Englewood Cliffs, NJ, 1976).

Donaldson, R.J., and L.J. Donaldson, *Essential Community Medicine* (MTP Press Ltd, 1983).

Duvall, Evelyn, *Family Development* (J.B. Lippincott Co., fifth edition, Philadelphia, 1977).

Freese, Arthur, 'Only $100 Trillion a Gram: Interferon Has a Future!' *Science Digest*, vol. 87 no. 4 (1980) pp. 49–53.

Friedman, M., and R.J. Rosenman, *Type A Behaviour and Your Heart* (Wildwood House, London, 1974).

Hall, Joanne, and Barbara Weaver, *Nursing of Families in Crisis* (J.B. Lippincott Company, Philadelphia, 1974).

Hamilton, Michael, ed., *The New Genetics and the Future of Man* (William B. Eerdmans Publishing Co., Grand Rapids MI, 1972).

Korner, E., chairperson, *Accountability in the NHS* (HMSO, 1983–7, reports 1–9).

Leaf, Alexander, MD, 'Every Day is a Gift When You Are Over 100', *National Geographic,* vol. 143 no. 1 (1973) pp. 93–119.

Martin, C., 'Marital and Coital Factors in Cervical Cancer', *American Journal of Public Health,* vol. 57 (1967) pp. 803–14.

McFarlane, J.A., *Child Health* (Grant McIntyre, 1980).

O'Donnell, Mike, *A New Introduction to Sociology* (Harrap Ltd, London, 1981).

Parker, William, 'Medication Histories', *American Journal of Nursing,* vol. 76 no. 12 (1976), pp. 1969–71.

Ponte, Lowell, 'How a Change in the Weather Changes You', *Reader's Digest,* March 1982, pp. 55–62.

Roy, Sr. Callista, *Introduction to Nursing: An Adaptation Model* (Prentice Hall Inc., Englewood Cliffs, NJ, 1976).

Saxton, Dolores, and Patricia Hyland, *Planning and Implementing Nursing Intervention* (The C.V. Mosby Company, St Louis, 1975).

Schmitt, Florence E., and Powhatan J. Wolldridge, 'Psychological Preparation of Surgical Patients', *Nursing Research,* vol. 22 no. 2 (1973), pp. 108–15.

Schulz, David, *The Changing Family* (Prentice Hall Inc., Englewood Cliffs, NJ, 1975).

Sparacino, Jack Don Ronchi, Marilyn Brenner, James Kuhn and Arthur Flesch, 'Psychological Correlates of Blood Pressure. A Closer Examination of Hostility, Anxiety and Engagement', *Nursing Research,* vol. 31 no. 3 (1982), pp. 143–9.

Sutherland, Ian, *Health Education, Perspectives and Choices* (Allen and Unwin, London, 1979).

Upton, Arthur, 'The Biological Effects of Low-Level Ionising Radiation', *Scientific American,* vol. 246 no. 2 (1982), pp. 41–9.

van Sickle, Derek, *The Ecological Citizen* (Harper & Row Publishers Inc., New York, 1971).

Walker, H.B., 'Why Medicine Needs Religion', *International Surgery,* vol. 56 no. 8 (1971) pp. 373–480.

Webb, Christine ed., *Feminist Practice in Women's Health Care* (Wiley, 1986).

Wright, Beatrice, *Physical Disability, A Psychological Approach* (Harper & Row, New York, 1960).

# Index

subjectivity in self-definition of illness, 4
suicide attempter in hospital, 181
sulphur oxides, 212
 definition of, 213
sulphuric acid, 214
 definition of, 213
summarizing points of discussion, 55
support groups in group education, 120−1
supportive intervention and adaptation, 158
surgery, study of patients on night before,
 119−20
survival of fittest, 152
susceptibility to illness, 190−2, 254
suspended particles in air, 212, 213
Sutherland, I., 188
syndrome, adaptation, 132
synthetic chemicals polluting water, 217
systematic
 approach, 71
 assessment of functional areas, 75−9
 observation, 39
systems
 definition of, 7
 framework, 12
 *see also* general systems theory; social
  system
Systems Developmental-Stress Model, 69

T lymphocytes, 143
taboos about nonverbal behaviour, 40, 44
Talmud, 111
 definition of, 267
Tao, definition of, 265
Taoism, 260, 264−5
Te, definition of, 265
teacher-learner, nurse as, 104−5
teaching
 definition of, 103
 machine, 118
 *see also* health teaching
teenagers, 311
television and health education, 25, 105, 120
temperature
 body, 131
 core, regulation of, 138−9
 climatic, variations in, 14−15
 heat
  need for, 62
  pollution of water, 217−18
  production, 138
teratogenic changes, 234
termination phase of nurse-client
 relationship, 98
territoriality, definition of, 36−7
tertiary prevention of crisis, definition of, 178
therapeutic communication, 52−62
 barriers to, 56, 58−62
 client with difficulties, 56, 57−8

effective methods, 52−6
 *see also* communication
therapeutic intervention and adaptation, 158
therapeutic milieu, 235
 definition of, 234
Theravada branch of Buddhism, definition of,
 263
thermal stimuli, definition of, 14−15
thermogenesis, chemical, 138−9
thinking, teaching method as way of, 117
third phase
 of crisis, 168−9, 171
 of nurse-client relationship, 97
Thomas, 201
thought *see* mind
thoughtful silence, 45, 52
Three Mile Island accident, 225
time
 language of, 35−6
 orientation, 255
 sequence, placing events in, 53
Tisha bab, definition of, 269
tissue histocytes, 142
tabacco *see* smoking
Toffler, A., 154, 246
tools
 of assessment in nursing process, 74−9
 of communication, 34−47
  eye behaviour, 40−2
  language, 34−8
  listening, 45−7
  nonverbal behaviour, 40
  observation and perception, 38−9
  silence, 45
  touch, 43−4
 for evaluating nursing effectiveness, 89−91
Torah, definition of, 267
total approach *see* holistic approach
touch, 42, 43−4
toxoids, 144
 *see also* chemicals; pollution
traditions, 241
 beliefs in families, 156
transmitting device, 30−1
travel and transport, 243−4
Travelbee, J., 69
treyfe, definition of, 268
trite expressions as barrier to
 communication, 59
Turnbull, 25
twins, 298−9

UKCC
 code of ethics, 68−9
 curriculum guidelines, 127
ultradian rhythmic processes, definition of,
 17−18
umpire role in family, 156−7